Diagnosis and Therapy of Hepatocellular Carcinoma: Status Quo and a Glimpse at the Future

Guest Editor

ADRIAN REUBEN, BSc, MBBS, FRCP, FACG

CLINICS IN LIVER DISEASE

www.liver.theclinics.com

Consulting Editor
NORMAN GITLIN, MD

May 2011 • Volume 15 • Number 2

SAUNDERS an imprint of ELSEVIER, Inc.

W.B. SAUNDERS COMPANY

A Division of Elsevier Inc.

1600 John F. Kennedy Boulevard, Suite 1800 • Philadelphia, PA 19103-2899

http://www.theclinics.com

CLINICS IN LIVER DISEASE Volume 15, Number 2
May 2011 ISSN 1089-3261, ISBN-13: 978-1-4557-0465-1

Editor: Kerry Holland
Developmental Editor: Donald Mumford

Clinics in Liver Disease (ISSN 1089-3261) is published quarterly by Elsevier Inc., 360 Park Avenue South, New York, NY 10010-1710. Months of issue are February, May, August, and November. Business and Editorial Offices: 1600 John F. Kennedy Blvd., Ste. 1800, Philadelphia, PA 19103-2899. Customer Service Office: 3251 Riverport Lane, Maryland Heights, MO 63043. Periodicals postage paid at New York, NY and additional mailing offices. Subscription prices are $251.00 per year (U.S. individuals), $124.00 per year (U.S. student/resident), $343.00 per year (U.S. institutions), $333.00 per year (foreign individuals), $171.00 per year (foreign student/resident), $413.00 per year (foreign instituitions), $290.00 per year (Canadian individuals), $171.00 per year (Canadian student/resident), and $413.00 per year (Canadian institutions). Foreign air speed delivery is included in all *Clinics* subscription prices. All prices are subject to change without notice. **POSTMASTER:** Send address changes to *Clinics in Liver Disease*, Elsevier Health Sciences Division, Subscription Customer Service, 3251 Riverport Lane, Maryland Heights, MO 63043. **Customer Service: Telephone: 1-800-654-2452 (U.S. and Canada); 314-447-8871 (outside U.S. and Canada). Fax: 314-447-8029. E-mail: journalscustomer service-usa@elsevier.com (for print support); journalsonlinesupport-usa@elsevier.com (for online support).**

Reprints. For copies of 100 or more of articles in this publication, please contact the Commercial Reprints Department, Elsevier Inc., 360 Park Avenue South, New York, NY 10010-1710. Tel.: 212-633-3812; Fax: 212-462-1935; E-mail: reprints@elsevier.com.

Clinics in Liver Disease is covered in *MEDLINE/PubMed (Index Medicus)*, Science Citation Index Expanded, Journal Citation Reports/Science Edition, and Current Contents/Clinical Medicine.

Printed and bound by CPI Group (UK) Ltd, Croydon, CR0 4YY

Transferred to Digital Print 2011

Contributors

CONSULTING EDITOR

NORMAN GITLIN, MD, FRCP(LONDON), FRCPE(EDINBURGH), FACG, FACP
Formerly, Professor of Medicine; Chief of Hepatology, Emory University; Currently, Consultant, Atlanta Gastroenterology Associates, Atlanta, Georgia

GUEST EDITOR

ADRIAN REUBEN, BSc, MBBS, FRCP, FACG
Professor of Medicine, Chief, Liver Service, Division of Gastroenterology and Hepatology, and Liver Transplant Program, Department of Medicine, Medical University of South Carolina, Charleston, South Carolina

AUTHORS

MUNAZZA ANIS, MD
Assistant Professor, Department of Radiologic Sciences, Medical University of South Carolina, Charleston, South Carolina

WILLIAM C. CHAPMAN, MD
Professor of Surgery and Chief, Section of Transplantation, Department of Surgery, Washington University School of Medicine, Washington University, St Louis, Missouri

KENNETH D. CHAVIN, MD, PhD
Division of Transplant Surgery, Department of Surgery, Medical University of South Carolina (MUSC), Charleston, South Carolina

T. MARK EARL, MD
Section of Transplantation, Department of Surgery, Washington University School of Medicine, Washington University, St Louis, Missouri

MILTON J. FINEGOLD, MD
Professor of Pathology and Pediatrics, Baylor College of Medicine, Texas Children's Hospital, Houston, Texas

CATHERINE FRENETTE, MD
Medical Director of Liver Transplantation; Director of Liver Cancer Program, The Methodist Center for Liver Disease, J.C. Walter Transplant Center, Department of Medicine, The Methodist Hospital, Houston, Texas

ROBERT G. GISH, MD
Chief of Clinical Hepatology; Clinical Professor of Medicine; Medical Director, Center for Hepatobiliary Disease and Abdominal Transplantation, University of California, San Diego, California

STEVAN A. GONZALEZ, MD, MS
Attending Physician, Division of General and Transplant Hepatology, Baylor Regional Transplant Institute, Baylor All Saints Medical Center at Fort Worth, Baylor University Medical Center at Dallas, Fort Worth, Texas

MARCELO GUIMARAES, MD
Assistant Professor, Division of Vascular and Interventional Radiology, Medical University of South Carolina, Charleston, South Carolina

NEDIM HADZIC, MD, MSc
Consultant and Honorary Reader in Paediatric Hepatology, Paediatric Liver Service, King's College Hospital Denmark Hill, London, United Kingdom

ABID IRSHAD, MD
Associate Professor, Department of Radiologic Sciences, Medical University of South Carolina, Charleston, South Carolina

ASSAF ISSACHAR, MD
Department of Medicine D and the Liver Institute, Rabin Medical Center, Beilinson Hospital, Molecular Hepatology Research Laboratory, Felsenstein Medical Research Center, Sackler School of Medicine, Tel Aviv University, Petah-Tikva, Israel

EMMET B. KEEFFE, MD
Professor of Medicine Emeritus, Division of Gastroenterology and Hepatology, Department of Medicine, Stanford University Medical Center, Palo Alto, California

KRIS V. KOWDLEY, MD, FACP
Director, Center for Liver Disease, Virginia Mason Medical Center, Digestive Disease Institute, Seattle, Washington

W. THOMAS LONDON, MD
Senior Member, Fox Chase Cancer Center, Philadelphia, Pennsylvania

HOWARD C. MASUOKA, MD, PhD
Instructor, Division of Gastroenterology and Hepatology, William J. von Liebig Transplant Center, Mayo Clinic and Mayo Clinic College of Medicine, Rochester, Minnesota

JOHN W. MCGILLICUDDY, MD
Division of Transplant Surgery, Department of Surgery, Medical University of South Carolina (MUSC), Charleston, South Carolina

KATHERINE A. MCGLYNN, PhD
Senior Investigator, Division of Cancer Epidemiology and Genetics, National Cancer Institute, Rockville, Maryland

JENS MITTLER, MD
Division of Transplant Surgery, Department of Surgery, Medical University of South Carolina (MUSC), Charleston, South Carolina

CHARLES B. ROSEN, MD
Professor and Chair, Division of Transplantation Surgery, William J. von Liebig Transplant Center, Mayo Clinic and Mayo Clinic College of Medicine, Rochester, Minnesota

TANIA ROSKAMS, MD, PhD
Professor of Pathology, Anatomy and Histology, University of Leuven; Department of Pathology, Head Liver Research Unit, Laboratory of Morphology and Molecular Pathology, University Hospitals of Leuven, Leuven, Belgium

MORRIS SHERMAN, MB BCh, PhD, FRCP(C)
Department of Medicine, University of Toronto, Toronto General Hospital, Toronto, Ontario, Canada

ASMA SIDDIQUE, MD
Fellow in Hepatology, Center for Liver Disease, Virginia Mason Medical Center, Digestive Disease Institute, Seattle, Washington

MARIO STRAZZABOSCO, MD, PhD
Professor of Medicine, Department of Internal Medicine, Section of Digestive Diseases, Yale University School of Medicine; Deputy Director, Yale Liver Center, Department of Internal Medicine, Yale University, New Haven, Connecticut; Chief, Section of Digestive Diseases, University of Milan-Bicocca, Monza, Italy

TAMAR H. TADDEI, MD
Assistant Professor of Medicine, Department of Internal Medicine, Section of Digestive Diseases, Yale University School of Medicine, New Haven; Co-Director, Veterans Affairs Connecticut Healthcare System, Hepatitis C Resource Center (HCRC), West Haven, Connecticut

RAN TUR-KASPA, MD
Department of Medicine D and the Liver Institute, Rabin Medical Center, Beilinson Hospital, Molecular Hepatology Research Laboratory, Felsenstein Medical Research Center, Sackler School of Medicine, Tel Aviv University, Petah-Tikva, Israel

†RENAN UFLACKER, MD
Professor and Director, Division of Vascular and Interventional Radiology, Medical University of South Carolina, Charleston, South Carolina

STEPHEN H. WRZESINSKI, MD, PhD
Assistant Professor of Medicine, Yale Comprehensive Cancer Center, Yale University School of Medicine, New Haven; Veterans Affairs Connecticut Healthcare System, Comprehensive Cancer Center, West Haven, Connecticut

ROMY ZEMEL, PhD
Department of Medicine D and the Liver Institute, Rabin Medical Center, Beilinson Hospital, Molecular Hepatology Research Laboratory, Felsenstein Medical Research Center, Sackler School of Medicine, Tel Aviv University, Petah-Tikva, Israel

---

† Deceased

Contents

The global risk of hepatocellular carcinoma (HCC) has been largely driven by hepatitis B virus (HBV) infection for the past century, along with hepatitis C virus (HCV), aflatoxin, excessive alcohol consumption, and obesity/diabetes. The dominant effect of HBV on global HCC risk should decline as the population vaccinated against HBV grows older. Infection with HCV is also expected to decline. Projections of HCV-related HCC rates remaining high for another 30 years may be overly pessimistic. Alcohol may be less of a factor in HCC in coming years. However, obesity and diabetes may become even more important risk factors for HCC.

A better understanding of signaling pathways in HCC pathogenesis has led to targeted therapies against HCC. Identification of liver cancer stem cell markers and their related pathways is one of the most important goals of liver cancer research. New therapies should ideally target cancer stem cells and not normal stem/progenitor cells, because the latter are very important in regeneration and repair. Individualized HCC therapy will require better definition of patient subgroups that benefit most or should be protected from therapy failure and unwanted side effects. Tumor tissue acquisition should be mandatory, reversing the practice that was established years ago when targeted HCC therapy was but a pope dream.

HBV and HCV have major roles in hepatocarcinogenesis. More than 500 million people are infected with hepatitis viruses and, therefore, HCC is highly prevalent, especially in those countries endemic for HBV and HCV. Viral and host factors contribute to the development of HCC. The main viral factors include the circulating load of HBV DNA or HCV RNA and specific genotypes. Various mechanisms are involved in the host-viral interactions that lead to HCC development, among which are genetic instability, self-sufficiency in growth signals, insensitivity to antigrowth signals, evasion of apoptosis, limitless replicative potential, sustained angiogenesis, and tissue invasiveness. Prevention of HBV by vaccination, as well as antiviral therapy against HBV and for HCV seem able to inhibit the development of HCC.

Coinciding with the increased incidence of hepatocellular carcinoma (HCC),
there has been a significant increase in the global incidence of obesity and
diabetes mellitus (DM), the two major risk factors for nonalcoholic steatohepatitis (NASH). There are many causes of HCC, and nonalcoholic fatty liver
disease/NASH is now emerging as a leading risk factor owing to the
epidemic of obesity and type 2 DM. The mechanisms leading to HCC in
obesity and type 2 DM likely involve interactions between several signaling
pathways, including oxidative stress, inflammation, oncogenes, adiponectins, and insulin resistance associated with visceral adiposity and diabetes.

Early diagnosis of hepatocellular carcinoma (HCC) has a significant impact
on survival by implementation of effective treatment strategies, including
hepatic resection, locoregional ablative therapy, and liver transplantation.
The use of serum tumor markers and biopsy are particularly important for
diagnosis of small hepatic lesions with atypical features on imaging studies. α-Fetoprotein remains the most frequently used tumor marker for the
diagnosis of HCC. The development of novel serum biomarkers for HCC,
identification of molecular markers for tissue immunohistochemistry, and
emergence of new diagnostic techniques such as proteomic profiling
may improve the early detection rate of HCC in the future.

Understanding of the genetic changes and molecular signaling pathways
that are active in hepatocellular carcinoma has improved substantially
over the last decade. As more information becomes available, it is clear
that the prognostication of hepatocellular carcinoma will soon include molecular and genomic "fingerprints" that are unique to each cancer, which
will allow more personalized treatment plans for patients as more targeted
therapies become available. This article discusses the molecular and
genomic changes that are important in hepatocellular carcinoma in order
for clinicians to understand the current and forthcoming treatment options
for patients with liver cancer.

Active screening of patients at risk for HCC has led to the identification of
early HCCs that are amenable to treatment with a high rate of cure. This
requires high-quality ultrasound examinations at 6-month intervals. If
widely applied, screening has the potential to substantially reduce the
mortality from this disease. The application of the Barcelona Cancer of
the Liver Clinic (BCLC) staging system should standardize assessment
of prognosis and determination of the most effective treatments for each

stage. With new molecular targeted agents coming, it is critical that studies are performed in patients stratified by stage into homogeneous groups. Because it is linked with therapy, the BCLC is ideally suited to this purpose.

Hepatocellular carcinoma (HCC) is most commonly seen in patients with cirrhosis. Criteria for diagnosis include arterial-phase enhancement, venous-phase washout, and a capsule on delayed sequences. Tiny HCC are best detected with magnetic resonance imaging using the new hepatocyte-specific gadolinium agents; otherwise, short-term follow up versus biopsy is considered. Diffuse HCC can be difficult to diagnose because of the inherent heterogeneous hepatic parenchyma in cirrhosis, however, portal vein expansion due to thrombosis is a helpful sign.

Liver resection remains the standard therapy for solitary hepatocellular carcinoma in patients with preserved hepatic function. In well-selected patients, 5-year survival rates are good and can approach that of liver transplantation for early-stage disease. Patient selection is critical to optimizing therapeutic benefit, and the health of the native liver must be considered in addition to tumor characteristics. Hepatic recurrence after resection is common. The difficulty lies in deciding which patients with chronic liver disease and small solitary tumors are best served by resection and which should proceed with transplant evaluation; this is the focus of this article.

Laparoscopic liver resection is an emerging technique in liver surgery. Although laparoscopy is well established for several abdominal procedures and is considered by some the preferred approach, laparoscopic hepatic resection has been introduced into clinical practice more widely since 2000. These procedures are performed only in experienced centers and only in a select group of patients. While initially performed only for benign hepatic lesions, the indications for laparoscopic resection have gradually broadened to encompass all kinds of malignant hepatic lesions, including hepatocellular carcinoma in patients with cirrhosis, for whom the advantages of the minimally invasive approach may be most evident.

Despite significant advances in nonsurgical treatments of hepatocellular carcinoma, these approaches rarely result in cure. Surgery remains the mainstay of curative therapy for hepatocellular carcinoma. Liver transplantation, in particular, has emerged as one of the most beneficial therapeutic

RELATED INTEREST

Medical Clinics of North America, July 2009 (Vol. 93, No. 4)
Care of the Cirrhotic Patient
David A. Sass, MD, *Guest Editor*

THE CLINICS ARE NOW AVAILABLE ONLINE!

Access your subscription at:
www.theclinics.com

Preface

Hepatocellular Carcinoma: Its Past, Present, and Future

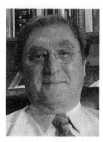

Adrian Reuben, MBBS, FRCP, FACG
Guest Editor

Hepatocellular carcinoma, commonly acronymized as HCC, is a scourge and a tragedy. Who would argue against the sentiment that HCC, for which the incidence and mortality virtually par and the global death toll is over half a million annually, is a blight on humanity. The tragedy is that HCC is largely preventable, theoretically at least. The major risk factors for HCC, namely chronic hepatitis B and C infection, are avoidable and treatable. Aflatoxin, which synergizes with hepatitis B in hepatocarcinogenesis, could be eradicated if cereals, nuts, and legumes were stored below 50°F at less than 17% humidity. Whether or not the pandemic of obesity and diabetes is due to a "Thrifty Gene" that evolved to conserve bodily energy in lean times, but is detrimental in our "obesogenic" environment,[1] is still debated. Yet, as obesity and insulin resistance proliferate, cancer becomes more prevalent, and that includes HCC too. Although the Old Testament tells us that there were flesh pots[a] in Egypt,[3] and cirrhosis was diagnosed in Egyptian mummies,[4] HCC was not discovered, although other cancers were found.[5,6] Even dinosaurs had cancer,[7] as did our human ancestors.[8] Readers who wish to learn more about the history and semantics of cancer are referred to a scholarly essay that was recently published on this topic.[9]

The history of HCC is both interesting and confusing, because early observers were bewildered too. Yet, Aretæus of Cappadocia, a second Century CE contemporary of Galen (who in turn popularized the term cancer that Hippocrates coined as *karkinoma*,

---

[a] Myles Coverdale, the 16th Century bible translator, explains in the first complete printed translation of the Bible in English[2] that he wrote, that flesh pots were metal caldrons used by luxuriating Egyptians for boiling meat.

Clin Liver Dis 15 (2011) xiii–xvii
doi:10.1016/j.cld.2011.04.001
1089-3261/11/$ – see front matter © 2011 Elsevier Inc. All rights reserved.

from the Greek word for crab), deduced the sequence of steps from inflammation through scarring and cirrhosis that led to HCC.[10] Frierichs, the patriarch of modern hepatology, credited Gaspard-Laurent Bayle in Paris with the first accurate account of liver cancer, together with an estimate of its prevalence.[11] George Budd, the father of English hepatology, reasoned that cancer was the commonest organic disease of the liver in mid-19th century Britain, among patients who were never hard drinkers. Budd was likely dealing primarily with metastatic liver cancer.[12] Virchow, the renowned anatomist and pathologist whose proposal that "organs commonly affected by metastases are rarely the site of primary neoplasia,"[13] was responsible for the delay in the recognition of HCC until the second half of the 20th century. Even William Osler perpetuated the view that primary liver cancer was rare, because "among the first three thousand patients admitted to the wards of the Johns Hopkins Hospital there were 7 cases of cancer of the liver."[14] The ghastly truth of the prevalence of HCC nowadays is comprehensively detailed by Catherine McGlynn and Thomas London, in the first article of the current issue of Clinics in Liver Disease.

Before highlighting the remaining articles in this issue, it is worth commenting on the nomenclature of liver cancer that until recently was an obfuscation. Hepatocyte-based tumors have been called cancer trabéculaire,[15] adenocarcinoma,[16] malignant adenomas,[17] carcinoma hepatocellulaire,[18] and hepatoma.[19] Whereas the term hepatoma trips off the tongue compared to hepatocellular carcinoma, the former term has been applied to benign hepatocyte-derived tumors, to tumors that are intermediate between benign and malignant, and to both.[20] The authors of the current monograph dutifully toed the party line, and I had to edit out the term hepatoma only twice—the identity of the nonconformist is privileged information.

The current issue of Clinics in Liver Disease is organized fairly conventionally, but it is the structure of the articles and their content in which authors have excelled to produce an unconventionally comprehensive and topical volume of the burgeoning and rapidly evolving topic that is HCC.

Catherine McGlynn's and Thomas London's encyclopedic yet lucid account of the global epidemiology of HCC nicely sets the stage for the players who follow. In her article on Anatomic Pathology of HCC, Tania Roskams—the "Hercules Poirot"[b] of hepatocarcinogenesis investigation—describes not only the histology of HCC, but also clarifies the stages of dysplasia that proceed it, focusing on the nature of HCC precursor lesions, and the cellular and molecular markers that will prove to have not only diagnostic but prognostic and therapeutic significance. Dr Roskams makes a case for universal acquisition of tumor tissue in clinical trials of HCC treatment, which should also extend to the care of individual patients. This position is supported by the Consensus Conference in Liver Transplantation for HCC, held in Zurich in December 2010, as well as by other distinguished hepatopathologists. Other authors in this volume make mention of the need for tissue examination, but none are as forthright in their demand for cancer samples.

The articles by Romy Zemel, Assef Isaschar, and Ran Tur-Kaspa on oncogenic viruses, and by Asma Siddique and Kris Kowdley on the molecular pathogenesis of the metabolic syndrome as a cause of HCC, deal thoroughly with their difficult topics at both the basic science and the clinical levels. Here, as in the articles on molecular biology and genomics by Catherine Frenette and Robert Gish, and on tumor markers

---

[b] Both are Belgian sleuths.

by Stevan Gonzalez and Emmett Keefe, the theme of the pivotal importance of cell receptors, signal transduction, cytokines, and a host of other molecular events is emphasized repeatedly. We make no apology for presenting the bewildering alphabet soup that permeates these and other articles, because knowledge of these will be critical soon, in both diagnosis and therapy. We have attempted, however, to define each acronym. The article by Stephen Wrzesinski, Tamar Taddei, and Mario Strazzabosco shows elegantly how molecular targets can be attacked in systemic chemotherapy regimens.

Morris Sherman, the guru of screening philosophy and strategy, gives the current view on the approach to screening. His contribution is complemented by those from Frenette and Gish, and Gonzalez and Keefe, which focus on diagnosis of the individual case. The diagnostic section for HCC is rounded out by the graphic and comparative account of various imaging modalities that are available for the diagnosis of liver lesions, by Munazza Anis and Abid Irshad.

Treatment of HCC ranges from curative attempts by resection and liver transplantation to palliation. The pros and cons of resection are covered admirably by Mark Earl and William Chapman, who emphasize the criteria and limitations for performing surgical resection, whereas Jens Mittler, John McGillicuddy, and Kenneth Chavin describe and assess thoroughly the still limited *tour de force* that is laparoscopic resection. Howard Masuoka and Charles Rosen discuss the efforts to extend the limits of transplantation by downstaging tumors; they pose many germane questions about exceeding conventional criteria, which still need answers. The feasibility of ablation without surgery, performed by talented interventional radiologists, is described vividly by Marcello Guimaraes and Renan Uflacker. Their ingenuity and bravado are seemingly boundless. As mentioned earlier, Wrzesinski, Taddei, and Strazzabosco discuss extensively systemic chemotherapy, which is based on molecular targeting derived from knowledge gained in hepatocarcinogenesis research, which has blossomed since the introduction of the tumor kinase inhibitor, sorafenib. Finally, the article on liver tumors in children embodies many of the principles of histopathology, immunohistochemistry, and molecular pathogenesis described earlier for adults. Nedim "Dino" Hadzic and Milton Finegold skillfully lift the veil from the myriad liver tumors that pediatricians know well, to make them more comprehensible to adult physicians (ie, physicians of adults).

For my part, this has been a delightful journey of enlightenment into the world of HCC with guides of exquisite expertise. It has also been a privilege to have been allowed by our Consulting Editor, Norman Gitlin, to have had a hand in author selection and to have been permitted to tinker with their offerings. Kerry Holland, Senior Editor at Elsevier, has the patience of Job, for which I am grateful.

Adrian Reuben, MBBS, FRCP, FACG
Division of Gastroenterology and Hepatology
and Liver Transplant Program
Department of Medicine
Medical University of South Carolina
ART 7100-A, MSC 290
25 Courtenay Drive
Charleston, SC 29425, USA

E-mail address:
reubena@musc.edu

REFERENCES

1. Neel JV. Diabetes mellitus: a "thrifty genotype rendered detrimental by 'progress'?" Am J Hum Genet 1962;14:353–62.
2. The Coverdale Bible (1535).
3. Exodus 16:3 (King James Version).
4. Zimmerman M. The paleopathology of the liver. Ann Clin Lab Sci 1990;20:301–6.
5. Halperin EC. Paleo-oncology: the role of ancient remains in the study of cancer. Persp Biol Med 2004;47:1–14.
6. Zimmerman MR. A possible histiocytoma in an Egyptian mummy. Arch Dermatol 1981;117:364–5.
7. Rothschild BM, Tanke DM, Heibling M II, et al. Epidemiologic study of tumors in dinasours. Natur Wissenschaffen 2003;90:495–500.
8. Capasso L, Constantini RM. [Paleopathology of human tumours]. Med Secol 1994;6:1–52 [in Italian].
9. Reuben A. The crab, the turkey and a malignant tale from the year of the rooster. Hepatology 2005;41:944–50.
10. Aretæus the Cappadocian. The extant works of Aretæus the Cappadocian. In: Adams F, editor. London: Publications of the Sydenham Society; 1856. p. 34.
11. Frerichs FT. VII Cancer of the liver (carcinoma hepatis). 1. Historical account. In: Murchison C, editor, A clinical treatise of diseases of the liver, vol. III. New York: W. Wood and Co; 1879. p. 41–3.
12. Budd G. Diseases which result from some growth foreign to the natural structure. Section 1. Cancer of the liver—Origin of cancerous tumors of the liver—Their growth, dissemination, and effects—Encysted, knotty tubera of the liver. In: On diseases of the liver. London: John Churchill; 1845. p. 299. Chapter IV.
13. Virchow R. Die krankhaften Geschwülste: Dreissig Vorlesungen, gehalten während des Wintersemesters 1862-1863, an der Universitat zu Berlin, vol. 1. Berlin: Augustus Hirschwald; 1863. p. 69.
14. Osler W. Section III. Diseases of the digestive system. VIII. Diseases of the liver. 6. New growths in the liver. In: The principles and practice of medicine. New York: D. Appleton and Company; 1892. p. 451.
15. Hanot VC, Gilbert A. Études sur les maladies du foie. Paris: Asselin et Houzean; 1888. p. 1–158.
16. Wegelin K. Über das Adenokarzinom and Adenom der Leber. Virchows Arch 1905;179:95–193.
17. Ribbert H. Das maligne Adenoma der Leber. Dtsch Med Wochenschr 1909;35:1607–9.
18. Goldziehr M, von Bókay Z. Der primäre. Leber Krebs. Virchows Arch 1911;203:75–131.
19. Yamagiwa K. Zur Kenntis. Des Primarën parenchymatösen Leberkarzinoms ("hepatoma"). Virchows Arch 1911;206:437–67.
20. Ewing J. Epithelial hyperplasia and tumors of the liver. In: Neoplastic diseases. 4th edition. Philadelphia: WB Saunders; 1940. p. 735–61. Chapter XXXIII.

Dedication

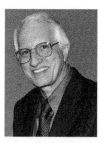

Renan Uflacker, MD
March 16th 1949 – June 12th 2011

Renan Uflacker passed away today after a brief and tragic illness. He is survived by his wife, Dr Helena Becker Uflacker, and his two children, Andre and Alice, both of whom graduated very recently in Medicine. Renan was born, raised and educated in Brazil, where he obtained his medical degree in 1974. He was appointed Professor of Radiology and Director of the Division of Interventional Radiology in 1993, at the Medical University of South Carolina, in Charleston SC. Aside from his unsurpassed skill and ingenuity as an interventional radiologist, he was a prolific scientific author, a talented and prodigious photographer, a student of world affairs and a champion of freedom and human rights. Above all, he was a devoted and doted upon family man, and a steadfast colleague and friend of the highest integrity, who will be missed by family, friends and colleagues worldwide.

The Editor thanks, with deepest gratitude, Kerry Holland and her colleagues in publishing at Elsevier, for graciously and generously allowing the dedication of this issue to the memory of Renan Uflacker, MD, whose article (written with his protégé, Marcello S. Guimaraes, MD) is included in this volume.

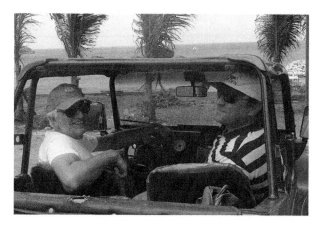

Adrian Reuben, MBBS, FRCP, FACG
Charleston SC, June 12th, 2011

The Global Epidemiology of Hepatocellular Carcinoma: Present and Future

Katherine A. McGlynn, PhD[a],*, W. Thomas London, MD[b]

KEYWORDS

• Incidence • Hepatitis B virus • Hepatitis C virus • Aflatoxin
• Alcohol • Diabetes

On the global scale, primary liver cancer is a major contributor to both cancer incidence and mortality. It is the sixth most commonly occurring cancer in the world and the third largest cause of cancer mortality.[1] The most common histologic type of primary liver cancer, hepatocellular carcinoma (HCC), is a malignant tumor arising from hepatocytes, the liver's parenchymal cells. HCCs have not been reported in autopsies of well-preserved Egyptian mummies, although Zimmerman and Auferheide[2] found evidence of cirrhosis of the liver. By the nineteenth century, HCCs were accurately described in European pathology journals, but they were believed to be uncommon.[3] In agreement, in the early twentieth century, William Osler and McCrae[4] in the United States also reported that primary liver cancer was rare. These views probably reflected the pronounced geographic disparity in incidence, because HCCs are common in Asia and Africa, but are uncommon in Europe and North America.

INCIDENCE AND MORTALITY

Because diagnostic confirmation of HCC is not routine worldwide, it is easier to examine incidences of primary liver cancer than incidences of HCC. However,

This work was supported by funding of the NCI Intramural Research Program.
The authors have nothing to disclose.
[a] Division of Cancer Epidemiology and Genetics, National Cancer Institute, EPS-5020, 6120 Executive Boulevard, Rockville, MD 20852–7234, USA
[b] Fox Chase Cancer Center, 333 Cottman Avenue, Philadelphia, PA 19111–2497, USA
* Corresponding author.
E-mail address: mcglynnk@mail.nih.gov

because HCC is the most common histology in most countries, primary liver cancer rates are a close approximation of HCC rates. An exception is northeast Thailand, which has high rates of primary liver cancer (male incidence = 88/100,000; female incidence = 35/100,000)[5] because of the exceptionally high incidence of intrahepatic cholangiocarcinoma.

The highest liver cancer incidences in the world are reported by registries in Asia and Africa. Approximately 85% of all liver cancers occur in these areas, with Chinese registries alone reporting more than 50%.[5] In addition to registries in China (eg, Hong Kong, Shanghai), other Asian registries with rates greater than 20/100,000 persons include those of Seoul, Korea and Osaka, Japan (**Fig. 1**). Registries in Africa that report incidences greater than 20/100,000 include those of Harare, Zimbabwe (African ancestry) and Gharbiah, Egypt. In contrast with these high-rate HCC areas, low-rate areas include northern Europe as well as North and South America. In general, registries in

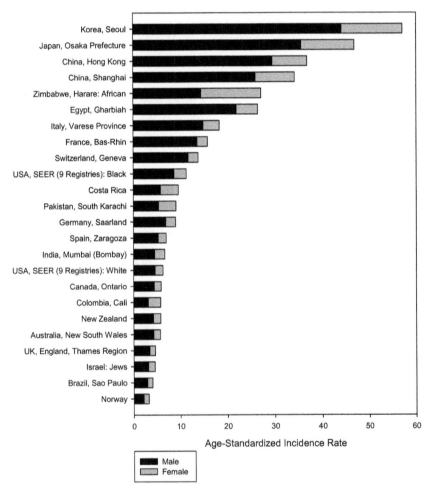

Fig. 1. Age-adjusted incidences per 100,000 of liver cancer by region, 1998–2002. Age adjusted to world standard. (*Data from* Ferlay J, Parkin DM, Curado MP, et al. Cancer incidence in five continents, volumes I to IX: IARC CANCERBase No. 9 [Internet]. Available at: http://ci5.iarc.fr.)

these areas report incidences of less than 10/100,000 (see **Fig. 1**). Intermediate-rate HCC areas, where the incidences are typically between 10/100,000 and 20/100,000, are principally located in central Europe (eg, Italy, France, Switzerland, Greece). Regardless of the magnitude of the incidence, almost all areas report rates in men that are twofold to threefold higher than rates in women (see **Fig. 1**). Notable exceptions to this gender disparity are the approximately equal incidences reported by registries in Harare, Zimbabwe (African ancestry); Costa Rica; Cali, Colombia; and South Karachi, Pakistan. The greatest gender disparity in incidence is reported by registries in central Europe, where the male/female ratio is greater than 4. Examples of this male/female disparity occur in the registries of Varese Province, Italy (M/F ratio = 4.4), Geneva, Switzerland (5.6) and Bas-Rhin, France (6.0).[5] The reasons that men have higher rates of liver cancer than women are not completely understood, but may be partly explained by the sex-specific prevalence of risk factors. Men are more likely to be chronically infected with hepatitis B virus (HBV) and hepatitis C virus (HCV), consume alcohol, smoke cigarettes, and have increased iron stores. Men have also been reported to have higher levels of aflatoxin markers in their blood than do women.[6] Whether androgenic hormones or increased genetic susceptibility also predispose men to the development of liver cancer is not clear.

In addition to variability by gender, many areas report incidence disparities by race/ethnicity. In the United States, for example, HCC incidence is highest among Asians/Pacific Islanders (11.7/100,000) and lowest among white persons (3.9/100,000).[7] Intermediate to these rates are those of Hispanic people (8.0/100,000), black persons (7.0/100,000), and American Indians/Alaska Natives (6.6/100,000).[7] Just as divergent as the rates among various ethnic groups residing in one area are the rates among members of a single ethnic group living in various locations. For example, incidences among Chinese populations are notably lower in the United States than they are in either China or in Singapore (**Fig. 2**). As with gender differences, race/ethnic differences in risk are likely to be related to the prevalence of major risk factors in each groups.

During the intervals from 1983 to 1987 and 1998 to 2002, liver cancer incidence increased in many areas of the world. Increases were notable in northern Europe, North and South America, Oceania, as well as in most countries of southern Europe, India, and Israel (**Fig. 3**).[5] In contrast, incidences declined in most Far East Asian countries and in Spain. Although the reasons for the increase in incidence in some areas are not clear, factors such as HCV infection, increasing rates of obesity and diabetes, and improved survival from cirrhosis are likely to be related. The reasons for the declining rates in some Far East Asian countries are likely to be several. In Japan, the cohort of individuals infected with HCV in the 1930s and 1940s is becoming smaller and thus the rate of HCV-related HCC is declining.[8] The declining HCC rates in China and Singapore, areas where HBV is the major risk factor, are more likely caused by the elimination of other HCC cofactors. Although HBV vaccination began in these areas in the mid-1980s, the vaccine was given to newborns. Thus, the vaccinated population is only in their mid-20s at the present time and would have contributed little to the current HCC incidence in the population.

Even in developed countries, the prognosis of liver cancer is unfavorable. In the United States, the 1-year survival is less than 50%, and the 5-year survival only 10%.[7] Survival is even less favorable in developing countries. As a result, mortalities in all locations are roughly equivalent to, or sometimes higher than, the incidences. Higher mortalities than incidences can seem to exist because the liver is a preferred site of metastasis for many cancers, and it is not always easy to distinguish these secondary liver cancers from primary liver cancers.

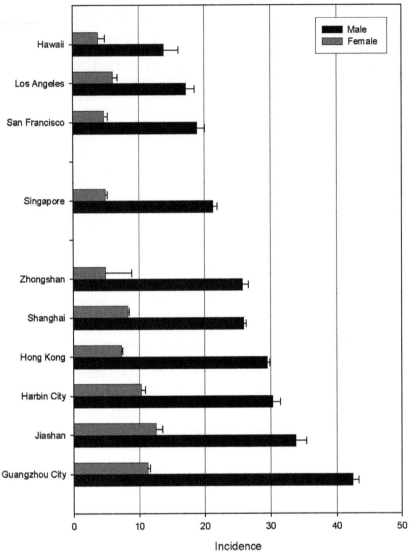

Fig. 2. Age-adjusted incidences per 100,000 of liver cancer among selected Chinese populations, 1998–2002. Age adjusted to world standard. (*Data from* Ferlay J, Parkin DM, Curado MP, et al. Cancer incidence in five continents, volumes I to IX: IARC CANCERBase No. 9 [Internet]. Available at: http://ci5.iarc.fr.)

RISK FACTORS

At least 80% of HCCs are associated with chronic infection with either of 2 viruses, HBV and HCV. Of these, HBV infections account for 75% to 80% of virus-associated HCCs, with HCV responsible for 10% to 20%.[9] Other risk factors include consumption of aflatoxin B_1 (AFB_1) contaminated foodstuffs, excessive consumption of alcohol, diabetes/obesity, and certain rare metabolic disorders, such as hemochromatosis, α-1 antitrypsin deficiency, tyrosinemia, and several porphyrias. Although persons with these rare metabolic disorders have increased risks of HCC, the rarity

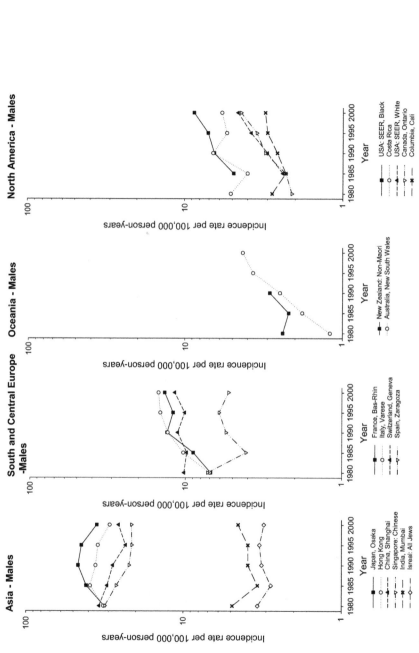

Fig. 3. Age-adjusted trends in liver cancer incidence among men by region, 1978–1982 to 1998–2002. Age adjusted to world standard. (*Data from* Ferlay J, Parkin DM, Curado MP, et al. Cancer incidence in five continents, volumes I to IX: IARC CANCERBase No. 9 [Internet]. Available at: http://ci5.iarc.fr.)

of the disorders in the population results in the disorders not being major risk factors. The dominant risk factors tend to vary in high-risk and low-risk HCC regions. In most high-risk countries of Asia and Africa, chronic HBV infection and AFB_1 exposure are the major risk factors. In contrast, HCV infection, excessive alcohol consumption, and diabetes/obesity play more important roles in low-risk HCC areas. Exceptions to these patterns are seen in Japan and Egypt where the dominant risk factor is HCV infection.

The global pattern of HCC incidence is related to the history of these major HCC risk factors and the length of time the factors have been present in human populations. Although fossils of hepadnaviruses in avian genomes date back at least 19 million years,[10] evidence suggests that HBV has been in human populations for about 6000 years, based on the divergence of human HBV from other primate HBVs.[11] In contrast, HCV dates back less than 1000 years and only became widely dispersed around the world during the twentieth century.[12] Alcohol consumption has been a common exposure among humans during all recorded history, whereas high rates of obesity and diabetes are phenomena of the late twentieth century.

HBV

Several pathologists proposed in the 1950s that chronic virus infections of the liver could lead to liver cancer.[13–15] They also noted the strong association between cirrhosis and liver cancer, because at least 80% of liver cancers occurred in cirrhotic livers. The cirrhosis-liver cancer link was suggested to be stronger in Asia and Africa, where 5% to 50% of men with cirrhosis developed liver cancer, whereas the percentage in the United States and Western Europe was 3% to 10%.[15] In most high-risk HCC regions, HBV infection is associated with most cases of cirrhosis and at least 80% of the cases of HCC.

In 1994, the International Agency for Research on Cancer classified HBV, a member of the Hepadnavirus family, as carcinogenic to humans.[16] Currently, about 5% of the world's population (350 million people) is chronically infected with HBV. The evidence supporting the causal association of HBV with HCC is substantive. Areas of the world with high incidence and mortality for HCC have high prevalences of chronic HBV infection (**Fig. 4**). The reverse is also true. Countries with prevalences of chronic HBV infection of greater than 2% have increased incidence and mortality of HCC.[17–19] Case-control studies in all regions of the world have consistently shown that chronic HBV infection (seropositivity for hepatitis B surface antigen [HBsAg]) is significantly more common among cases than controls. Odds ratios have ranged from 5:1 to 65:1.[16] Prospective studies of persons chronically infected with HBV have consistently shown high relative risks for HCC, ranging from 5 to 103.[16,20–24] In a seminal study of male government workers in Taiwan, the age-adjusted annual incidence of HCC was 474 per 100,000 in HBsAg(+) men compared with 6 per 100,000 in HBsAg(−) men.[20] Similarly, in an 8-year follow-up of a very high-risk cohort in China, the cumulative risks of HCC mortality were 8% in HBsAg(+) men and 0.5% in HBsAg(−). Among women, the cumulative risks were 2.0% in HBsAg(+) persons and 0.1% among HBsAg(−) persons.[22]

In areas of the world with high incidences of HCC and high prevalences of chronic HBV infection, approximately 70% of HBV infections are acquired in the perinatal period or in early childhood.[19,25–27] Thus, among HBV carriers in endemic areas, those born to HBsAg(+) mothers are likely to have been infected longest and are at higher risk of HCC than are HBV carriers with HBsAg(−) mothers.[28–30] HBV DNA is integrated into the genome of liver tissues in almost all HCC cases from patients with HBsAg in

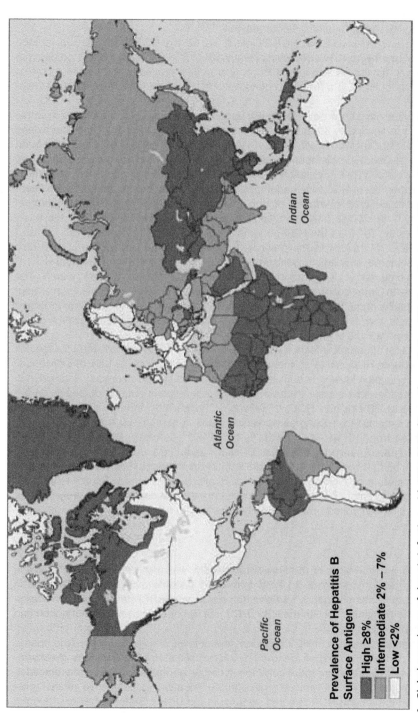

Fig. 4. Global prevalence of chronic infection with HBV, 2006. (*From* Chaves S. Hepatitis B. In: Centers for Disease Control and Prevention: CDC Health Information for International Travel 2010. Atlanta: U.S. Department of Health and Human Services, Public Health Service, 2009. Availalbe at: http://wwwnc.cdc.gov/travel/yellowbook/2010/chapter-5/hepatitis-b.htm. Accessed December 15, 2010.)

their serum. Investigators have also detected HBV DNA sequences in 10% to 20% of HCC tumors from patients who were seronegative for HBsAg, but positive for antibodies to HBsAg or hepatitis B core antigen.[31–33]

Among individuals with chronic HBV infections, risks of HCC vary by several factors, the major one being HBV DNA levels (viral load).[23,34,35] Although there is no discrete cutoff level, having greater than 10^5/mL viral copies confers a 2.5-fold to threefold greater risk of HCC, in a follow-up period of 8 to 10 years, than does having a lower viral load.

Genotypes have been defined as HBV genomes that differ from each other in whole genome sequencing by 8% or more. By those criteria, 8 genotypes, A to H, have been identified; subgenotypes, differing by 4% to 8% within genotypes, have also been reported.[36] Genotype distribution varies by geography, response to treatment, and HCC risk. In multiple population-based studies, genotype C has been associated with a higher risk of HCC than genotypes A2, Ba, Bj, and D. Genotype C is also associated with delayed clearance of hepatitis virus e antigen (HBeAg), a marker of infectivity.[37] In studies that controlled for genotype, double mutations in the basal core promoter (BCP) of the HBV genome were independent predictors of increased risk of HCC. Mutations in the precore (PC) region of the viral genome have also been associated, although inconsistently, with increased risks of cirrhosis and HCC.[38]

The lifetime risk of HCC among HBV carriers is estimated to be 10% to 25%. The World Health Organization and the Centers for Disease Control and Prevention project that, annually, some 600,000 chronically infected people die from HCC and chronic liver disease and, eventually, 35 million to 87 million of the 350 million prevalent global HBV carriers will die of HCC.[39]

Prevention of chronic infection with HBV via vaccination drastically reduces the risk of subsequent HCC, although the vaccine is ineffective in 5% to 10% of individuals. On the population level, it is anticipated that the widespread neonatal vaccination in many countries that started in the mid-1980s will result in notable decreases in the incidence of HBV-related HCC. In Taiwan, 20 years after the initiation of universal newborn vaccination, HBsAg seropositivity rates in persons younger than 20 years have fallen from 10% to 17% to 0.7% to 1.7%.[40] Currently, 92% of all countries have integrated newborn hepatitis B vaccination into their routine vaccination programs and 70% are now delivering 3 immunization doses.[39] However, vaccination is not routine in all high-risk countries, particularly those in sub-Saharan Africa. In these areas, control of aflatoxin is critically important because there is a synergistic effect of aflatoxin consumption and HBV infection on risk of HCC.

HCV

The HCV, an RNA virus of the Flaviviridae family, was identified in 1989.[41] Reliable serologic tests for antibody to HCV (anti-HCV) became available in 1990, and in 1994 the International Agency for Research on Cancer (IARC) classified HCV as carcinogenic to humans.[16] Unlike the HBV, HCV has not been shown to infect nonhuman hosts in the wild.

Phylogenetic analysis of HCV has identified at least 6 major genotypes (numbered 1–6) and numerous subtypes (denoted by lowercase letters).[42,43] Particular genotype-subtype combinations are more common in certain geographic areas and are associated with the mode of viral transmission. By location, genotype 1a is the most common type among HCV-infected persons in the United States, whereas 1b is the most common in Japan and 4a is the most common in Egypt. By mode of transmission, in Europe, genotypes 1b and 2 are more common in older persons, whereas genotypes 1a and 3a are more common among injecting drug users.[12] Coalescent theory studies of HCV genotypes have determined that genotypes 1a and 1b originated approximately 100 years ago, whereas genotypes 4 (found predominantly in Africa and the Middle East) and 6 (found predominantly in southeast Asia) arose 350 and 700 years ago, respectively.[44] Evidence indicates that HCV existed as a long-term, low-level, endemic virus before the twentieth century, but spread worldwide starting around 1900 via several transmission routes including pooling of blood products, widespread blood transfusion, and injection drug use.[45] How HCV was maintained as an endemic infection before the twentieth century is not well understood at present.[46]

As seen on the map shown in **Fig. 5**, the highest rates of chronic HCV infection in the world occur in northern Africa, particularly Egypt, where the rate has been estimated at 18%.[47] In Asia, Mongolia reports rates (10%) considerably higher than those of Vietnam (6%), Cambodia (4%), China (3%–4%), or Japan (2%).[47] European rates of 0.5% to 2.5% are similar to the rate of 1.8% in the United States, but higher than the Canadian rate of 0.1% to 0.8%, which is one of the lowest in the world.

Using genetic evolutionary analysis of HCV in Japan, molecular clock studies have suggested that HCV first appeared in that country in the early 1880s and became more widely disseminated throughout the population in the 1930s and 1940s.[48] The population dispersal times are consistent with the introduction of antischistosomal therapy using intravenous antimony sodium tartrate, which began in the 1920s.[48,49] HCV infection may have become more widespread during World War II because of the use of intravenous stimulants,[48] the liberal use of blood transfusions to treat anemias,[50] and the use of blood from paid donors.[51] The spread of HCV 1b in Japan began to decline around 1995.[52]

Molecular clock studies have also examined HCV in Egypt, a country with high rates of chronic HCV infection. As in Japan, evidence suggests that HCV was spread in the population by the use of intravenous antischistosomal therapy.[53] Although the antischistosomal campaigns began in the 1920s, they were particularly widespread between 1961 and 1986.[54] In addition to spreading HCV, the campaigns were also likely to have spread HBV. However, the risk of an adult becoming a chronic HBV carrier after infection is fairly low (~10%) compared with the risk of an adult becoming a chronic HCV carrier after infection (~80%).

Molecular analysis of HCV genotype 1a in the United States suggests that the virus first entered the population around 1910 and became more widely disseminated in the 1960s.[48] The introduction may have come as a result of US soldiers becoming infected while abroad during the Spanish-American War.[55] The reason for dissemination of HCV more widely in the 1960s is less clear, but the timing of the dissemination is consistent with the estimates derived from mathematical modeling.[56,57] Using National Health and Nutrition Examination Survey III (NHANES III) HCV prevalence data, it was estimated that HCV infection rates rapidly increased from the late 1960s to the early 1980s, then began to decline sharply in the early 1990s.[56] Another modeling effort reached similar conclusions, noting an increase in HCV infection starting in the mid-1960s that hit a peak in the mid-1980s, before starting to decline.[57] Implications for the future incidence of HCC in the United States are not clear. Although several models suggest that HCC incidence could hit the high levels seen earlier in Japan, other studies suggest that the long-term risk of HCC among HCV-infected Americans is low compared with HCV-infected Japanese.[58] Because HCV circulated in the US blood supply for fewer years than it did in Japan, and newer antiviral agents are being developed to treat HCV infection, the long-term effect of HCV on HCC rates may be less dramatic in the United States than in Japan.

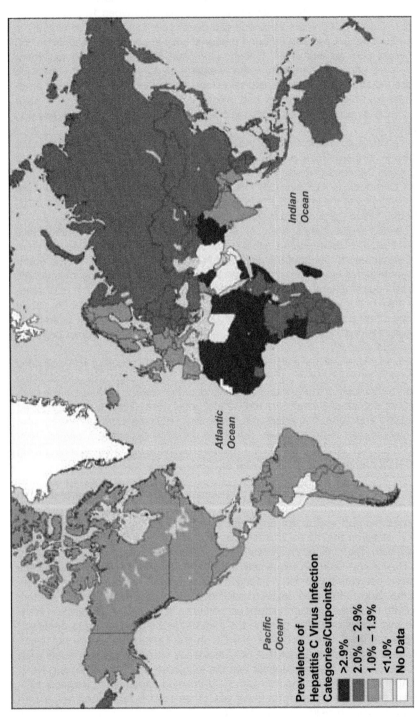

Fig. 5. Global prevalence of HCV infection, 2004. (*From* Holmberg S. Hepatitis C. In: Centers for Disease Control and Prevention. CDC Health Information for International Travel 2010. Atlanta: U.S. Department of Health and Human Services, Public Health Service, 2009. Available at: http://wwwnc.cdc.gov/travel/yellowbook/2010/chapter-5/hepatitis-c.htm. Accessed December 15, 2010.)

AFLATOXIN

Aflatoxin, a mycotoxin produced by molds of *Aspergillus* species (*Aspergillus flavus* and *Aspergillus parasiticus*), contaminates maize, groundnuts, and tree nuts in warm, humid environments and is a well-established hepatic carcinogen.[59] Aflatoxin exposure has likely been prevalent in human populations throughout history. There are 4 principal aflatoxins (B_1, B_2, G_1, and G_2), of which aflatoxin B_1 (AFB_1) has been shown to be the most potent in animal studies.[59] Based largely on the indisputable animal data, IARC determined that there was sufficient evidence to classify aflatoxin as a group 1 human carcinogen.[59]

Many ecological studies of AFB_1 contamination of food stores conducted in the 1970s and 1980s were compatible with a role for the carcinogen in human HCC. Person-specific epidemiologic studies performed subsequently provided strong evidence that AFB_1 was a causal factor or cofactor in the development of HCC. These studies were made possible by the development of assays for aflatoxin metabolites in urine, AFB_1-albumin adducts in serum, and detection of a signature aflatoxin DNA mutation in tissues. The mutation occurs in a hotspot region of the p53 cancer suppressor gene at the third base of codon 249 (p53 249ser mutation). The G-to-T transversion, observed in 30% to 60% of tumors arising in persons living in aflatoxin-rich environments,[60–62] is postulated to result from the reaction of the 8,9 epoxide activated form of AFB_1 with the N-7 guanine in DNA.

The regions of the world with the highest levels of aflatoxin exposure are sub-Saharan Africa, southeast Asia, and China. Within these areas, higher levels are found among rural populations than among urban populations,[63] among men rather than women,[6,64] and among persons chronically infected with HBV.[6]

The synergistic effect of AFB_1 and chronic HBV infection on HCC risk was revealed in short-term prospective studies in Shanghai, China. Compared with persons without aflatoxin or HBV exposure, the risk of HCC was fourfold greater among persons with increased levels of aflatoxin metabolites in urine, sevenfold greater among persons chronically infected with HBV and 60-fold greater among individuals with both risk factors.[65,66] More current evidence suggests that there is also a synergistic effect between AFB_1 and HCV infection.[67] However, AFB_1 contamination is more common in areas where HBV is the dominant virus. Using data on aflatoxin levels in food, consumption of aflatoxin-contaminated foods, and prevalence of chronic infection with HBV, a recent risk assessment found that aflatoxin is associated with between 4.6% and 28.2% of HCCs worldwide.[68]

In general, in areas of the world where AFB_1 exposure is high, chronic HBV infection is highly prevalent. Because little can be done to alter the HBV chronic infection state, eradicating AFB_1 from the food supply would be one way to bring down the HCC incidence.[69] However, simply avoiding foods contaminated with AFB_1 is not a practical solution in areas afflicted with chronic malnutrition.

ALCOHOL

In 1988, IARC concluded that there was a causal relationship between alcohol consumption and liver cancer.[70] In 2007, the World Cancer Research Fund and American Institute for Cancer Research, in a review of diet and physical activity studies, concluded that alcohol consumption was probably a direct cause of liver cancer.[71]

Most studies in low-risk HCC populations have found alcohol to be a significant risk factor,[72–80] whereas the evidence from earlier studies in high-risk populations has been more equivocal.[81–86] The disparity between low-risk and high-risk regions may have been caused by lower mean alcohol consumption in high-risk populations and/or difference in the interaction between alcohol with HBV and HCV and/or other risk factors. However, evidence suggests that both HBV and HCV, in conjunction with alcohol, have synergistic effects on HCC risk.[87–89] In addition, the same studies find that alcohol consumption is significantly associated with HCC in the absence of viral infection (odds ratios between 2.4 and 7.0), although higher levels of alcohol consumption are likely required to increase risk in the absence of viral infection. Whether risk is increased with low or moderate levels of alcohol consumption in the absence of other factors is not well understood.

Whether alcohol is more strongly associated with HCC in women than in men has been difficult to study given that women are less likely to be heavy drinkers and less likely to develop HCC than men. A greater effect of alcohol on women has been hypothesized based on differences in alcohol dehydrogenase activity[90] and evidence of a greater association between alcohol and cirrhosis among women.[91,92] However, no substantial gender difference in risk of HCC with alcohol consumption was reported by at least 1 study.[87] Results of some studies have suggested that alcohol in combination with smoking may be more risk-producing than alcohol alone[93] and that women may be particularly affected by the combination.[94] Recent evidence also suggests that there is a synergistic effect of alcohol consumption and obesity on HCC.[95] Although women are as likely as men to be obese,[96] they are less likely than men to either drink or smoke at high levels.

The mechanism by which alcohol increases HCC risk is not clear. Animal and human studies provide little evidence that ethanol is a carcinogen.[97] Some of the mechanisms by which alcohol might increase risk include the production of acetaldehyde and free radicals during alcohol metabolism, cytochrome P4502E1 induction, modulation of cell regeneration, promotion or exacerbation of nutritional deficiencies, and alterations of the immune system.[98] It is certain that alcohol induces cirrhosis, and cirrhosis is a factor in 60% to 90% of HCCs. Whether alcohol is related to HCC independently of cirrhosis is less clear.

Worldwide, alcohol consumption is highest in European countries and lowest in eastern Mediterranean countries.[99] However, between 1960 and 2000, per capita consumption declined in European, North American, and African countries after reaching peak levels in the early 1980s. During the same interval, consumption increased in southeast Asian and, even more notably, in western Pacific countries. During the same period, eastern Mediterranean countries maintained very low levels of consumption. Because excessive alcohol consumption has historically been a more important HCC risk factor in low-risk HCC areas such as Europe and North America, downward trends in consumption suggest a favorable effect on HCC rates in those areas. However, increasing consumption in southeast Asia and the western Pacific countries, areas with already high rates of HCC, may be a future concern.

OBESITY, DIABETES MELLITUS AND NONALCOHOLIC STEATOHEPATITIS

A significant relationship between diabetes and liver cancer was first reported in 1986.[100] Although several early epidemiology studies[101,102] did not confirm the relationship, later studies, with a few exceptions,[103,104] were confirmatory. The bulk of the literature, summarized in systematic reviews[105,106] and meta-analyses,[107] now provides strong evidence from low-risk, intermediate-risk, and high-risk countries that HCC and diabetes are significantly associated.

Many of the studies in individuals with diabetes also noted a relationship between diabetes and cirrhosis.[108–111] Because insulin resistance is known to be associated with cirrhosis, it is possible that the diabetes-cirrhosis and diabetes-HCC relationships are a consequence of the cirrhotic process. Cohort studies, which have found increased risks of HCC among diabetics and persons with hyperinsulinemia, suggest that diabetes usually precedes the development of cirrhosis and HCC.[112–114] In support of these observations are results of studies showing that hepatic steatosis is common among persons with type II diabetes.[115] Similarly, it has been suggested that the diabetes-HCC relationship is a result of HCV infection[116] because of impaired glucose and insulin metabolism.[117] HCV status has been determined in several studies that examined the diabetes-HCC relationship. Although some of these studies reported that the effect of diabetes was dependent on HCV infection,[103,104] others found that the effect of diabetes effect was independent.[118,119]

Obesity is a major risk factor for the development of type II diabetes. In a recent analysis of data from the US NHANES, it was reported that 80.3% of NHANES participants with diabetes were overweight (body mass index [BMI, calculated as weight in kilograms divided by the square of height in meters] ≥ 25 kg/m^2) and, conversely, the prevalence of diabetes rose linearly with weight class from 8% of persons with normal BMI to 43% of persons with obese BMI.[120] Several studies have reported that obesity is related to liver cancer, as summarized in a recent review.[121] In comparing normal weight persons with overweight and obese persons, a meta-analysis of 11 cohort studies found that the risk of liver cancer was 1.17 (95% CI = 1.0–1.3) in overweight persons and 1.87 (95% CI = 1.5–2.4) in obese persons.[122] However, whether obesity is an independent risk factor is not yet clear. At the present time, there are more studies from low-risk than high-risk populations and many studies have not adjusted their analyses for other known risk factors. One study that did examine the joint effects of obesity and alcohol consumption on risk of liver diseases, including cancer, found a synergistic effect on risk.[95]

With relative risks of approximately 2.5 for diabetes and approximately 1.5 for obesity, neither factor is associated with HCC as strongly as are HCV or HBV. However, the prevalence of diabetes and obesity in developed countries are far greater than HCV and HBV, and the prevalence of diabetes in developing countries is growing faster than it is in developed countries.[123] It has been estimated that there are currently 285 million persons in the world, or 6.4% of the global population, with diabetes.[123] The prevalence is projected to increase by 69% in developing countries, and 20% in developed countries, by the year 2030. Similarly, increases in BMI have been documented in many countries since 1980.[124] In the United States, the prevalence of obesity was stable between 1960 and 1980.[125] However, during the interval between the years 1976 to 1980 and 1988 to 1994, the prevalence of obesity increased approximately 8%, then further increased during the interval between 1988 to 1994 and 1999 to 2000.[126] More encouraging results came from a comparison of rates between 1999 to 2000 and 2007 to 2008.[96] During the most recent 10-year period, obesity prevalence did not increase among US women. Although prevalence did increase among men, the most recent data were flat, suggesting that the prevalence of obesity may not be continuing to increase at the same rate as previously.

In 1980, Ludwig and colleagues[127] coined the term nonalcoholic steatohepatitis (NASH) to describe a condition among nondrinkers, characterized by morphologic evidence of fatty changes in the liver with lobular hepatitis. Although subsequent definitions have varied, Brunt and colleagues[128] proposed that NASH be defined by the presence of steatosis, inflammation, hepatocellular degenerative changes, and variable fibrosis. Now recognized as the most severe form of nonalcoholic fatty liver disease, NASH is estimated to be the third most common liver disorder in North America,[129] and the most common in Australia and New Zealand.[130]

Although most of the patients described in the initial report of Ludwig and colleagues[127] were women, subsequent reports have found that NASH occurs equally among men and women.[131] Conditions frequently found in association with NASH include insulin resistance, impaired glucose tolerance, type II diabetes mellitus, hypertriglyceridemia, age greater than 45 years, and obesity; particularly central obesity.[130] Evidence for a possible genetic component to risk has come from a family study that found an unexpectedly high occurrence of NASH-related conditions in relatives of NASH probands.[132]

Although some early reports suggested that NASH was a nonprogressive disorder, it is now recognized that severe fibrosis occurs in 15% to 50% of patients with NASH, and cirrhosis in 7% to 25%.[133] It has also been suggested that burned-out NASH is the cause of many cases of cryptogenic cirrhosis because many of the same comorbid conditions are equally present in NASH and cryptogenic cirrhosis.[134–136] The incidence of HCC is increased in most forms of cirrhosis,[137] and NASH is proving to be no exception.[133,138–142] A recent analysis of risk factors for HCC in the United States between 2002 and 2008 reported that nonalcoholic fatty liver disease/NASH is already the most common risk factor (59%), followed by diabetes (36%).[143]

SUMMARY

The global risk of HCC has been largely driven by HBV infection for the past century. Contributions to risk have also been made by other factors, including HCV, aflatoxin, excessive alcohol consumption, and obesity/diabetes. The dominant effect of HBV on global HCC risk should decline in future generations as the population vaccinated against HBV advances in years. Infection with HCV should also decline as a major cause of HCC in future generations because HCV was removed from the blood supply of most countries in the early 1990s. Although projections of HCV-related HCC rates have suggested high rates for another 30 years, the projections may be overly pessimistic. Declining levels of alcohol consumption in many areas also suggest that alcohol may be less of a factor in HCC in coming years. However, high global prevalence rates of obesity and diabetes may ensure that they become even more important risk factors for HCC as the prevalence of other risk factors declines.

REFERENCES

1. Ferlay J, Shin H, Bray F, et al. GLOBOCAN 2008, Cancer incidence and mortality worldwide: IARC CANCERBase no. 10 [Internet]. Available at: http://globocan.iarc.fr. Accessed November 25, 2010.
2. Zimmerman M, Aufderheide AC. Paleopathology Newsletter 2010;150:16–23.
3. Frerichs FT. A clinical treatise on diseases of the liver. New York: Wood; 1879.
4. Osler W, McCrae T. The principles and practice of medicine: designed for the use of practitioners and students of medicine. 8th edition. New York: D. Appleton and Company; 1912.
5. Ferlay J, Parkin DM, Curado MP, et al. Cancer incidence in five continents, volumes I to IX: IARC CANCERBase No. 9 [Internet]. Available at: http://ci5.iarc.fr. Accessed November 9, 2010.
6. Sun CA, Wu DM, Wang LY, et al. Determinants of formation of aflatoxin-albumin adducts: a seven-township study in Taiwan. Br J Cancer 2002;87:966–70.
7. Altekruse SF, McGlynn KA, Reichman ME. Hepatocellular carcinoma incidence, mortality, and survival trends in the United States from 1975 to 2005. J Clin Oncol 2009;27:1485–91.

8. Tanaka H, Imai Y, Hiramatsu N, et al. Declining incidence of hepatocellular carcinoma in Osaka, Japan, from 1990 to 2003. Ann Intern Med 2008;148: 820–6.

9. Perz JF, Armstrong GL, Farrington LA, et al. The contributions of hepatitis B virus and hepatitis C virus infections to cirrhosis and primary liver cancer worldwide. J Hepatol 2006;45:529–38.

10. Gilbert C, Feschotte C. Genomic fossils calibrate the long-term evolution of hepadnaviruses. PLoS Biol 2010;8(9):e1000495, pii.

11. Fares MA, Holmes EC. A revised evolutionary history of hepatitis B virus (HBV). J Mol Evol 2002;54:807–14.

12. Simmonds P. Reconstructing the origins of human hepatitis viruses. Philos Trans R Soc Lond B Biol Sci 2001;356:1013–26.

13. Edmondson HA, Steiner PE. Primary carcinoma of the liver: a study of 100 cases among 48,900 necropsies. Cancer 1954;7:462–503.

14. Higginson J, Grobbelaar BG, Walker AR. Hepatic fibrosis and cirrhosis in man in relation to malnutrition. Am J Pathol 1957;33:29–44.

15. Edmondson HA. Tumors of the liver and intrahepatic bile duct. Washington, DC: Armed Forces Institute of Pathology; 1958.

16. IARC. Working Group on the Evaluation of Carcinogenic Risks to Humans, International Agency for Research on Cancer. Hepatitis viruses. Lyon (France): International Agency for Research on Cancer; 1994.

17. Parkin DM, Bray F, Ferlay J, et al. Global cancer statistics, 2002. CA Cancer J Clin 2005;55:74–108.

18. Schutte K, Bornschein J, Malfertheiner P. Hepatocellular carcinoma–epidemiological trends and risk factors. Dig Dis 2009;27:80–92.

19. CDC. Hepatitis B. Available at: http://wwwnc.cdc.gov/travel/yellowbook/2010/chapter-2/hepatitis-b.aspx. Accessed December 15, 2010.

20. Beasley RP, Hwang LY, Lin CC, et al. Hepatocellular carcinoma and hepatitis B virus. A prospective study of 22 707 men in Taiwan. Lancet 1981;2:1129–33.

21. Heyward WL, Lanier AP, McMahon BJ, et al. Early detection of primary hepatocellular carcinoma. Screening for primary hepatocellular carcinoma among persons infected with hepatitis B virus. JAMA 1985;254:3052–4.

22. Evans AA, Chen G, Ross EA, et al. Eight-year follow-up of the 90,000-person Haimen City cohort: I. Hepatocellular carcinoma mortality, risk factors, and gender differences. Cancer Epidemiol Biomarkers Prev 2002;11:369–76.

23. Chen CJ, Iloeje UH, Yang HI. Long-term outcomes in hepatitis B: the REVEAL-HBV study. Clin Liver Dis 2007;11:797–816, viii.

24. Ijima T, Saitoh N, Nobutomo K, et al. A prospective cohort study of hepatitis B surface antigen carriers in a working population. Gann 1984;75:571–3.

25. Stevens CE, Beasley RP, Tsui J, et al. Vertical transmission of hepatitis B antigen in Taiwan. N Engl J Med 1975;292:771–4.

26. Okada K, Kamiyama I, Inomata M, et al. e Antigen and anti-e in the serum of asymptomatic carrier mothers as indicators of positive and negative transmission of hepatitis B virus to their infants. N Engl J Med 1976;294:746–9.

27. Marinier E, Barrois V, Larouze B, et al. Lack of perinatal transmission of hepatitis B virus infection in Senegal, West Africa. J Pediatr 1985;106:843–9.

28. Larouze B, Saimot G, Lustbader ED, et al. Host responses to hepatitis-B infection in patients with primary hepatic carcinoma and their families. A case/control study in Senegal, West Africa. Lancet 1976;2:534–8.

29. Hann HW, Kim CY, London WT, et al. Hepatitis B virus and primary hepatocellular carcinoma: family studies in Korea. Int J Cancer 1982;30:47–51.

30. Beasley RP. Hepatitis B virus. The major etiology of hepatocellular carcinoma. Cancer 1988;61:1942–56.
31. Shafritz DA, Shouval D, Sherman HI, et al. Integration of hepatitis B virus DNA into the genome of liver cells in chronic liver disease and hepatocellular carcinoma. Studies in percutaneous liver biopsies and post-mortem tissue specimens. N Engl J Med 1981;305:1067–73.
32. Brechot C, Degos F, Lugassy C, et al. Hepatitis B virus DNA in patients with chronic liver disease and negative tests for hepatitis B surface antigen. N Engl J Med 1985;312:270–6.
33. Ming L, Thorgeirsson SS, Gail MH, et al. Dominant role of hepatitis B virus and cofactor role of aflatoxin in hepatocarcinogenesis in Qidong, China. Hepatology 2002;36:1214–20.
34. Chen G, Lin W, Shen F, et al. Past HBV viral load as predictor of mortality and morbidity from HCC and chronic liver disease in a prospective study. Am J Gastroenterol 2006;101:1797–803.
35. Chen CJ, Yang HI, Iloeje UH. Hepatitis B virus DNA levels and outcomes in chronic hepatitis B. Hepatology 2009;49:S72–84.
36. McMahon BJ. The natural history of chronic hepatitis B virus infection. Hepatology 2009;49:S45–55.
37. McMahon BJ. Natural history of chronic hepatitis B. Clin Liver Dis 2010;14: 381–96.
38. Sumi H, Yokosuka O, Seki N, et al. Influence of hepatitis B virus genotypes on the progression of chronic type B liver disease. Hepatology 2003;37:19–26.
39. WHO. Hepatitis B. Available at: http://www.who.int/immunization/topics/hepatits_b/en/index.html. Accessed November 20, 2010.
40. Chang MH, You SL, Chen CJ, et al. Decreased incidence of hepatocellular carcinoma in hepatitis B vaccinees: a 20-year follow-up study. J Natl Cancer Inst 2009;101:1348–55.
41. Choo QL, Kuo G, Weiner AJ, et al. Isolation of a cDNA clone derived from a blood-borne non-A, non-B viral hepatitis genome. Science 1989;244:359–62.
42. Simmonds P. Genetic diversity and evolution of hepatitis C virus–15 years on. J Gen Virol 2004;85:3173–88.
43. Simmonds P, Holmes EC, Cha TA, et al. Classification of hepatitis C virus into six major genotypes and a series of subtypes by phylogenetic analysis of the NS-5 region. J Gen Virol 1993;74(Pt 11):2391–9.
44. Pybus OG, Charleston MA, Gupta S, et al. The epidemic behavior of the hepatitis C virus. Science 2001;292:2323–5.
45. Pybus OG, Barnes E, Taggart R, et al. Genetic history of hepatitis C virus in East Asia. J Virol 2009;83:1071–82.
46. Pybus OG, Markov PV, Wu A, et al. Investigating the endemic transmission of the hepatitis C virus. Int J Parasitol 2007;37:839–49.
47. Bostan N, Mahmood T. An overview about hepatitis C: a devastating virus. Crit Rev Microbiol 2010;36:91–133.
48. Tanaka Y, Hanada K, Mizokami M, et al. Inaugural article: a comparison of the molecular clock of hepatitis C virus in the United States and Japan predicts that hepatocellular carcinoma incidence in the United States will increase over the next two decades. Proc Natl Acad Sci U S A 2002;99:15584–9.
49. Iida F, Iida R, Kamijo H, et al. Chronic Japanese schistosomiasis and hepatocellular carcinoma: ten years of follow-up in Yamanashi Prefecture, Japan. Bull World Health Organ 1999;77:573–81.

50. Primary liver cancer in Japan. The Liver Cancer Study Group of Japan. Cancer 1984;54:1747–55.
51. Chung H, Ueda T, Kudo M. Changing trends in hepatitis C infection over the past 50 years in Japan. Intervirology 2010;53:39–43.
52. Moriya T, Koyama T, Tanaka J, et al. Epidemiology of hepatitis C virus in Japan. Intervirology 1999;42:153–8.
53. Frank C, Mohamed MK, Strickland GT, et al. The role of parenteral antischistosomal therapy in the spread of hepatitis C virus in Egypt. Lancet 2000;355:887–91.
54. Tanaka Y, Agha S, Saudy N, et al. Exponential spread of hepatitis C virus genotype 4a in Egypt. J Mol Evol 2004;58:191–5.
55. Mizokami M, Tanaka Y. Tracing the evolution of hepatitis C virus in the United States, Japan, and Egypt by using the molecular clock. Clin Gastroenterol Hepatol 2005;3:S82–5.
56. Armstrong GL, Alter MJ, McQuillan GM, et al. The past incidence of hepatitis C virus infection: implications for the future burden of chronic liver disease in the United States. Hepatology 2000;31:777–82.
57. Salomon JA, Weinstein MC, Hammitt JK, et al. Empirically calibrated model of hepatitis C virus infection in the United States. Am J Epidemiol 2002;156:761–73.
58. Seeff LB, Miller RN, Rabkin CS, et al. 45-year follow-up of hepatitis C virus infection in healthy young adults. Ann Intern Med 2000;132:105–11.
59. IARC. In: Working Group on the Evaluation of Carcinogenic Risks to Humans, International Agency for Research on Cancer. Some traditional herbal medicines, some mycotoxins, naphthalene and styrene, vol. 2010. Lyon (France): International Agency for Research on Cancer; 2002.
60. Ozturk M. p53 mutation in hepatocellular carcinoma after aflatoxin exposure. Lancet 1991;338:1356–9.
61. Bressac B, Kew M, Wands J, et al. Selective G to T mutations of p53 gene in hepatocellular carcinoma from southern Africa. Nature 1991;350:429–31.
62. Hsu IC, Metcalf RA, Sun T, et al. Mutational hotspot in the p53 gene in human hepatocellular carcinomas. Nature 1991;350:427–8.
63. Wild CP, Hall AJ. Primary prevention of hepatocellular carcinoma in developing countries. Mutat Res 2000;462:381–93.
64. Plymoth A, Viviani S, Hainaut P. Control of hepatocellular carcinoma through hepatitis B vaccination in areas of high endemicity: perspectives for global liver cancer prevention. Cancer Lett 2009;286:15–21.
65. Qian GS, Ross RK, Yu MC, et al. A follow-up study of urinary markers of aflatoxin exposure and liver cancer risk in Shanghai, People's Republic of China. Cancer Epidemiol Biomarkers Prev 1994;3:3–10.
66. Ross RK, Yuan JM, Yu MC, et al. Urinary aflatoxin biomarkers and risk of hepatocellular carcinoma. Lancet 1992;339:943–6.
67. Kuang SY, Lekawanvijit S, Maneekarn N, et al. Hepatitis B 1762T/1764A mutations, hepatitis C infection, and codon 249 p53 mutations in hepatocellular carcinomas from Thailand. Cancer Epidemiol Biomarkers Prev 2005;14:380–4.
68. Liu Y, Wu F. Global burden of aflatoxin-induced hepatocellular carcinoma: a risk assessment. Environ Health Perspect 2010;118:818–24.
69. Wild CP, Gong YY. Mycotoxins and human disease: a largely ignored global health issue. Carcinogenesis 2010;31:71–82.
70. IARC. Working Group on the Evaluation of Carcinogenic Risks to Humans, International Agency for Research on Cancer. Alcohol drinking. Lyon (France): International Agency for Research on Cancer; 1988.

71. World Cancer Research Fund/American Institute for Cancer Research. Food, nutrition, physical activity, and the prevention of cancer: a global perspective. Washington, DC: American Institute for Cancer Research; 2007.

72. Aizawa Y, Shibamoto Y, Takagi I, et al. Analysis of factors affecting the appearance of hepatocellular carcinoma in patients with chronic hepatitis C. A long term follow-up study after histologic diagnosis. Cancer 2000;89:53–9.

73. Corrao G, Bagnardi V, Zambon A, et al. Exploring the dose-response relationship between alcohol consumption and the risk of several alcohol-related conditions: a meta-analysis. Addiction 1999;94:1551–73.

74. Kono S, Ikeda M, Tokudome S, et al. Cigarette smoking, alcohol and cancer mortality: a cohort study of male Japanese physicians. Jpn J Cancer Res 1987;78:1323–8.

75. Hirayama TA. large-scale cohort study on risk factors for primary liver cancer, with special reference to the role of cigarette smoking. Cancer Chemother Pharmacol 1989;23(Suppl):S114–7.

76. Roudot-Thoraval F, Bastie A, Pawlotsky JM, et al. Epidemiological factors affecting the severity of hepatitis C virus-related liver disease: a French survey of 6,664 patients. The Study Group for the Prevalence and the Epidemiology of Hepatitis C Virus. Hepatology 1997;26:485–90.

77. Shibata A, Hirohata T, Toshima H, et al. The role of drinking and cigarette smoking in the excess deaths from liver cancer. Jpn J Cancer Res 1986;77:287–95.

78. Tanaka K, Hirohata T, Takeshita S. Blood transfusion, alcohol consumption, and cigarette smoking in causation of hepatocellular carcinoma: a case-control study in Fukuoka, Japan. Jpn J Cancer Res 1988;79:1075–82.

79. Tsukuma H, Hiyama T, Oshima A, et al. A case-control study of hepatocellular carcinoma in Osaka, Japan. Int J Cancer 1990;45:231–6.

80. Ikeda K, Saitoh S, Suzuki Y, et al. Disease progression and hepatocellular carcinogenesis in patients with chronic viral hepatitis: a prospective observation of 2215 patients. J Hepatol 1998;28:930–8.

81. Chen CJ, Liang KY, Chang AS, et al. Effects of hepatitis B virus, alcohol drinking, cigarette smoking and familial tendency on hepatocellular carcinoma. Hepatology 1991;13:398–406.

82. Oshima A, Tsukuma H, Hiyama T, et al. Follow-up study of HBs Ag-positive blood donors with special reference to effect of drinking and smoking on development of liver cancer. Int J Cancer 1984;34:775–9.

83. Lam KC, Yu MC, Leung JW, et al. Hepatitis B virus and cigarette smoking: risk factors for hepatocellular carcinoma in Hong Kong. Cancer Res 1982;42:5246–8.

84. Lu SN, Lin TM, Chen CJ, et al. A case-control study of primary hepatocellular carcinoma in Taiwan. Cancer 1988;62:2051–5.

85. Goodman MT, Moriwaki H, Vaeth M, et al. Prospective cohort study of risk factors for primary liver cancer in Hiroshima and Nagasaki, Japan. Epidemiology 1995;6:36–41.

86. Yu MW, Hsu FC, Sheen IS, et al. Prospective study of hepatocellular carcinoma and liver cirrhosis in asymptomatic chronic hepatitis B virus carriers. Am J Epidemiol 1997;145:1039–47.

87. Donato F, Tagger A, Gelatti U, et al. Alcohol and hepatocellular carcinoma: the effect of lifetime intake and hepatitis virus infections in men and women. Am J Epidemiol 2002;155:323–31.

88. Kuper H, Tzonou A, Kaklamani E, et al. Tobacco smoking, alcohol consumption and their interaction in the causation of hepatocellular carcinoma. Int J Cancer 2000;85:498–502.

89. Yuan JM, Govindarajan S, Arakawa K, et al. Synergism of alcohol, diabetes, and viral hepatitis on the risk of hepatocellular carcinoma in blacks and whites in the U.S. Cancer 2004;101:1009–17.

90. Frezza M, di Padova C, Pozzato G, et al. High blood alcohol levels in women. The role of decreased gastric alcohol dehydrogenase activity and first-pass metabolism. N Engl J Med 1990;322:95–9.

91. Tuyns AJ, Pequignot G. Greater risk of ascitic cirrhosis in females in relation to alcohol consumption. Int J Epidemiol 1984;13:53–7.

92. Corrao G, Arico S, Zambon A, et al. Female sex and the risk of liver cirrhosis. Collaborative groups for the study of liver diseases in Italy. Scand J Gastroenterol 1997;32:1174–80.

93. Mukaiya M, Nishi M, Miyake H, et al. Chronic liver diseases for the risk of hepatocellular carcinoma: a case-control study in Japan. Etiologic association of alcohol consumption, cigarette smoking and the development of chronic liver diseases. Hepatogastroenterology 1998;45:2328–32.

94. Hassan MM, Spitz MR, Thomas MB, et al. Effect of different types of smoking and synergism with hepatitis C virus on risk of hepatocellular carcinoma in American men and women: case-control study. Int J Cancer 2008;123:1883–91.

95. Hart CL, Morrison DS, Batty GD, et al. Effect of body mass index and alcohol consumption on liver disease: analysis of data from two prospective cohort studies. BMJ 2010;340:c1240.

96. Flegal KM, Carroll MD, Ogden CL, et al. Prevalence and trends in obesity among US adults, 1999–2008. JAMA 2010;303:235–41.

97. McKillop IH, Schrum LW. Role of alcohol in liver carcinogenesis. Semin Liver Dis 2009;29:222–32.

98. Seitz HK, Poschl G, Simanowski UA. Alcohol and cancer. Recent Dev Alcohol 1998;14:67–95.

99. WHO. WHO global status report on alcohol 2004. Available at: http://www.who.int/substance_abuse/publications/global_status_report_2004_overview.pdf. Accessed October 20, 2010.

100. Lawson DH, Gray JM, McKillop C, et al. Diabetes mellitus and primary hepatocellular carcinoma. Q J Med 1986;61:945–55.

101. Kessler II. Cancer mortality among diabetics. J Natl Cancer Inst 1970;44:673–86.

102. Ragozzino M, Melton LJ 3rd, Chu CP, et al. Subsequent cancer risk in the incidence cohort of Rochester, Minnesota, residents with diabetes mellitus. J Chronic Dis 1982;35:13–9.

103. El-Serag HB, Richardson PA, Everhart JE. The role of diabetes in hepatocellular carcinoma: a case-control study among United States Veterans. Am J Gastroenterol 2001;96:2462–7.

104. Hadziyannis S, Tabor E, Kaklamani E, et al. A case-control study of hepatitis B and C virus infections in the etiology of hepatocellular carcinoma. Int J Cancer 1995;60:627–31.

105. Beasley RP. Diabetes and hepatocellular carcinoma. Hepatology 2006;44:1408–10.

106. Gao C, Yao SK. Diabetes mellitus: a "true" independent risk factor for hepatocellular carcinoma? Hepatobiliary Pancreat Dis Int 2009;8:465–73.

107. El-Serag HB, Hampel H, Javadi F. The association between diabetes and hepatocellular carcinoma: a systematic review of epidemiologic evidence. Clin Gastroenterol Hepatol 2006;4:369–80.

108. Adami HO, McLaughlin J, Ekbom A, et al. Cancer risk in patients with diabetes mellitus. Cancer Causes Control 1991;2:307–14.

109. Koskinen SV, Reunanen AR, Martelin TP, et al. Mortality in a large population-based cohort of patients with drug-treated diabetes mellitus. Am J Public Health 1998;88:765–70.
110. Weiderpass E, Gridley G, Nyren O, et al. Cause-specific mortality in a cohort of patients with diabetes mellitus: a population-based study in Sweden. J Clin Epidemiol 2001;54:802–9.
111. Sasaki A, Uehara M, Horiuchi N, et al. 15-year follow-up study of patients with non-insulin-dependent diabetes mellitus (NIDDM) in Osaka, Japan. Factors predictive of the prognosis of diabetic patients. Diabetes Res Clin Pract 1997;36:41–7.
112. Adami HO, Chow WH, Nyren O, et al. Excess risk of primary liver cancer in patients with diabetes mellitus. J Natl Cancer Inst 1996;88:1472–7.
113. Wideroff L, Gridley G, Mellemkjaer L, et al. Cancer incidence in a population-based cohort of patients hospitalized with diabetes mellitus in Denmark. J Natl Cancer Inst 1997;89:1360–5.
114. Balkau B, Kahn HS, Courbon D, et al. Hyperinsulinemia predicts fatal liver cancer but is inversely associated with fatal cancer at some other sites: the Paris Prospective Study. Diabetes Care 2001;24:843–9.
115. Clark JM, Diehl AM. Hepatic steatosis and type 2 diabetes mellitus. Curr Diab Rep 2002;2:210–5.
116. Mason AL, Lau JY, Hoang N, et al. Association of diabetes mellitus and chronic hepatitis C virus infection. Hepatology 1999;29:328–33.
117. Petrides AS, DeFronzo RA. Glucose and insulin metabolism in cirrhosis. J Hepatol 1989;8:107–14.
118. Hassan MM, Hwang LY, Hatten CJ, et al. Risk factors for hepatocellular carcinoma: synergism of alcohol with viral hepatitis and diabetes mellitus. Hepatology 2002;36:1206–13.
119. Lagiou P, Kuper H, Stuver SO, et al. Role of diabetes mellitus in the etiology of hepatocellular carcinoma. J Natl Cancer Inst 2000;92:1096–9.
120. Nguyen NT, Nguyen XM, Lane J, et al. Relationship between obesity and diabetes in a US adult population: findings from the National Health and Nutrition Examination Survey, 1999–2006. Obes Surg 2011;21:351–5.
121. Saunders D, Seidel D, Allison M, et al. Systematic review: the association between obesity and hepatocellular carcinoma - epidemiological evidence. Aliment Pharmacol Ther 2010;31:1051–63.
122. Larsson SC, Wolk A. Overweight, obesity and risk of liver cancer: a meta-analysis of cohort studies. Br J Cancer 2007;97:1005–8.
123. Shaw JE, Sicree RA, Zimmet PZ. Global estimates of the prevalence of diabetes for 2010 and 2030. Diabetes Res Clin Pract 2010;87:4–14.
124. James WP. The epidemiology of obesity: the size of the problem. J Intern Med 2008;263:336–52.
125. Flegal KM, Carroll MD, Kuczmarski RJ, et al. Overweight and obesity in the United States: prevalence and trends, 1960–1994. Int J Obes Relat Metab Disord 1998;22:39–47.
126. Flegal KM, Carroll MD, Ogden CL, et al. Prevalence and trends in obesity among US adults, 1999–2000. JAMA 2002;288:1723–7.
127. Ludwig J, Viggiano TR, McGill DB, et al. Nonalcoholic steatohepatitis: Mayo Clinic experiences with a hitherto unnamed disease. Mayo Clin Proc 1980;55:434–8.
128. Brunt EM, Janney CG, Di Bisceglie AM, et al. Nonalcoholic steatohepatitis: a proposal for grading and staging the histological lesions. Am J Gastroenterol 1999;94:2467–74.

129. Byron D, Minuk GY. Clinical hepatology: profile of an urban, hospital-based practice. Hepatology 1996;24:813–5.
130. Farrell GC. Non-alcoholic steatohepatitis: what is it, and why is it important in the Asia-Pacific region? J Gastroenterol Hepatol 2003;18:124–38.
131. Bacon BR, Farahvash MJ, Janney CG, et al. Nonalcoholic steatohepatitis: an expanded clinical entity. Gastroenterology 1994;107:1103–9.
132. Struben VM, Hespenheide EE, Caldwell SH. Nonalcoholic steatohepatitis and cryptogenic cirrhosis within kindreds. Am J Med 2000;108:9–13.
133. Bugianesi E, Leone N, Vanni E, et al. Expanding the natural history of nonalcoholic steatohepatitis: from cryptogenic cirrhosis to hepatocellular carcinoma. Gastroenterology 2002;123:134–40.
134. Caldwell SH, Oelsner DH, Iezzoni JC, et al. Cryptogenic cirrhosis: clinical characterization and risk factors for underlying disease. Hepatology 1999;29:664–9.
135. Poonawala A, Nair SP, Thuluvath PJ. Prevalence of obesity and diabetes in patients with cryptogenic cirrhosis: a case-control study. Hepatology 2000;32: 689–92.
136. Powell EE, Cooksley WG, Hanson R, et al. The natural history of nonalcoholic steatohepatitis: a follow-up study of forty-two patients for up to 21 years. Hepatology 1990;11:74–80.
137. Schafer DF, Sorrell MF. Hepatocellular carcinoma. Lancet 1999;353:1253–7.
138. Cotrim HP, Parana R, Braga E, et al. Nonalcoholic steatohepatitis and hepatocellular carcinoma: natural history? Am J Gastroenterol 2000;95:3018–9.
139. Shimada M, Hashimoto E, Taniai M, et al. Hepatocellular carcinoma in patients with non-alcoholic steatohepatitis. J Hepatol 2002;37:154–60.
140. Zen Y, Katayanagi K, Tsuneyama K, et al. Hepatocellular carcinoma arising in non-alcoholic steatohepatitis. Pathol Int 2001;51:127–31.
141. Sorensen HT, Mellemkjaer L, Jepsen P, et al. Risk of cancer in patients hospitalized with fatty liver: a Danish cohort study. J Clin Gastroenterol 2003;36:356–9.
142. Ertle J, Dechene A, Sowa JP, et al. Nonalcoholic fatty liver disease progresses to HCC in the absence of apparent cirrhosis. Int J Cancer 2011;128(10):2436–43.
143. Sanyal A, Poklepovic A, Moyneur E, et al. Population-based risk factors and resource utilization for HCC: US perspective. Curr Med Res Opin 2010;26: 2183–91.

Anatomic Pathology of Hepatocellular Carcinoma: Impact on Prognosis and Response to Therapy

Tania Roskams, MD, PhD

KEYWORDS

- Dysplastic nodules • Early HCC • Hepatic progenitor cells
- Liver biopsy • K19 • Glypican 3 • HSP70
- Glutamine synthetase

The diagnosis of a malignant tumor usually requires histologic confirmation before a curative or palliative treatment is considered. Recent guidelines published by the professional associations for the study of the liver and liver disease, in Europe and the United States, have challenged this paradigm in patients with cirrhosis.[1] The proposed current decision tree in patients with cirrhosis and liver lesions is as follows.[1]

1. Lesions smaller than 1 cm: Repeat ultrasound at 3 months.
2. Lesions larger than 1 cm: Arterial hypervascularity and venous or delayed washout confirms a diagnosis of hepatocellular carcinoma (HCC).
3. Lesions larger than 1 cm: No arterial hypervascularity and venous or delayed washout requires second contrast-enhanced imaging study or biopsy. If the second imaging study shows arterial hypervascularity and venous or delayed washout, then the diagnosis of HCC is confirmed. If not, proceed to biopsy.

In recent years, noninvasive imaging techniques for the diagnosis of HCC before liver transplantation have been widely used in different centers. In the study by Hayashi and colleagues,[2] 27% of 30 patients with a pretransplantation diagnosis of HCC had no evidence of tumor in the explanted liver, and this led to incorrect organ allocation in 7% of their patients. Wiesner and colleagues[3] reported that in 31% and 9% of the patients who underwent liver transplantation for stage 1 (1 nodule ≤1.9 cm) and stage 2 HCC (1 nodule 2.0–5.0 cm or 2–3 nodules all ≤3 cm) respectively, there was no evidence of tumor in the explanted liver. Similar results were also reported from a recent study in France, where a false positive preoperative

Department of Pathology, Laboratory of Morphology and Molecular Pathology, University Hospitals of Leuven, Minderbroederstraat 12, B-3000 Leuven, Belgium
E-mail address: tania.roskams@uz.kuleuven.ac.be

Clin Liver Dis 15 (2011) 245–259
doi:10.1016/j.cld.2011.03.004
1089-3261/11/$ – see front matter © 2011 Elsevier Inc. All rights reserved.

diagnosis of HCC was made in 20% of the patients.[4] Results from these studies suggest that the noninvasive diagnosis of HCC is associated with a significant false positive rate. Nevertheless, a correct pretransplant diagnosis of HCC is not only of utmost importance for the patient, but also has a major impact on organ allocation. In several countries, for example the United States, patients with stage 2 HCC are awarded extra Model for Endstage Liver Disease (MELD) points to allow for transplantation in a timely manner, whereas for patients with stage 1 HCC (1 nodule ≤1.9 cm), no extra points are assigned.

With the current guidelines, HCC is the only clinically significant malignant tumor that does not require histologic examination and confirmation to establish the diagnosis. Because for HCC diagnosis, tissue analysis is not mandatory in clinical trials, this can have a deleterious effect on the interpretation of the trial results. Currently, it is impossible to determine whether certain molecularly defined tumor subgroups show better responses than other tumors to experimental therapies. Targeted therapy with a priori tissue-based histopathological and/or molecular evaluation before treatment is decided and given, is a reality for other cancers: eg, carcinoma of the breast, lung, and colon. If this standard diagnostic certainly is not applied soon to HCC, clinical trial reliability will lag further behind the standards expected and achieved in other branches of oncology. Individualized HCC therapy requires definition of patient subgroups that could benefit most, and/or should be protected from therapy failure and unwarranted side effects. The decision not to make biopsy of HCC mandatory was made decades ago, when no customized systemic therapy seemed feasible or imminent. This decision clearly must be revisited urgently in the light of modern therapeutic options. Ultimately, it is also an ethical necessity to design clinical trials in a way that optimizes data interpretation for the sake of future generations of patients.

From histopathological and molecular points of view, it is now clear that primary liver cancer is even more heterogeneous than we previously thought.

The discipline of pathology should now take advantage of molecular techniques, so that a diagnosis of primary liver carcinoma is not based solely on classical histologic staining methods, but also on immunohistochemistry and characterization of molecular markers and signaling pathways. According to the current guidelines described earlier, pathologists preferentially receive for diagnosis biopsies from small lesions that have an atypical vascularization pattern. In this context, differentiating between a high-grade dysplastic nodule (HGDN) and early HCC is the first challenge.[5]

HGDNS VERSUS EARLY HCC

Hepatocarcinogenesis in the human liver is a stepwise process in which a small monoclonal focus (dysplastic focus, <1 mm) expands into a larger than 1 mm dysplastic nodule (DN). Low-grade dysplastic nodules (LGDNs) evolve into HGDNs.[6] The evolution into true carcinoma includes the recruitment of an arterial blood supply, stromal invasion, venous invasion, and, finally, metastasis (**Fig. 1**).[6,7] In the early stages of HCC, the typical arterial hypervascular pattern is not yet present. In 1995, the International Working Party Classification rationalized the nomenclature of early hepatocellular neoplasia by referring to premalignant neoplastic nodules as LGDNs and HGDNs.[8] This terminology has been widely accepted. To obtain international consensus on the pathologic diagnosis of equivocal lesions, such as DNs and early HCC, an International Consensus Group for Hepatocellular Neoplasia (ICGHN) was convened in April 2002 in Kurume, Japan. The group met several times subsequently up to July 2007 in Leuven, Belgium; Bordeaux, France; and Tessaloniki, Greece, culminating in the release of a consensus document that was reported in *Hepatology* in 2009.[5]

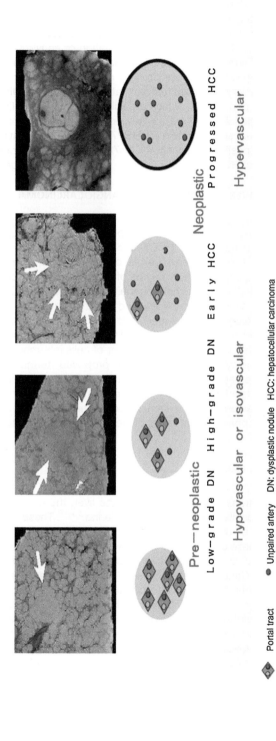

Fig. 1. Clinicopathologic consensus on the evolution from preneoplastic nodular lesions to hepatocellular carcinoma in cirrhotic liver.

In the skin, gastrointestinal tract, and other organs, epithelia are lined by a basement membrane. In these organs, cancer is defined as lesions that invade the basement membrane. Lesions that exhibit cellular characteristics of malignancy, but do not invade the basement membrane, are defined as high-grade dysplasia and in situ carcinoma. In the normal liver, however, there is no structured basement membrane present along the sinusoids. This makes the differentiation of early invasive cancer from HGDN very difficult. Therefore, it took several years of exchanging slides among pathologists and correlation with molecular profiling results before a clinically useful consensus was reached. A very important feature that distinguishes HGDN from early HCC is stromal invasion in portal tracts, which are still present in early HCC, albeit at low number. A panel of molecular markers is now also used for the diagnosis of early HCC, namely glypican 3, heat shock protein 70 (HSP70), and glutamine synthetase. If 2 of these 3 markers are positive, a sensitivity of 72% and specificity of 100% is reached for the diagnosis of HCC.

DIAGNOSIS OF PRIMARY LIVER CANCER: HCC, CHOLANGIOCARCINOMA, OR MIXED PHENOTYPES

Once the diagnosis of malignancy is established, primary liver cancer is classically classified as hepatocellular carcinoma (HCC) or cholangiocarcinoma (CC) as the main categories, and according to degree of cellular differentiation or extent of nuclear abnormalities. Although this differentiation may be of prognostic relevance, problems remain because of the marked degree of heterogeneity in both HCC and CC. Although a mixed HCC/CC category is recognized in the World Health Organization (WHO) classification, confusing terminology has been generated to describe different overlapping entities (eg, intermediate cell tumors, progenitor cell tumors, mixed tumors, small cell HCC, CCs), showing features of both HCC and CC or of cells intermediate between hepatocytes and cholangiocytes. The variety of proposed terms reflects our increasing knowledge of the pathogenesis of liver cancer and possible cellular precursors. In fact, there is growing evidence for the concept of a stem cell or progenitor cell origin of liver cancer, as was proposed in animal models and human tumors showing a whole range of immunophenotypical traits of hepatocytes, cholangiocytes, and progenitor cells (**Fig. 2**).[9–12]

ORIGIN OF PRIMARY LIVER CARCINOMA
Liver Progenitor Cells

In humans, the so-called transit amplifying cells of the liver, the hepatic progenitor cells (HPCs), have been localized in the canals of Hering.[13–16] These are cells that have a higher probability of undergoing terminal differentiation than self-renewal. Among other properties, these cells have been shown to be capable of differentiating into both hepatocytes and cholangiocytes, and of expressing multidrug-resistant proteins, including Breast Cancer–Related Protein (BCRP). The latter confers resistance to various disadvantageous survival conditions, including toxic drugs.[17,18] These cells are activated in most chronic human liver diseases.[19–21] Chronic liver disease, and specifically cirrhosis, is a major risk factor for HCC development. In the cirrhotic stage of chronic liver disease, mature hepatocytes are known to become senescent.[22] Inhibition of replication of hepatocytes is the perfect trigger for activation of progenitor cells.[16,19,23,24] As such, activated progenitor cells may form target cells for subsequent initiation of carcinogenesis.[10,11,25,26]

Results from several studies have shown that liver carcinomas are monoclonal, ie, derived from a single cell. The question is, of course, which cell: hepatocytes,

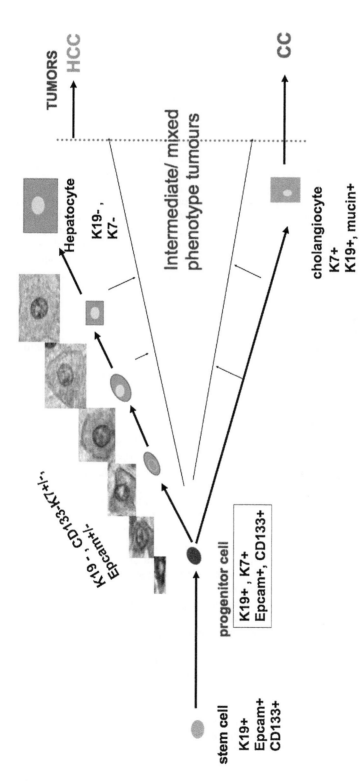

Fig. 2. Mature epithelial cell types: hepatocytes and cholangiocytes can give rise to hepatocellular and cholangiocellular carcinoma; maturation arrest of hepatic progenitor cells on their way to hepatocytes/cholangiocytes can give rise to tumors with a range of immature and mixed phenotypes.

cholangiocytes, HPC, or all 3, as all these different cell types have the required longevity and long-term repopulating potential.

Animal Studies

Results of animal models show that hepatocytes are implicated in some models of HCC, whereas other models that use direct injury to the essentially unipotent cholangiocytes induce CC. Progenitor cells (oval cells in rodents) are activated in many animal models, just as they are in many instances of human liver damage, irrespective of etiology, making such cells very likely carcinogen targets. If progenitor cells do give rise to cancer during their process of maturation/differentiation (maturation arrest theory), one would expect a range of neoplastic phenotypes recapitulating stages in normal development. This prediction is supported experimentally,[27] as well as in human liver tumors (see later in this article). One of the earliest tests of this hypothesis was by Valeer Desmet in 1963.[28] He studied rats intoxicated by Butter Yellow. Using detailed microscopy and enzyme histochemistry, he saw that a variety of premalignant changes and associated tumors evolved in this model (**Fig. 3**). He hypothesized that mature hepatocytes could give rise to HCC and mature cholangiocytes to CC. In addition, he observed an "oval cell reaction" (in humans, the equivalent is called ductular reaction or progenitor cell activation), with differentiation either into hepatocytes to create HCC, or directly giving rise to immature "anaplastic" tumors. The same variety of tumors is seen in humans (see **Fig. 2**).

Direct evidence for the involvement of oval cells (progenitor cells) in the histogenesis of HCC was obtained by Dumble and colleagues,[29] who isolated oval cells from p53 null mice. When these cells were transplanted into athymic nude mice, they produced HCCs.

Evidence for Progenitor Cells in Human Liver Cancer

In humans, chronic viral hepatitis B and C, alcoholic and nonalcoholic steatohepatitis, metabolic diseases, and mutagens, such as aflatoxins (toxic metabolites of the food mold *Aspergillus* sp), are the most important risk factors for the development of HCC. Chronic inflammatory biliary diseases, such as primary sclerosing cholangitis, hepatolithiasis (intraductal gallstones), and liver fluke infestation by *Opisthorchis viverrini* and *Clonorchis sinensis*, are known risk factors for the development of CCs. This underscores the notion that oxidative stress and chronic inflammation form common carcinogenic risk factors in all primary liver cancers.

In adult humans, the 2 major primary liver cancers are HCC and CC. In addition, mixed forms of HCC and CC are described. When more detailed immunohistochemical phenotyping of a liver carcinoma is performed, a whole range of phenotypical traits of hepatocytes, cholangiocytes, and progenitor cells can be seen, which strongly suggests that progenitor cells can give rise to the primary cancers, HCC and CC, and to mixed forms that contain both hepatocytic and cholangiocytic traits, as well as intermediate cells.[10]

The presence of progenitor cell features in a tumor can be explained in 2 ways: either the cell of origin is a progenitor cell (maturation arrest theory) or alternatively, tumors dedifferentiate and acquire progenitor cell features during carcinogenesis (dedifferentiation theory). When progenitor cells are the cells of origin of a subtype of primary liver tumors, one would expect that the earlier premalignant precursor lesions would also consist of progenitor cells and their progeny. This is indeed the case: 55% of small-cell dysplastic foci (smaller than 1 mm), the earliest premalignant lesions known to date in humans, consist of progenitor cells and intermediate

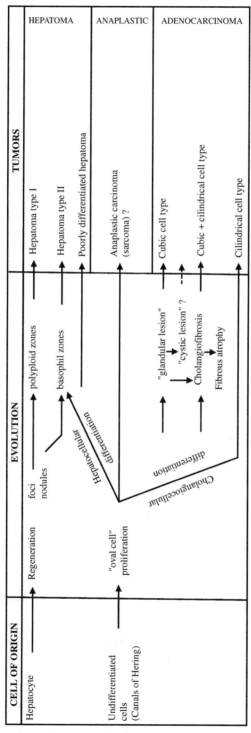

Fig. 3. Origin of liver carcinoma according to V. Desmet in 1963, based on rat experiments.

hepatocytes.[30] This is a very strong argument in favor of the progenitor cell origin of at least some HCCs.

An often emphasized concept is that of the cancer stem cell, which is the cell renewal source of a neoplasm and the seed for metastasis,[31] and which expresses similar toxic drug-exporting protein pumps as non-neoplastic stem cells. According to this concept, a tumor consists of a hierarchy of cell populations, of which the very small cancer stem cell population is the one that has the growth and metastatic potential of the tumor. The other neoplastic cells are offspring of the cancer stem cells and each can differentiate a little differently, according to the local microenvironment in different parts of the tumor. This explains the enormous heterogeneity of the phenotype of a neoplasm in different areas (**Figs. 4** and **5**). How do liver stem cells drive cancer initiation? By using microdissection and analysis of the molecular pathways of activated progenitor cells, we could show that Wnt signaling plays a pivotal role in the expansion of non-neoplastic human progenitor cells, whereas notch activation is important for biliary differentiation and notch inhibition is necessary to have hepatocyte differentiation (see **Fig. 1**).[32] An excessive and persistent self-renewal signal, involving Wnt/beta-catenin and BMI-1, is also one of the key events in early carcinogenesis.[33–36] Therefore, targeting the liver cancer stem cell should be the ideal treatment for liver cancer.

IMMUNOPHENOTYPE OF PRIMARY LIVER CARCINOMA

Mature hepatocytes express keratins (K)8 and 18 in the cytoplasm, CD10 and CD66e (detectable by polyclonal anti–carcinoembryonic antigen [CEA] antibody) in canaliculi (**Fig. 6A**), and Hep-Par-1 Ag in cytoplasmic granules. This profile contrasts with that of mature cholangiocytes, which express K7 and K19, in addition to K8 and K18. HPCs present K19, a very early hepatoblast marker (see **Fig. 1**), and K7, K8, and K18, whereas some subpopulations express epithelial cell adhesion molecule (EpCAM), CD133, c-kit, CD34, and CD90.

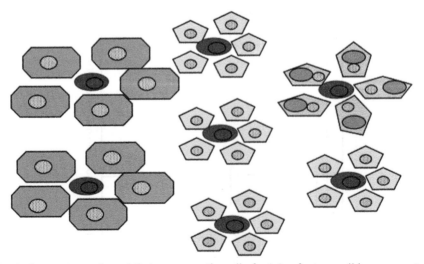

Fig. 4. Cancer stem cells and their progeny: the cell of origin of a tumor (*blue cancer stem cell*), expands clonally. When the tumor grows, the offspring can differentiate differently according to the local microenvironment of the tumor cells: eg, into hepatocytes (*large orange cells left*), biliary cells (*center*), or mucin-producing cells (*right*).

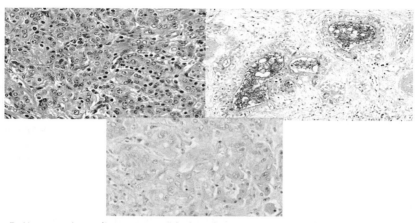

Fig. 5. Human primary liver cancer with ductular areas, mucin-producing glands, and hepatocytic areas, within the same tumor. *Left upper and lower panel*: hematoxylin-eosin stain, *right upper panel*: PAS diastase staining.

As in rodents, HCC and CC evolve from focal precursor lesions that reflect the stages of multistep carcinogenesis.[6,7,37] Most tumors still show phenotypical features of their cell of origin and the histopathological classification of tumors is largely based on this. A considerable number of human HCCs (diagnosed according to WHO criteria on hematoxylin-eosin [HE] staining) express markers of progenitor/biliary cells such as K7, K19, and OV6 (see **Fig. 6**B–D).[9,38–45] Morphologically, these tumors consist of cells with a very immature phenotype, as well as a range of cells with intermediate

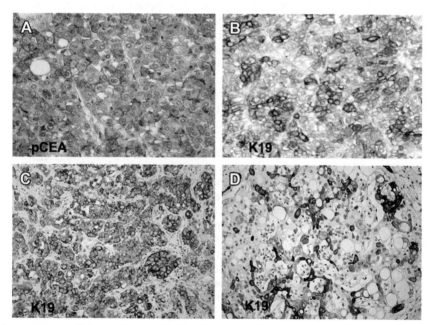

Fig. 6. Hepatocellular carcinoma (HCC) with (*A*) canalicular staining pattern on polyclonal CEA staining and (*B*) positivity for K19 in small and intermediate cells, (*C*) HCC with K19 in intermediate cells throughout the tumor, and (*D*) HCC with K19 reactivity in strands of small cells in continuity with intermediate cells.

phenotypes between progenitor cells and hepatocytes. One common feature of all these tumors was decreased survival of patients; in fact, the survival of patients with these tumors was close to the known poor survival of patients with CC.

Prognostic Significance of Keratin 19

Results of several recent studies using diverse methods, in different centers and among different ethnic groups, have shown that K19 expression may be used as an independent prognostic marker of HCC that is associated with short survival times and fast recurrence after surgical treatment or liver transplantation.[9,38–43,45]

Wu and colleagues[41] observed a significantly shorter survival of patients with HCCs expressing AE1-AE3 and K19 without any treatment, than in patients with AE1-AE3 and K19 negative tumors. Uenishi and colleagues[39] reported that HCCs expressing K19 and K7 have a lower tumor-free survival rate after nominally curative resection (than for K19 and K17 negative lesions) and demonstrated that K19 expression was an independent predictor of postoperative recurrence. In a study by Ding and colleagues,[46] overexpression of K19 correlated with HCC metastasis. In a consecutive series of 109 HCCs in Caucasians, K19-positive tumors (K19+ in more than 5% of tumor cells) had a higher rate of tumor recurrence after liver transplantation, compared with patients with K19-negative HCCs.[42] K19 expression was significantly associated with elevated serum alpha-fetoprotein (AFP>400 ng/mL), and expression of AFP by the tumor. The investigators concluded that the association with AFP, a marker of hepatic progenitor cells, is compatible with a progenitor cell origin of these tumors. Aishima and colleagues[47] studied 35 small (<3 cm) HCCs with biliary differentiation based on morphology, K19 immunoexpression, and mucin secretion and compared them with 61 ordinary HCCs. They found that extrahepatic recurrence was more common in K19(+) than in K19(–) HCC, and that patients with K19(+)/mucin(+) HCCs had the worst survival. More recently, Zhuang and colleagues[43] recognized 2 pathologic types of HCC in terms of lymph node metastasis, based on their K19 immunophenotype. They studied 172 HCCs with or without positive lymph nodes, and showed that K19 immunoreactivity was an independent prognostic factor for development of lymph node metastasis. Moreover, in the subgroup of lymph node metastatic HCC, patients with K19-expressing HCC had shorter overall survivals.

The prognostic value of K19 expression in HCC was further supported by microarray-based gene expression profiling. A study of the global gene expression pattern in 91 HCCs from China and Belgium revealed 2 distinctive subclasses (A and B) that were highly associated with patient survival.[48] A subsequent integrative functional genomics study compared the gene expression data of an independent set of 61 HCCs with rat fetal hepatoblasts and adult hepatocytes, and with mouse HCCs from different experimental models. Individuals with HCC who shared a gene expression pattern with fetal hepatoblasts (hepatoblast signature) belonged to subclass A with a poor prognosis, and the profile that included markers of hepatic progenitor cells (K19, K7, vimentin), suggested that HCC of this subtype may arise from progenitor cells.[49] Yamashita and colleagues,[44] using cDNA microarrays to study 238 HCCs, identified a subset of EpCAM-positive HCCs with a bad prognosis that displayed a unique molecular signature of features of HPCs, including the presence of K19 expression. In the current WHO guidelines, K19 is therefore included as a prognostic marker.

POTENTIAL LIVER CANCER STEM CELL MARKERS

Several liver stem cell markers have been proposed. Given the similarities between normal stem cells and cancer stem cells, it is reasonable to assume that the phenotype of liver cancer stem cells resembles that of normal stem/progenitor cells.

As described previously, K19 is a very early hepatoblast marker and marker of normal adult liver progenitor cells and is associated with a poor prognosis for HCC. OV6, a rodent progenitor cell marker, recognizes K19 and K14 in the rat and as such is the rodent equivalent of K19. Yang and colleagues[36] demonstrated that OV6(+) HCC cells posses greater tumorigenic ability and chemoresistance to standard chemotherapy than OV6(–) cells. The Wnt/beta-catenin pathway plays a key role in the expansion of progenitor cells in human HCC, similar to its role in expansion of non-neoplastic progenitor cells in acute and chronic liver diseases.[32]

Ma and colleagues[50] discovered that prominin-1, the murine homolog of human CD133, was significantly upregulated in liver regeneration. In subsequent functional studies on sorted HCC cells, CD133+ cells displayed cancer stem cell properties. CD133+ cells had greater tumorigenicity than CD133– cells in immunodeficient mice, higher colony-forming capacity, and proliferation ability in vitro, and could be induced into nonhepatocytelike lineages, showing multipotency. The expression of "stemness" genes was higher in CD133+ cells than in CD133– cells. Further studies showed that CD133+ cells are resistant to conventional chemotherapy.[51]

CD90 has been suggested as a putative marker for liver cancer stem cells. This marker is expressed by hepatic progenitor cells during development[52] and CD90 expression correlates with tumorigenic potential in a panel of liver cell lines.[53] Further characterization with cell sorting for CD45 resulted in a population of CD90+CD45– cells of which most also expressed CD44.[54] CD44 is a cell surface receptor for hyaluronic acid and its blockade with neutralizing antibodies induces apoptosis of CD90+ cells and prevents tumor formation in mice.[54]

EpCAM has been suggested as a cancer stem cell marker, because EpCAM+ HCC cells were found to be more tumorigenic than EpCAM– cells.[55] Interestingly, EpCAM is a direct transcriptional target in the Wnt/beta-catenin pathway and hence could serve as a biomarker for the activation of this pathway.[56]

Normal human progenitor cells have certain subtypes of active transmembrane adenosine triphosphate-binding cassette (ABC) transporters, such as MDR1, ABCG2, and ABCC2,[17,18,57] which render them resistant to oxidative stress and toxic substances, including chemotherapy agents. These transporters also efflux the DNA-binding dye Hoechst 33342 and hence "side sort" in fluorescence-activated cell sorting. It was shown that side population cells from HCC cell lines harbor cancer stem cell–like properties: they were highly proliferative and chemoresistant in vitro,[58] whereas nonside population cells did not. The increased tumorigenic potential of side population cells was shown in vivo in SCID mice where 10^3 side population cells consistently led to tumor formation, whereas 10^6 nonside population cells did not. In addition, it was found that side population cells isolated from HCC cell lines may be related to the metastatic potential of HCC.[59] MRP1 expression correlated with a more aggressive tumor phenotype and with K19 expression.[60] High expression of ABC transporters renders the cells resistant to chemotherapy, including cisplatin and doxorubicin. Inhibition of MDR1,[61] ABCG2,[62] and ABCC2[63] by inhibitors or using an antisense approach, can reverse this chemoresistance.

SUMMARY

A better understanding of signaling pathways in HCC pathogenesis has led to targeted therapies against HCC, using drugs like sorafenib, erlotinib, and bevacizumab.[63] These therapies target the major cell populations of rapidly growing differentiated tumor cells.[64,65] However, increasing evidence for the existence of cancer stem cells suggests the possibility of targeting the undifferentiated cancer stem cells that constitute only a small proportion of the tumor. Identification of liver cancer stem cell markers and their related pathways is one of the most important goals of liver cancer research. Understanding the mechanisms of activation and differentiation of non-neoplastic stem/progenitor cells and especially the differences from their malignant counterparts should therefore also be a top priority. New therapies should ideally target cancer stem cells and NOT normal stem/progenitor cells, because the latter are very important in regeneration and repair. Individualized HCC therapy will require better definition of patient subgroups that benefit most or should be protected from therapy failure and unwanted side effects, eg, biliary/progenitor cell features in an HCC render these tumors more resistant to chemotherapy. For all these reasons, tumor tissue acquisition should be mandatory, reversing the practice that was established years ago when targeted HCC therapy was but a pope dream.

REFERENCES

1. Bruix J, Llovet JM. Two decades of advances in hepatocellular carcinoma research. Semin Liver Dis 2010;30:1–2.
2. Hayashi PH, Trotter JF, Forman L, et al. Impact of pretransplant diagnosis of hepatocellular carcinoma on cadaveric liver allocation in the era of MELD. Liver Transpl 2004;10:42–8.
3. Wiesner RH, Freeman RB, Mulligan DC. Liver transplantation for hepatocellular cancer: the impact of the MELD allocation policy. Gastroenterology 2004;127: S261–7.
4. Compagnon P, Grandadam S, Lorho R, et al. Liver transplantation for hepatocellular carcinoma without preoperative tumor biopsy. Transplantation 2008;86: 1068–76.
5. International Concensus Group for Hepatocellular Neoplasia. International consensus on the pathologic diagnosis of early hepatocellular carcinoma: a report of the International Concensus Group for Hepatocellular Neoplasia. Hepatology 2009;49:658–64.
6. Kojiro M, Roskams T. Early hepatocellular carcinoma and dysplastic nodules. Semin Liver Dis 2005;25:133–42.
7. Roskams T, Kojiro M. Pathology of early hepatocellular carcinoma: conventional and molecular diagnosis. Semin Liver Dis 2010;30:17–25.
8. Terminology of nodular hepatocellular lesions. International Working Party. Hepatology 1995;22:983–93.
9. Yoon DS, Jeong J, Park YN, et al. Expression of biliary antigen and its clinical significance in hepatocellular carcinoma. Yonsei Med J 1999;40:472–7.
10. Roskams T. Liver stem cells and their implication in hepatocellular and cholangio-carcinoma. Oncogene 2006;25:3818–22.
11. Alison MR, Lovell MJ. Liver cancer: the role of stem cells. Cell Prolif 2005;38: 407–21.
12. Theise ND, Yao JL, Harada K, et al. Hepatic 'stem cell' malignancies in adults: four cases. Histopathology 2003;43:263–71.
13. Theise ND, Saxena R, Portmann BC, et al. The canals of Hering and hepatic stem cells in humans. Hepatology 1999;30:1425–33.
14. Kuwahara R, Kofman AV, Landis CS, et al. The hepatic stem cell niche: identification by label-retaining cell assay. Hepatology 2008;47(6):1994–2002.

15. Roskams TA, Theise ND, Balabaud C, et al. Nomenclature of the finer branches of the biliary tree: canals, ductules, and ductular reactions in human livers. Hepatology 2004;39:1739–45.
16. Roskams T. Different types of liver progenitor cells and their niches. J Hepatol 2006;45:1–4.
17. Ros JE, Libbrecht L, Geuken M, et al. High expression of MDR1, MRP1, and MRP3 in the hepatic progenitor cell compartment and hepatocytes in severe human liver disease. J Pathol 2003;200:553–60.
18. Vander Borght S, Libbrecht L, Katoonizadeh A, et al. Breast cancer resistance protein (BCRP/ABCG2) is expressed by progenitor cells/reactive ductules and hepatocytes and its expression pattern is influenced by disease etiology and species type: possible functional consequences. J Histochem Cytochem 2006; 54:1051–9.
19. Falkowski O, An HJ, Ianus IA, et al. Regeneration of hepatocyte 'buds' in cirrhosis from intrabiliary stem cells. J Hepatol 2003;39:357–64.
20. Libbrecht L, Desmet V, Van Damme B, et al. Deep intralobular extension of human hepatic 'progenitor cells' correlates with parenchymal inflammation in chronic viral hepatitis: can 'progenitor cells' migrate? J Pathol 2000;192:373–8.
21. Roskams T. Progenitor cell involvement in cirrhotic human liver diseases: from controversy to consensus. J Hepatol 2003;39:431–4.
22. Wiemann SU, Satyanarayana A, Tsahuridu M, et al. Hepatocyte telomere shortening and senescence are general markers of human liver cirrhosis. FASEB J 2002;16:935–42.
23. Lowes KN, Brennan BA, Yeoh GC, et al. Oval cell numbers in human chronic liver diseases are directly related to disease severity. Am J Pathol 1999;154: 537–41.
24. Lowes KN, Croager EJ, Olynyk JK, et al. Oval cell-mediated liver regeneration: role of cytokines and growth factors. J Gastroenterol Hepatol 2003;18:4–12.
25. Roskams TA, Libbrecht L, Desmet VJ. Progenitor cells in diseased human liver. Semin Liver Dis 2003;23:385–96.
26. Roskams T, Yang SQ, Koteish A, et al. Oxidative stress and oval cell accumulation in mice and humans with alcoholic and nonalcoholic fatty liver disease. Am J Pathol 2003;163:1301–11.
27. Hixson DC, Brown J, McBride AC, et al. Differentiation status of rat ductal cells and ethionine-induced hepatic carcinomas defined with surface-reactive monoclonal antibodies. Exp Mol Pathol 2000;68:152–69.
28. Desmet V. Experimentele levercarcinogenese: Histochemische studie. Brussels: Presses Academiques Europeennes; 1963.
29. Dumble ML, Croager EJ, Yeoh GC, et al. Generation and characterization of p53 null transformed hepatic progenitor cells: oval cells give rise to hepatocellular carcinoma. Carcinogenesis 2002;23:435–45.
30. Libbrecht L, Desmet V, Van Damme B, et al. The immunohistochemical phenotype of dysplastic foci in human liver: correlation with putative progenitor cells. J Hepatol 2000;33:76–84.
31. Hamburger AW, Salmon SE. Primary bioassay of human tumor stem cells. Science 1977;197:461–3.
32. Spee B, Carpino G, Schotanus BA, et al. Characterisation of the activated liver progenitor cell niche, potential involvement of Wnt and Notch signalling. Gut 2010;59(2):247–57.
33. Wicha MS, Liu S, Dontu G. Cancer stem cells: an old idea—a paradigm shift. Cancer Res 2006;66:1883–90 [discussion: 1895–6].

34. Taniguchi H, Chiba T. Stem cells and cancer in the liver. Dis Markers 2008;24: 223–9.

35. Armengol C, Cairo S, Fabre M, et al. Wnt signaling and hepatocarcinogenesis: the hepatoblastoma model. Int J Biochem Cell Biol 2011;43(2):265–70.

36. Yang W, Yan HX, Chen L, et al. Wnt/beta-catenin signaling contributes to activation of normal and tumorigenic liver progenitor cells. Cancer Res 2008;68: 4287–95.

37. Libbrecht L, Desmet V, Roskams T. Preneoplastic lesions in human hepatocarcinogenesis. Liver Int 2005;25:16–27.

38. Hsia CC, Evarts RP, Nakatsukasa H, et al. Occurrence of oval-type cells in hepatitis B virus-associated human hepatocarcinogenesis. Hepatology 1992;16: 1327–33.

39. Uenishi T, Kubo S, Yamamoto T, et al. Cytokeratin 19 expression in hepatocellular carcinoma predicts early postoperative recurrence. Cancer Sci 2003;94:851–7.

40. Van Eyken P, Sciot R, Paterson A, et al. Cytokeratin expression in hepatocellular carcinoma: an immunohistochemical study. Hum Pathol 1988;12:562–8.

41. Wu PC, Lai VC, Fang JW, et al. Hepatocellular carcinoma expressing both hepatocellular and biliary markers also expresses cytokeratin 14, a marker of bipotential progenitor cells. J Hepatol 1999;31:965–6.

42. Durnez A, Verslype C, Nevens F, et al. The clinicopathological and prognostic relevance of cytokeratin 7 and 19 expression in hepatocellular carcinoma. A possible progenitor cell origin. Histopathology 2006;49:138–51.

43. Zhuang PY, Zhang JB, Zhu XD, et al. Two pathologic types of hepatocellular carcinoma with lymph node metastasis with distinct prognosis on the basis of CK19 expression in tumor. Cancer 2008;112(12):2740–8.

44. Yamashita T, Forgues M, Wang W, et al. EpCAM and alpha-fetoprotein expression defines novel prognostic subtypes of hepatocellular carcinoma. Cancer Res 2008;68:1451–61.

45. Aishima S, Kuroda Y, Nishihara Y, et al. Proposal of progression model for intrahepatic cholangiocarcinoma: clinicopathologic differences between hilar type and peripheral type. Am J Surg Pathol 2007;31:1059–67.

46. Ding SJ, Li Y, Tan YX, et al. From proteomic analysis to clinical significance: overexpression of cytokeratin 19 correlates with hepatocellular carcinoma metastasis. Mol Cell Proteomics 2004;3:73–81.

47. Aishima S, Nishihara Y, Kuroda Y, et al. Histologic characteristics and prognostic significance in small hepatocellular carcinoma with biliary differentiation: subdivision and comparison with ordinary hepatocellular carcinoma. Am J Surg Pathol 2007;31:783–91.

48. Lee JS, Chu IS, Heo J, et al. Classification and prediction of survival in hepatocellular carcinoma by gene expression profiling. Hepatology 2004;40:667–76.

49. Lee JS, Heo J, Libbrecht L, et al. A novel prognostic subtype of human hepatocellular carcinoma derived from hepatic progenitor cells. Nat Med 2006;12(4): 410–6.

50. Ma S, Chan KW, Hu L, et al. Identification and characterization of tumorigenic liver cancer stem/progenitor cells. Gastroenterology 2007;132:2542–56.

51. Ma S, Lee TK, Zheng BJ, et al. CD133+ HCC cancer stem cells confer chemoresistance by preferential expression of the Akt/PKB survival pathway. Oncogene 2008;27:1749–58.

52. Dan YY, Riehle KJ, Lazaro C, et al. Isolation of multipotent progenitor cells from human fetal liver capable of differentiating into liver and mesenchymal lineages. Proc Natl Acad Sci U S A 2006;103:9912–7.

53. Yang ZF, Ho DW, Ng MN, et al. Significance of CD90+ cancer stem cells in human liver cancer. Cancer Cell 2008;13:153–66.
54. Yang ZF, Ngai P, Ho DW, et al. Identification of local and circulating cancer stem cells in human liver cancer. Hepatology 2008;47:919–28.
55. Yamashita T, Ji J, Budhu A, et al. EpCAM-positive hepatocellular carcinoma cells are tumor-initiating cells with stem/progenitor cell features. Gastroenterology 2009;136:1012–24.
56. Yamashita T, Budhu A, Forgues M, et al. Activation of hepatic stem cell marker EpCAM by Wnt-beta-catenin signaling in hepatocellular carcinoma. Cancer Res 2007;67:10831–9.
57. Roskams T, Ros JE, Libbrecht L, et al. High Expression of MDR1, MRP1, and MRP3 in the hepatic progenitor cell compartment and hepatocytes in severe human liver disease. Hepatology 2001;34:479.
58. Chiba T, Kita K, Zheng YW, et al. Side population purified from hepatocellular carcinoma cells harbors cancer stem cell-like properties. Hepatology 2006;44:240–51.
59. Shi GM, Xu Y, Fan J, et al. Identification of side population cells in human hepatocellular carcinoma cell lines with stepwise metastatic potentials. J Cancer Res Clin Oncol 2008;134:1155–63.
60. Vander Borght S, Komuta M, Libbrecht L, et al. Expression of multidrug resistance-associated protein 1 in hepatocellular carcinoma is associated with a more aggressive tumour phenotype and may reflect a progenitor cell origin. Liver Int 2008;28:1370–80.
61. Wakamatsu T, Nakahashi Y, Hachimine D, et al. The combination of glycyrrhizin and lamivudine can reverse the cisplatin resistance in hepatocellular carcinoma cells through inhibition of multidrug resistance-associated proteins. Int J Oncol 2007;31:1465–72.
62. Hu C, Li H, Li J, et al. Analysis of ABCG2 expression and side population identifies intrinsic drug efflux in the HCC cell line MHCC-97L and its modulation by Akt signaling. Carcinogenesis 2008;29:2289–97.
63. Folmer Y, Schneider M, Blum HE, et al. Reversal of drug resistance of hepatocellular carcinoma cells by adenoviral delivery of anti-ABCC2 antisense constructs. Cancer Gene Ther 2007;14:875–84.
64. Siegel A. Moving targets in hepatocellular carcinoma: hepatic progenitor cells as novel targets for tyrosine kinase inhibitors. Gastroenterology 2008;135:733–5.
65. Schirmacher P, Bedossa P, Roskams T, et al. Fighting the bushfire in HCC trials. J Hepatology 2011, in press.

The Role of Oncogenic Viruses in the Pathogenesis of Hepatocellular Carcinoma

Romy Zemel, PhD, Assaf Issachar, MD, Ran Tur-Kaspa, MD*

KEYWORDS

- Hepatocellular carcinoma (HCC) • Hepatitis B virus (HBV)
- Hepatitis C (HCV) • Cirrhosis

Hepatocarcinogenesis in humans is a multistep process, which reflects the genetic alterations that drive the progressive transformation of normal human cells into malignant cells.[1] Viruses may use diverse approaches that contribute to cancer development; however, additional factors such as host immunity and chronic inflammation, and host cellular mutations also play a role in the transformation process. More than 75% of all cases of hepatocellular carcinoma (HCC) are related to virus-induced hepatitis, mainly hepatitis B virus (HBV) and hepatitis C virus (HCV), leading to a 20-fold increased risk for the development of HCC in patients with chronic viral hepatitis.[2] Approximately 350 million people are chronically infected with HBV and 170 million with HCV worldwide; HBV infection is responsible for two-thirds of all HCC cases. The geographic distribution of HCC coincides with the distribution of HBV and HCV infections in those areas.[3]

A variety of viral and host factors contribute to HCC development in chronic HBV infection. Host factors include male gender, age older than 50 years, family history of HCC, and the presence of cirrhosis.[4] Other environmental and personal cofactors include excessive alcohol intake, cigarette smoking, obesity, and aflatoxin B1 (AFB1) exposure. The mycotoxin aflatoxin B1 (AFB1), produced by several fungal species of the *Aspergillus* genus, has strong hepatocarcinogenic potential and potentiates the carcinogenic effect of HBV infection.[5] That individuals infected with HBV who are exposed to aflatoxin have a higher risk of liver cancer than with either alone,

All authors have no financial disclosures and/or conflicts of interest.

Department of Medicine D and the Liver Institute, Rabin Medical Center, Beilinson Hospital, Molecular Hepatology Research Laboratory, Felsenstein Medical Research Center, Sackler School of Medicine, Tel Aviv University, 39 Jabotinsky Street, Petah-Tikva 49100, Israel

* Corresponding author.

E-mail address: turkaspa@post.tau.ac.il

suggests a synergistic effect between HBV and AFB1,[6] which has been reviewed comprehensively recently.[5] There is synergism between HBV and AFB1 in inducing oxidative stress and subsequently increasing the risk for HCC.[7] Wild and Montesano[5] suggested that HBV could predispose hepatocytes to carcinogenic activity based on the observation that cells expressing wild-type p53 transfected with HBx gene were more sensitive to the cytotoxic effects of AFB1 metabolites than were the parent cells.[8]

Among the viral factors that contribute to hepatocarcinogenesis are the level of HBV DNA in serum, hepatitis B e-antigen (HBeAg)-positive status, mutations in the viral genome, such as basal core promoter mutations (BCP T1762/A1764), genotype C, especially genotype C2 in Asia,[9,10] and genotype D.[11] Chronic infection with hepatitis virus D (HDV) is considered as a risk factor for HCC. However, a direct involvement of HDV in HCC development was not reported and it is believed that it might reflect the increasing severity of the disease in patient coinfected with HBV and HDV.[12] In addition, co-infection with other viruses such as HCV and HIV also increases the risk of HCC.[13]

HCV is a major cause of HCC worldwide owing to the high prevalence of HCV infection and the high rate of HCC occurrence in patients with HCV cirrhosis. In Japan, HCV is currently the main cause of HCC, accounting for more than 70% of cases. A similar rate is observed in Southern Europe, such as Italy or Spain. There are several risk factors for developing HCC in HCV-infected individuals, including cirrhosis and possibly even advanced hepatic fibrosis, heavy alcohol use, diabetes mellitus, obesity, low platelet count, male gender, older age, and increased hepatic iron stores.[14] A meta-analysis of 21 studies of age-adjusted risk showed that patients infected with HCV genotype 1b have an almost double risk for HCC development compared with other genotypes with a relative risk (RR) of 1.78.[15] Ishikawa and colleagues[16] showed, in a retrospective study of patients with positive HCV antibody, that male gender and a high titer of HCV-RNA were predictive factors for the development of HCC.

MECHANISM OF HEPATOCARCINOGENESIS

HCV-related HCC is generally agreed to occur on a background of cirrhosis and possibly severe fibrosis as well. Immune-mediated destruction of viral-infected hepatocytes induces liver regeneration that may lead to accumulation of mutations and subsequent selection of cells with a carcinogenic phenotype.[17–19] In HBV-related HCC, approximately 70% of cases occur in association with cirrhosis, which favors the hypothesis that HBV-related HCC may occur not only via cirrhosis.[20]

Both HBV and HCV viruses share many common features promoting cancer development. Although the mechanisms have not been completely clarified, they are believed to be different for each virus. The pattern of genetic alterations in viral-related HCC has been found to be quite discretely different for the 2 viruses. Gene expression, using microarray analysis, shows distinctively different patterns between HBV- and HCV-related HCC.[21] However, common pathogenetic pathways among the different etiological factors that induce HCC are suggested to contribute to the mechanisms of hepatocarcinogenesis, in particular, p53 inactivation or mutation and inflammation followed by continual rounds of necrosis and regeneration, and oxidative stress.[22]

Inflammation

The cross-talk between inflammatory cells and hepatocytes in the development of HCC is described in a detailed review published recently.[23] Emerging data suggest that the inflammatory milieu represents a favorable condition for genetic mutations.

The critical components linking inflammation and liver cancer are the expression and activity of different cytokines, such as interleukin (IL)-6 and IL-1α, and their signaling systems in cirrhosis and HCC.[23] Both hepatotropic viruses promote inflammatory reactions, which eventually contribute to HCC development.[23,24]

Oxidative Stress

Extensive oxidative DNA damage has been observed in hepatocytes from HBV-positive transgenic mice and HBV-infected humans.[25,26] Chronic HCV infection is also characterized by increased oxidative stress, and patients with chronic HCV infection show an increase in serum or liver content of oxidative stress markers, such as lipid peroxidation products, superoxide dismutase, and 8-isoprostane.[27] HCV-specific proteins, namely NS5A, NS3, and core protein, have been linked to the induction of endoplasmic reticulum (ER) stress and the production of reactive oxygen species (ROS). ROS in turn may modulate gene expression, cell adhesion, cell metabolism, cell cycle, and cell death and induce oxidative DNA damage, which leads to increased chromosomal aberrations associated with cell transformation.[28] A direct correlation between oxidative DNA damage and hepatic inflammation is observed in patients with both chronic HBV and HCV, which suggests direct involvement of hepatic oxidative stress in the pathogenesis and progression of liver cell injury in chronic viral hepatitis. However, oxidative DNA damage in HCV-infected livers seems to be significantly higher than in HBV-infected livers, suggesting that HCV may cause more advanced oxidative stress in the liver during chronic infection than does HBV.[27]

HCC without Cirrhosis

Epidemiologically, as already mentioned, the development of HCC is closely related to cirrhosis, regardless of the underlying cause(s).[29] However, almost 20% of HCCs develop in noncirrhotic livers,[30] raising the interesting question of the role of viral hepatitis in these cases.

That HCC can develop in noncirrhotic HBV-infected patients, favors a direct role for HBV in carcinogenesis. This direct carcinogenic effect of HBV, which is a DNA virus, is primarily attributed to its ability to integrate into the human genome. Integrated HBV sequences have been found in the host chromosome of 80% to 90% of HBV-related HCC.[18,31–34] This integration can cause rearrangement of host genomic DNA, which might confer a selective growth advantage on target cells, leading to the development of preneoplastic nodules, or provide an additional step in tumor progression.[32] HBV integrations appear to be partially preferential to particular genomic regions that encode cellular regulatory genes of importance in cell proliferation, differentiation, and viability.

HCV, as a positive-stranded RNA virus with a completely cytoplasmic-replicating life cycle, is not integrated into the host genome. However, its close association with HCC qualifies it as the only positive-stranded RNA virus to be included among the human oncogenic viruses.[18] Because most HCV-related HCC occurs on a background of cirrhosis or severe fibrosis, it is thought that the mechanism of carcinogenesis probably involves an interplay between the activities of viral proteins that modulate cell signal transduction pathways and the host immune response mechanism, chronic inflammation, cell death, and proliferation.

Establishment of Persistent Infection

One key feature of oncogenic viruses is the establishment of persistent infection, in which the virus develops strategies for evading the host immune response that sets the stage for a variety of molecular events contributing to eventual virus-mediated tumorigenesis.[18] As a DNA virus, the direct carcinogenic effect of HBV is primarily attributable to its ability to integrate into the human genome. HBV integration, although not necessary for viral replication, allows for long-term persistence.[31] HBV integration in the host genome results in decreased viral DNA replication, leading to a reduction in HBV expression,[35] which facilitates escape recognition of the infected cells by the immune system.[36] Although integrated viral sequences are defective for replication,[37] they might contribute to the tumorigenic phenotype by integrating and mutating key regulatory cellular genes. Moreover, the long-term expression of viral gene products, whether expressed from the HBV-integrated DNA or from the virus itself, might participate in tumorigenesis, supporting the notion of a direct oncogenic contribution of HBV to hepatocarcinogenesis.[38]

The selection of quasispecies that escape the host immune response contributes to the persistence of HCV infection.[39] HCV viral-specific proteins can disrupt the host antiviral cellular immune response by directly interacting with host cell defense regulatory pathways, such as the interferon-signaling pathway.[39] Another mechanism that may contribute to impairing the immune system, is the ability of HCV to downregulate the proteasome peptidase activities, thereby interfering with the processing of viral antigens for presentation by MHC class I molecules, in turn allowing persistent viral infection.[40]

Genetic Instability

Integration of HBV DNA may enhance chromosomal instability that is associated with large inverted duplications, deletions, amplifications, or chromosomal translocations.[33] Of interest, the integrated HBx gene product was demonstrated to contribute directly to chromosomal instability. HBx could stimulate centrosome duplication and increase the numbers of multinucleated and micronuclei cells, which results in abnormal numbers of centrosomes.[41] HBx protein expression could also interfere in the mitotic checkpoint, by interacting with a component of the mitotic checkpoint complex (BubR1).[42] Recently, HBx was reported to inhibit pituitary tumor–transforming gene 1 (PTTG1) ubiquitination, which in turn impaired its degradation by the proteasome, leading to accumulation of PTTG1, a protein implicated in inhibition of sister chromatid separation during mitosis.[43] Genomic instability was also demonstrated to result from the expression of defective HBV genomes that are frequently associated with HBV-mediated HCC. Deletion mutants of HBV envelope proteins in the 3' of pre-S1 and the 5' of pre-S2 result in intracellular retention that causes ER stress[32,44] and leads to oxidative stress and DNA damage, which may contribute to HCC formation.[26]

Genomic instability was also reported in HCV infection, and involves the HCV core protein. It was shown that constitutive expression of HCV core protein in NIH 3T3 cells resulted in genomic instability, seen as disruption of the mitotic spindle cell checkpoint that increases ploidy and triggers malignant transformation.[45]

Molecular Mechanism of HCC Development

Common alterations in cell physiology are shared in most human tumors and are considered as the hallmarks of cancer development. The capacity for self-sufficiency in growth signals, insensitivity to growth-inhibitory (antigrowth) signals, evasion of programmed cell death (apoptosis), limitless replicative potential, sustained angiogenesis, and tissue invasion and metastasis, collectively dictate malignant growth.[46] The specific HCV and HBV viral-encoded proteins can exert pleiotropic effects by interacting with the host cell machinery, thereby promoting the alterations involved in HCC development. The expression of HBx was found to be preferentially maintained in HCCs.[32] HBx is considered as a potential oncogenic factor, as it plays an important regulatory role in controlling host processes by interacting with both virus and host factors, contributing to the development of HBV-related HCC. HBx may function, in the nucleus, as specific transcriptional activator and in the cytoplasm by affecting signal transduction pathways. It does not exploit its effect directly at the DNA level but, rather, a protein interaction is crucial for HBx transactivation. Defective HBV genomes, especially COOH-terminal deletion of HBx, truncated HBx, and HBV pre-S mutations, are frequent in HBV-associated HCC and might contribute to cell transformation.[33,44,47,48]

HCV proteins may also contribute directly to hepatic carcinogenesis, mediated via HCV core protein, NS3, and NS5A. HCV core protein functions as a modulator of cellular processes and may also interact directly with nuclear transcription factors.[49] Transgenic mice expressing core protein were shown to develop HCC without coexisting inflammation.[50] A direct involvement of NS3 protease activity in the induction of neoplastic transformation of the cells has been described.[51] NS5A has been shown to interact with a range of cellular proteins implicated in signal transduction, denoting the potential of the protein to affect the host-cell environment.[52]

Self-sufficiency in growth signal

Tumor cells generate many of their own growth signals, thereby reducing their dependence on stimulation from their normal tissue microenvironment. It is suspected that growth signaling pathways undergo deregulation in all human tumors.[46] Abundant research demonstrates that the HBx protein interferes with the epidermal growth factor (EGF) signaling pathway by directly increasing the mRNA level of the EGF receptor (EGFR) gene.[53] HBx was shown to induce activation of Ras,[54–57] to stimulate the Ras-Raf mitogen-activated protein (MAP) kinase cytosolic signal transduction pathway,[41,58,59] to activate the extracellular signal-regulated kinases (ERKs)[60,61] and c-Jun terminal kinases (JNKs),[61] to increase the activation of activated protein (AP)-1 DNA binding activity and the de novo synthesis of c-Fos and c-Jun proteins,[61,62] and to induce the janus kinase (JAK)/signal transducer and activator of transcription (STAT) signaling pathway to exert growth signals and promote cell proliferation.

HBx was shown to interfere directly with the regulation of cell growth by transactivating a number of cellular promoters and enhancers containing binding sites of nuclear transcription factor that regulate the expression of genes critical for cell growth, such as the activator protein 1 (AP-1), AP-2, nuclear factor kappa-B (NF-kB), cAMP response element-binding (CREB) protein, TATA box-binding protein (TBP), and CCAAT enhancer-binding protein (c-EBP).[32,33] The HBx truncated mutant was also reported to affect cell growth by modulating STAT/suppressor of cytokine signaling (SOCS) cellular signaling pathway.[63]

Deregulation of growth signaling pathways in the case of HCV infection is less well documented. Recently, HCV infection was demonstrated to increase the activation of the EGFR signaling pathway through proteolytic cleavage of tyrosine phosphatase T-cell protein (TC-PTP) by HCV NS3/4A protease, resulting in enhancement of ligand-induced EGFR activation and of the downstream signaling of the PI3K/Akt pathway.[64] HCV core protein was reported to activate the MAP kinase cascade and to prolong its activity in response to mitogenic stimuli in cells expressing HCV core gene, cooperatively with the v-H-ras.[65] Core protein was also shown to activate Map kinase kinase (MEK)1 and Erk1/2 MAP kinases.[66] ERK, JNK, p38 MAP kinases, and Map kinase phosphatase (MKP)-1 were activated by core when produced at low level in the HepG2 Tet-Off cell system[67] and also by HCV NS5A in response to oxidative stress.[68] MAP kinase signaling, through activation of JNK, was also implicated in HCV NS3 protein-mediated cell growth in infected cells.[69] However, there are conflicting observations of the ability of HCV to intervene in EGF signaling . It is suggested, rather, that HCV inhibits host-cell mitogenic signaling as a strategy to enhance viral replication and establish chronic infection.[70–72]

Insensitivity to antigrowth signal

HBV was documented to interfere with cell-cycle regulation, promoting the cell through the G1 state and, as with other effects of HBV, this is mostly mediated by the HBx protein.[17,33,73] HBx increases the levels of G1-phase proteins (p21, p27, cyclin D1, and cyclin E) and the activity of the G1-phase kinase, cyclin-dependent kinase 4 (CDK4), decreases the levels of p15 and p16 proteins that inhibit progression from G0 to G1, and inhibits the activation of the late-G1/S-phase CDK, CDK2 leading to enhanced cell proliferation.[17] HBx[74] and the pre-S2 mutant[75] inhibited the tumor suppressor retinoblastoma (pRb) signaling, which led to an increase in E2F1 activity, resulting in continuous growth of HBV-infected cells that promoted the development of HBV-related HCC. HBV infection also involves the deregulation of Myc, which is known to participate in cell growth and cell-cycle progression. HBx was shown to increase the stability of intracellular c-myc by blocking the ubiquitination of Myc through a direct interaction with the F box region of Skp2 and destabilization of the Skp-Cullin-F-box (SCF) Skp2 complex (a ubiquitin-conjugating enzyme E2 complex).[76] The expression of the HBx truncated mutant was reported to enhance the transforming ability of Myc, supporting the hypothesis that HBx mutants might be selected in tumor tissues and play a role in hepatocarcinogenesis.[77]

Deregulation of the cell cycle is also implicated in HCV infection. Studies performed on liver biopsies from patients with chronic HCV have shown an impairment of checkpoint of cell cycle.[78] Progression of cell cycle from G1-phase to S-phase was demonstrated in cells supporting the replication of subgenomic and genome length HCV RNA replicons as a result of negative regulation of pRb protein, occurring via the ubiquitin-proteasome system in an NS5B-dependent manner.[79,80] Activation of the pRb/E2F pathway by HCV core protein was also shown. HCV core suppresses p53 tumor suppressor protein and p21 CDK inhibitor expression, and enhances the activation of CDK2, phosphorylation of pRb, and activation and expression of E2F-1, which results in enhanced proliferation.[81] Repression of the CDK inhibitor p21 gene by HCV core and by NS5A proteins has been described in NIH 3T3, HeLa, and in human hepatoma-transfected cells.[82–84] NS5A protein activates the human proliferating cell nuclear antigen (PCNA) gene, leading to promotion of cell proliferation.[85] Deregulation of the cell cycle by activating c-myc expression was demonstrated in transgenic mice expressing HCV core protein.[86] In stable transfectant Rat-1 cell lines, HCV core was shown to promote cell proliferation through upregulation of the cyclin E expression levels.[87]

Increased b-catenin accumulation and gene mutations are observed in both HBV-associated and HCV-associated HCCs, although with higher frequencies in the case of HCV infection. HCV NS5A protein was shown to bind b-catenin, causing its stabilization, which results in an increase in b-catenin-dependent transcription levels.[88,89] In HBV infection, the increased cell proliferation can be linked to the ability of HBx to upregulate the cytoplasmic signaling of b-catenin through the Erk/RSK pathway.[90,91]

Evasion of apoptosis

Abundant data suggest that HBV alters the balance between programmed cell death and proliferation, by participating in the apoptotic and antiapoptotic pathways. These effects may be dependent on the experimental system and the status of the cells being examined. HBx was shown to inhibit transforming growth factor β-1 (TGFβ1)-induced apoptosis in transgenic mice.[92] Shih and colleagues[57] linked the protection from TGF-β–induced apoptosis to the ability of HBx to activate PI 3-kinase (PI3K) and Src. HBx was reported to activate PI3K through the PI3K-Akt-Bad pathway, thus inactivating caspase 3 in a p53-independent manner.[93] HBx also appears to interact with p53 and inhibit p53-mediated apoptosis by sequestering p53 in the cytosol.[94,95] HBx was demonstrated to promote the activation of NF-kB in different cell lines inhibiting tumor necrosis factor (TNF)-α–mediated and Fas-mediated stimulation of apoptotic pathways.[96–98] HBx was demonstrated both in vitro and in vivo to promote antiapoptotic function by interacting with hepsin and survivin.[99–102] A caspase-independent cell death pathway, in which the serine protease granzyme A (GzmA) induces apoptotic death of target cells as part of the immune response,[103] was shown to be modulated by HBV infection.[104]

Increasing evidence is emerging of HCV interaction with regulatory pathways that control apoptosis. HCV was suggested to act as a tumor accelerator by blocking apoptosis.[105] HCV transgenic mice were shown to inhibit Fas-mediated apoptosis, thereby suppressing the activation of caspase-9 and caspase-3/7.[105,106] HCV NS5A has been shown to play a major role in inhibiting apoptosis.[107] It blocks the activation of caspase-3 and inhibits proteolytic cleavage of the death substrate poly (ADP-ribose) polymerase in TNF-α–induced cells.[108] HCV NS5A was reported to bind p53[109] and the proapoptotic protein Bin1[110] and to interact with PI3K, thus promoting the PI3K-AKT cell survival pathway.[111] Recently, NS5A was shown to interact with the cellular protein FK-binding protein (FKBP) 38, impairing the interaction between the mammalian target of rapamycin (mTOR) and FKBP38 and, thus, inhibiting apoptosis through the mTOR pathway.[112,113] Inhibition of apoptosis is also mediated through HCV core expression, which inhibits caspase-8 activation by maintaining the expression of the cellular FADD-like interleukin-1 converting enzyme (c-FLIP), an endogenous caspase-8 inhibitor.[114] HCV core also inhibits deoxycholic acid-mediated apoptosis when expressed in Huh-7 cells and in HeLa cells, by increasing Bcl-x protein and decreasing Bax protein.[115] HCV core represses p53 activity, thereby inhibiting p-53–induced apoptosis.[116] It was also shown to interfere with the proapoptotic function of p53 by inhibiting tumor suppressor promyelocytic leukemia protein (PML)-induced apoptosis, a key regulator of p53 activity.[117] HCV E2 was reported to inhibit TNF-related apoptosis, inducing ligand (TRAIL)-induced apoptosis through inhibition of mitochondrial cytochrome C release.[118]

Limitless replicative potential
The intrinsic capacity for limitless replicative potential is a characteristic of cancer cells. Mammalian cells carry an intrinsic, cell-autonomous program that limits their multiplication. Deregulation of such pathways can contribute to the development of cancer. Telomere maintenance is a key component of the capability for unlimited replication.[46]

Short telomeres were present in HBV-positive tissues, although strong telomerase activity was observed.[119,120] Accumulation of cells containing chromosomes with shorter telomeres and telomeres of critical length was implied as playing a key role in tumorigenesis.[121] HBx[122] and preS2[123] were demonstrated to upregulate the expression and activity of telomerase reverse transcriptase (hTERT) in hepatoma cells, contributing to tumor development.

The effects of HCV core protein were demonstrated to be associated with increased telomerase activity in hepatoma cells and in core-mediated immortalized primary human hepatocytes.[124,125]

Sustained angiogenesis

HBV infection has been shown to modulate angiogenic factors. HBx was suggested to act as a modulator in hypoxia-induced angiogenesis of HCC. It has been demonstrated to induce the expression of inducible nitric oxide synthase (iNOS)[126] and to increase the transcriptional activity and protein level of hypoxia-inducible factor-1alpha (HIF-1alpha),[127] which is involved in angiogenesis. HBx was also shown to stimulate the induction of angiopoietin-2 (Ang2), a major mediator of angiogenic control that is upregulated in liver tissue from chronic hepatitis B– infected patients.[128] HBx can stimulate the transcription of vascular endothelial growth factor (VEGF) and induce angiogenesis in HBx-transfected cells.[129] Moreover, accumulation of pre-S mutants in the ER results in upregulation of VEGF-A. The enhanced expression and secretion of VEGF-A activates Akt/mTOR signaling and may promote HBV-related hepatocarcinogenesis through the VEGFR.[130] In a recently published study, Zhang and colleagues[131] used a proteomics-based analysis to evaluate the effects of HBV replication on liver angiogenesis. Their findings suggest that the angiogenesis-associated protein fumarate hydratase (FH) is affected by HBV replication.

Evidence for the induction of hepatic angiogenesis during HCV infection was provided by demonstrating the production of TGF-β2, VEGF, and expression of CD34 protein in liver biopsy specimens of HCV-infected patients. This hepatic angiogenesis was shown to be regulated by HCV core protein, as it triggered the production of TGF-β2 and VEGF proteins by many pathways including protein kinase C (PKC), RB/E2F1, apoptosis signal-regulating kinase (ASK)1-JNK/p38, and ERK.[132] The HCV infection leads to the stabilization of hypoxia-inducible factor 1 (HIF-1a) which subsequently stimulates the synthesis and secretion of VEGF. Moreover, HCV-infected cells were demonstrated to release angiogenic cytokines, which lead to neo-vascularization in vivo.[133] Recently, VEGF expression was connected to the activity of the androgen receptor (AR) signaling pathway. HCV infection or HCV core protein were shown to enhance AR activity and VEGF expression in the presence of androgen.[134]

Tissue invasion and metastasis

The ability of HBx to modulate the expression and activation of matrix metalloproteinases (MMPs) was also implicated in its capacity to enhance the invasive potential of HCC cells. HBx induces the expression of MMP-9 by ERKs and PI-3K signal pathways.[135] HBx also induces upregulation of membrane type (MT)1-MMP,[136] MMP-2, MMP-14,[137] and activation of MMP-3.[138]

HCV core protein was recently reported to shut down TGF-β–dependent tumor-suppressive activity in a JNK/pSmad3L pathway–dependent manner, leading to loss of epithelial homeostasis and acquisition of a migratory mesenchymal phenotype, essential for tumor invasion.[139,140]

PREVENTION

Viral hepatitis infection can be prevented either by vaccination or by avoiding the transmission of the virus in contaminated body fluids.

Vaccination

The benefit of HBV vaccination has been best documented in Taiwan, where a gradual decline of HCC incidence from 0.70 to 0.36 per 100,000 individuals was reported for children older than 6 years in the period between 1981 and 1994.[141] Similarly, a reduction of HCC has been demonstrated among Thai and native Alaskan children who received hepatitis B vaccination at birth.[142,143]

Antiviral Treatment

Interferon treatment in the prevention of HCC in HBV patients

A large case-controlled study in Taiwan of patients who received interferon (IFN)-α treatment of HBV, with 15 years of follow-up, showed significant benefit in terms of HBeAg seroconversion (75% vs 52%, P = .031), HBsAg clearance (3.0% vs 0.4%, P = .03), incidence of cirrhosis (18% vs 34%, P = .041), and HCC development (2.7% vs 13%, P = .011).[144]

A meta-analysis in 2001 examining the use of IFN in preventing HCC in hepatitis B–related cirrhosis, found only nonrandomized control studies. The pooled estimate was significantly in favor of IFN (risk difference –6.4; confidence interval [CI]: –2.8 to –10.0, P<.001), but there was significant heterogeneity among the studies and subgroup analysis showed consistent results only when data were pooled from European studies. Although heterogeneity was not significant in the European subanalysis, IFN did not show any efficacy.[145]

In a more recent meta-analysis, 12 controlled trials were selected that included 2082 patients and compared IFN with no treatment. There was a different incidence of cirrhosis and HCC between treated and untreated patients. Relative risks (RRs) of cirrhosis and HCC, respectively, were 0.65 (95% CI: 0.47–0.91) and 0.59 (95% CI: 0.43–0.81).[146] The quality of the studies was quite variable, with differences in types of patients and response rates, and wide variation in the IFN regimens. The impact of IFN appeared to be more significant in those with cirrhosis than in those with less severe liver disease.

Nucleoside analog treatment in the prevention of HCC in patients with HBV

The Food and Drug Administration (FDA)-approved medications that are currently in use for the management of HBV disease are lamivudine, adefovir, entecavir, telbivudine, tenofovir, emtricitabine and tenofivir/emtricitabine; emtricitabine and tenofivir/emtricitabine are not labeled for HBV treatment.

As noted before, high HBV DNA levels correlate with the development of HCC,[147] whereas low viral loads have been reported in association with reductions in HCC risk.[148]

In a meta-analysis published in 2008, 5 studies (n = 2289) compared patients treated with nucleoside analogs and controls. The risk of HCC after treatment was reduced by 78% (RR: 0.22, 95% CI: 0.10–0.50). HBeAg-positive patients showed more significantly reduced HCC risk with treatment. Patients without cirrhosis benefited more from nucleoside analogs than those with cirrhosis, but resistance to nucleoside analogs has obviated the benefit of the treatment.[149] In one of the few prospective randomized controlled clinical trials performed in patients with cirrhosis, lamivudine has been shown to reduce the development of complications, including HCC. A total of 651 patients with fibrosis scores of 4 or greater were randomized to receive lamivudine or placebo. The study was stopped after a median of 32 months because there was a significant benefit of lamivudine. Overall disease progression was 7.8% in the treated group versus 18.0% in the controls (hazard ratio [HR], 0.45; P = .001). Risk of HCC was also decreased by treatment: 3.9% in the lamivudine group versus 7.4% in controls (HR, 0.49; P = .047).[150] For patients with chronic HBV but without cirrhosis, a case-controlled study of 142 HBeAg-positive lamivudine-treated patients were compared with 124 untreated controls matched for age, HBeAg status, and absence of cirrhosis, and followed for a mean of 89 months. Controls developed HCC and/or cirrhosis at a significantly higher rate than lamivudine-treated patients without drug resistance (P = .03).[151]

IFN monotherapy or IFN with ribavirin, in the prevention of HCC in patients with HCV

Unlike with HBV infection, permanent viral eradication is possible in HCV infection. After acute HCV infection, spontaneous recovery occurs in 15% to 50% of cases (depending on age, genotype, and severity of initial hepatitis), or after successful IFN/ribavirin-based antiviral treatment of acute or chronic HCV infection. Yoshida and colleagues[152] reported results of a large-scale cohort study Inhibition of Hepato-carcinogenesis by IFN Therapy (IHIT). Of the total number of 2890 patients enrolled, 2400 received IFN. In multivariate analysis, the adjusted RR of HCC development with IFN treatment versus nontreatment was 0.52 (95% CI: 0.36–0.74), representing 50% with IFN therapy. In a meta-analysis, Camma and colleagues[145] selected 14 articles that reported HCC development after IFN therapy in patients with chronic hepatitis C with cirrhosis, together with untreated controls. The summary risk difference of HCC development was −13% (95% CI: −8.3 to −17.2) in the IFN treatment group compared with the nontreatment group. In a more recent meta-analysis of 20 studies that compared untreated patients with those given IFN alone or with ribavirin, the RR for HCC development was 0.43 (95% CI: 0.33–0.56; $P<.00001$) in favor of antiviral therapy. They also evaluated 14 studies that compared results when there was a sustained virologic response (SVR) versus a nonsustained virologic response; there was a significant reduction in the occurrence of HCC, favoring those who achieved SVR over nonresponders (RR, 0.35; 95% CI: 0.26–0.46; $P<.00001$). In a prospective study of 101 patients with HCV-related cirrhosis who were treated with IFN alone, IFN and ribavirin, or no treatment, the incidence of HCC was significantly lower in the treatment groups.[153]

In the Hepatitis C Antiviral Long-term Treatment against Cirrhosis (HALT-C),[154] the Colchicine versus Peg-Intron Long-Term (Co-Pilot),[155] and the Evaluation of PegIntron in Control of Hepatitis C Cirrhosis (EPIC 3)[156] trials, patients who failed to achieve SVRs with standard treatment were randomized to maintenance treatment with IFN versus no treatment. No significant difference in the cumulative rate of developing HCC was observed for patients who received pegylated-IFN maintenance therapy compared with those randomized to the control, no-treatment group. Maintenance treatment with IFN for nonresponders to IFN/ribavirin therapy does not appear to reduce the risk of HCC in patients with chronic hepatitis C.

SUMMARY

HBV and HCV have major roles in hepatocarcinogenesis. More than 500 million people in the world are infected with hepatitis viruses and, therefore, HCC is highly prevalent, especially in those countries that are endemic for HBV and HCV. Viral and host factors contribute to the development of HCC. The main viral factors include the circulating load of HBV DNA or HCV RNA and specific genotypes. Various mechanisms have been demonstrated to be involved in the host-viral interactions that lead to HCC development, among which are genetic instability, self-sufficiency in growth signals, insensitivity to antigrowth signals, evasion of apoptosis, limitless replicative potential, sustained angiogenesis, and tissue invasiveness. Prevention of HBV by vaccination, as well as antiviral therapy against HBV and for HCV seem able to inhibit the development of HCC.

ACKNOWLEDGMENTS

This work was supported in part by the Cesarman Chair for Research in Liver Diseases, Tel Aviv University incumbent, Ran Tur-Kaspa.

REFERENCES

1. Hanahan D, Bergers G, Bergsland E. Less is more, regularly: metronomic dosing of cytotoxic drugs can target tumor angiogenesis in mice. J Clin Invest 2000;105(8):1045–7.
2. Schutte K, Bornschein J, Malfertheiner P. Hepatocellular carcinoma—epidemiological trends and risk factors. Dig Dis 2009;27(2):80–92.
3. Franceschi S, Raza SA. Epidemiology and prevention of hepatocellular carcinoma. Cancer Lett 2009;286(1):5–8.
4. Marrero CR, Marrero JA. Viral hepatitis and hepatocellular carcinoma. Arch Med Res 2007;38(6):612–20.
5. Wild CP, Montesano R. A model of interaction: aflatoxins and hepatitis viruses in liver cancer aetiology and prevention. Cancer Lett 2009;286(1):22–8.
6. Nordenstedt H, White DL, El-Serag HB. The changing pattern of epidemiology in hepatocellular carcinoma. Dig Liver Dis 2010;42(Suppl 3):S206–14.
7. Liu ZM, Li LQ, Peng MH, et al. Hepatitis B virus infection contributes to oxidative stress in a population exposed to aflatoxin B1 and high-risk for hepatocellular carcinoma. Cancer Lett 2008;263(2):212–22.
8. Sohn S, Jaitovitch-Groisman I, Benlimame N, et al. Retroviral expression of the hepatitis B virus x gene promotes liver cell susceptibility to carcinogen-induced site specific mutagenesis. Mutat Res 2000;460(1):17–28.
9. Chan HL, Tse CH, Mo F, et al. High viral load and hepatitis B virus subgenotype ce are associated with increased risk of hepatocellular carcinoma. J Clin Oncol 2008;26(2):177–82.
10. Yen-Hsuan N, Mei-Hwei C, Kuan-Jan W, et al. Clinical relevance of hepatitis B virus genotype in children with chronic infection and hepatocellular carcinoma. Gastroenterology 2004;127(6):1733–8.
11. Cooksley WG. Do we need to determine viral genotype in treating chronic hepatitis B? J Viral Hepat 2010;17(9):601–10.
12. Romeo R, Del Ninno E, Rumi M, et al. A 28-year study of the course of hepatitis Delta infection: a risk factor for cirrhosis and hepatocellular carcinoma. Gastroenterology 2009;136:1629–38.
13. Lim SG, Mohammed R, Yuen MF, et al. Prevention of hepatocellular carcinoma in hepatitis B virus infection. J Gastroenterol Hepatol 2009;24(8):1352–7.
14. Ueno Y, Sollano JD, Farrell GC. Prevention of hepatocellular carcinoma complicating chronic hepatitis C. J Gastroenterol Hepatol 2009;24(4):531–6.
15. Raimondi S, Bruno S, Mondelli MU, et al. Hepatitis C virus genotype 1b as a risk factor for hepatocellular carcinoma development: a meta-analysis. J Hepatol 2009;50(6):1142–54.
16. Ishikawa T, Ichida T, Yamagiwa S, et al. High viral loads, serum alanine aminotransferase and gender are predictive factors for the development of hepatocellular carcinoma from viral compensated liver cirrhosis. J Gastroenterol Hepatol 2001;16(11):1274–81.
17. Gearhart TL, Bouchard MJ. The hepatitis B virus X protein modulates hepatocyte proliferation pathways to stimulate viral replication. J Virol 2010;84(6):2675–86.
18. McLaughlin-Drubin ME, Munger K. Viruses associated with human cancer. Biochim Biophys Acta 2008;1782(3):127–50.
19. Bartosch B, Thimme R, Blum HE, et al. Hepatitis C virus-induced hepatocarcinogenesis. J Hepatol 2009;51(4):810–20.
20. Di Bisceglie AM. Hepatitis B and hepatocellular carcinoma. Hepatology 2009;49(Suppl 5):S56–60.

21. Brechot C. Pathogenesis of hepatitis B virus-related hepatocellular carcinoma: old and new paradigms. Gastroenterology 2004;127(5 Suppl 1):S56–61.

22. Farazi PA, DePinho RA. Hepatocellular carcinoma pathogenesis: from genes to environment. Nat Rev Cancer 2006;6(9):674–87.

23. Berasain C, Castillo J, Perugorria MJ, et al. Inflammation and liver cancer: new molecular links. Ann N Y Acad Sci 2009;1155:206–21.

24. Chemin I, Zoulim F. Hepatitis B virus induced hepatocellular carcinoma. Cancer Lett 2009;286(1):52–9.

25. Hagen TM, Huang S, Curnutte J, et al. Extensive oxidative DNA damage in hepatocytes of transgenic mice with chronic active hepatitis destined to develop hepatocellular carcinoma. Proc Natl Acad Sci U S A 1994;91(26): 12808–12.

26. Hsieh YH, Su IJ, Wang HC, et al. Pre-S mutant surface antigens in chronic hepatitis B virus infection induce oxidative stress and DNA damage. Carcinogenesis 2004;25(10):2023–32.

27. Fujita N, Sugimoto R, Ma N, et al. Comparison of hepatic oxidative DNA damage in patients with chronic hepatitis B and C. J Viral Hepat 2008;15(7):498–507.

28. Tsai WL, Chung RT. Viral hepatocarcinogenesis. Oncogene 2010;29(16): 2309–24.

29. Caldwell S, Park SH. The epidemiology of hepatocellular cancer: from the perspectives of public health problem to tumor biology. J Gastroenterol 2009; 44(Suppl 19):96–101.

30. Madhoun MF, Fazili J, Bright BC, et al. Hepatitis C prevalence in patients with hepatocellular carcinoma without cirrhosis. Am J Med Sci 2010;339(2):169–73.

31. Feitelson MA, Lee J. Hepatitis B virus integration, fragile sites, and hepatocarcinogenesis. Cancer Lett 2007;252(2):157–70.

32. Cougot D, Neuveut C, Buendia MA. HBV induced carcinogenesis. J Clin Virol 2005;34(Suppl 1):S75–8.

33. Brechot C, Kremsdorf D, Soussan P, et al. Hepatitis B virus (HBV)-related hepatocellular carcinoma (HCC): Molecular mechanisms and novel paradigms. Pathol Biol (Paris) 2010;58(4):278–87.

34. Brechot C, Gozuacik D, Murakami Y, et al. Molecular bases for the development of hepatitis B virus (HBV)-related hepatocellular carcinoma (HCC). Semin Cancer Biol 2000;10(3):211–31.

35. Raimondo G, Burk RD, Lieberman HM, et al. Interrupted replication of hepatitis B virus in liver tissue of HBsAg carriers with hepatocellular carcinoma. Virology 1988;166(1):103–12.

36. Butel JS. Viral carcinogenesis: revelation of molecular mechanisms and etiology of human disease. Carcinogenesis 2000;21(3):405–26.

37. Paterlini-Brechot P, Saigo K, Murakami Y, et al. Hepatitis B virus-related insertional mutagenesis occurs frequently in human liver cancers and recurrently targets human telomerase gene. Oncogene 2003;22(25):3911–6.

38. Carrillo-Infante C, Abbadessa G, Bagella L, et al. Viral infections as a cause of cancer (review). Int J Oncol 2007;30(6):1521–8.

39. Gale M Jr, Foy EM. Evasion of intracellular host defence by hepatitis C virus. Nature 2005;436(7053):939–45.

40. Khu YL, Tan YJ, Lim SG, et al. Hepatitis C virus non-structural protein NS3 interacts with LMP7, a component of the immunoproteasome, and affects its proteasome activity. Biochem J 2004;384(Pt 2):401–9.

41. Yun C, Cho H, Kim SJ, et al. Mitotic aberration coupled with centrosome amplification is induced by hepatitis B virus X oncoprotein via the

Ras-mitogen-activated protein/extracellular signal-regulated kinase-mitogen-activated protein pathway. Mol Cancer Res 2004;2(3):159–69.

42. Kim S, Park SY, Yong H, et al. HBV X protein targets hBubR1, which induces dysregulation of the mitotic checkpoint. Oncogene 2008;27(24):3457–64.

43. Molina-Jimenez F, Benedicto I, Murata M, et al. Expression of pituitary tumor-transforming gene 1 (PTTG1)/securin in hepatitis B virus (HBV)-associated liver diseases: evidence for an HBV X protein-mediated inhibition of PTTG1 ubiquitination and degradation. Hepatology 2010;51(3):777–87.

44. Cao Z, Bai X, Guo X, et al. High prevalence of hepatitis B virus pre-S mutation and its association with hepatocellular carcinoma in Qidong, China. Arch Virol 2008;153(10):1807–12.

45. Smirnova IS, Aksenov ND, Kashuba EV, et al. Hepatitis C virus core protein transforms murine fibroblasts by promoting genomic instability. Cell Oncol 2006;28(4):177–90.

46. Hanahan D, Weinberg RA. The hallmarks of cancer. Cell 2000;100(1):57–70.

47. Gao ZY, Li T, Wang J, et al. Mutations in preS genes of genotype C hepatitis B virus in patients with chronic hepatitis B and hepatocellular carcinoma. J Gastroenterol 2007;42(9):761–8.

48. Lin CL, Liu CH, Chen W, et al. Association of pre-S deletion mutant of hepatitis B virus with risk of hepatocellular carcinoma. J Gastroenterol Hepatol 2007;22(7):1098–103.

49. Kasprzak A, Adamek A. Role of hepatitis C virus proteins (C, NS3, NS5A) in hepatic oncogenesis. Hepatol Res 2008;38(1):1–26.

50. Tsutsumi T, Suzuki T, Moriya K, et al. Hepatitis C virus core protein activates ERK and p38 MAPK in cooperation with ethanol in transgenic mice. Hepatology 2003;38(4):820–8.

51. Zemel R, Gerechet S, Greif H, et al. Cell transformation induced by hepatitis C virus NS3 serine protease. J Viral Hepat 2001;8(2):96–102.

52. Mankouri J, Griffin S, Harris M. The hepatitis C virus non-structural protein NS5A alters the trafficking profile of the epidermal growth factor receptor. Traffic 2008; 9(9):1497–509.

53. Miyaki M, Sato C, Sakai K, et al. Malignant transformation and EGFR activation of immortalized mouse liver epithelial cells caused by HBV enhancer-X from a human hepatocellular carcinoma. Int J Cancer 2000;85(4):518–22.

54. Bouchard M, Giannakopoulos S, Wang EH, et al. Hepatitis B virus HBx protein activation of cyclin A-cyclin-dependent kinase 2 complexes and G1 transit via a Src kinase pathway. J Virol 2001;75(9):4247–57.

55. Klein NP, Schneider RJ. Activation of Src family kinases by hepatitis B virus HBx protein and coupled signaling to Ras. Mol Cell Biol 1997;17(11):6427–36.

56. Yang SZ, Zhang LD, Zhang Y, et al. HBx protein induces EMT through c-Src activation in SMMC-7721 hepatoma cell line. Biochem Biophys Res Commun 2009; 382(3):555–60.

57. Shih WL, Kuo ML, Chuang SE, et al. Hepatitis B virus X protein activates a survival signaling by linking SRC to phosphatidylinositol 3-kinase. J Biol Chem 2003;278(34):31807–13.

58. Benn J, Schneider RJ. Hepatitis B virus HBx protein activates Ras-GTP complex formation and establishes a Ras, Raf, MAP kinase signaling cascade. Proc Natl Acad Sci U S A 1994;91(22):10350–4.

59. Wang HD, Trivedi A, Johnson DL. Regulation of RNA polymerase I-dependent promoters by the hepatitis B virus X protein via activated Ras and TATA-binding protein. Mol Cell Biol 1998;18(12):7086–94.

60. Shan C, Xu F, Zhang S, et al. Hepatitis B virus X protein promotes liver cell proliferation via a positive cascade loop involving arachidonic acid metabolism and p-ERK1/2. Cell Res 2010;20(5):563–75.

61. Twu JS, Lai MY, Chen DS, et al. Activation of protooncogene c-jun by the X protein of hepatitis B virus. Virology 1993;192(1):346–50.

62. Benn J, Su F, Doria M, et al. Hepatitis B virus HBx protein induces transcription factor AP-1 by activation of extracellular signal-regulated and c-Jun N-terminal mitogen-activated protein kinases. J Virol 1996;70(8):4978–85.

63. Bock CT, Toan NL, Koeberlein B, et al. Subcellular mislocalization of mutant hepatitis B X proteins contributes to modulation of STAT/SOCS signaling in hepatocellular carcinoma. Intervirology 2008;51(6):432–43.

64. Brenndorfer ED, Karthe J, Frelin L, et al. Nonstructural 3/4A protease of hepatitis C virus activates epithelial growth factor-induced signal transduction by cleavage of the T-cell protein tyrosine phosphatase. Hepatology 2009;49(6):1810–20.

65. Tsuchihara K, Hijikata M, Fukuda K, et al. Hepatitis C virus core protein regulates cell growth and signal transduction pathway transmitting growth stimuli. Virology 1999;258(1):100–7.

66. Giambartolomei S, Covone F, Levrero M, et al. Sustained activation of the Raf/MEK/Erk pathway in response to EGF in stable cell lines expressing the Hepatitis C Virus (HCV) core protein. Oncogene 2001;20(20):2606–10.

67. Erhardt A, Hassan M, Heintges T, et al. Hepatitis C virus core protein induces cell proliferation and activates ERK, JNK, and p38 MAP kinases together with the MAP kinase phosphatase MKP-1 in a HepG2 Tet-Off cell line. Virology 2002;292(2):272–84.

68. Qadri I, Iwahashi M, Capasso JM, et al. Induced oxidative stress and activated expression of manganese superoxide dismutase during hepatitis C virus replication: role of JNK, p38 MAPK and AP-1. Biochem J 2004;378(Pt 3):919–28.

69. Hassan M, Ghozlan H, Abdel-Kader O. Activation of c-Jun NH2-terminal kinase (JNK) signaling pathway is essential for the stimulation of hepatitis C virus (HCV) non-structural protein 3 (NS3)-mediated cell growth. Virology 2005;333(2):324–36.

70. Macdonald A, Chan JK, Harris M. Perturbation of epidermal growth factor receptor complex formation and Ras signalling in cells harbouring the hepatitis C virus subgenomic replicon. J Gen Virol 2005;86(Pt 4):1027–33.

71. Tan SL, Nakao H, He Y, et al. NS5A, a nonstructural protein of hepatitis C virus, binds growth factor receptor-bound protein 2 adaptor protein in a Src homology 3 domain/ligand-dependent manner and perturbs mitogenic signaling. Proc Natl Acad Sci U S A 1999;96(10):5533–8.

72. Georgopoulou U, Caravokiri K, Mavromara P. Suppression of the ERK1/2 signaling pathway from HCV NS5A protein expressed by herpes simplex recombinant viruses. Arch Virol 2003;148(2):237–51.

73. Qiao L, Leach K, McKinstry R, et al. Hepatitis B virus X protein increases expression of p21(Cip-1/WAF1/MDA6) and p27(Kip-1) in primary mouse hepatocytes, leading to reduced cell cycle progression. Hepatology 2001;34(5):906–17.

74. Choi BH, Choi M, Jeon HY, et al. Hepatitis B viral X protein overcomes inhibition of E2F1 activity by pRb on the human Rb gene promoter. DNA Cell Biol 2001;20(2):75–80.

75. Hsieh YH, Su IJ, Wang HC, et al. Hepatitis B virus pre-S2 mutant surface antigen induces degradation of cyclin-dependent kinase inhibitor p27Kip1 through c-Jun activation domain-binding protein 1. Mol Cancer Res 2007;5(10):1063–72.

76. Kalra N, Kumar V. The X protein of hepatitis B virus binds to the F box protein Skp2 and inhibits the ubiquitination and proteasomal degradation of c-Myc. FEBS Lett 2006;580(2):431–6.

77. Tu H, Bonura C, Giannini C, et al. Biological impact of natural COOH-terminal deletions of hepatitis B virus X protein in hepatocellular carcinoma tissues. Cancer Res 2001;61(21):7803–10.

78. Aileen M, Simon R, Susan ED, et al. Relation between hepatocyte G1 arrest, impaired hepatic regeneration, and fibrosis in chronic hepatitis C virus infection. Gastroenterology 2005;128(1):33–42.

79. Munakata T, Nakamura M, Liang Y, et al. Down-regulation of the retinoblastoma tumor suppressor by the hepatitis C virus NS5B RNA-dependent RNA polymerase. Proc Natl Acad Sci U S A 2005;102(50):18159–64.

80. Munakata T, Liang Y, Kim S, et al. Hepatitis C virus induces E6AP-dependent degradation of the retinoblastoma protein. PLoS Pathog 2007;3(9):1335–47.

81. Hassan M, Ghozlan H, Abdel-Kader O. Activation of RB/E2F signaling pathway is required for the modulation of hepatitis C virus core protein-induced cell growth in liver and non-liver cells. Cell Signal 2004;16(12):1375–85.

82. Ray RB, Steele R, Meyer K, et al. Hepatitis C virus core protein represses p21WAF1/Cip1/Sid1 promoter activity. Gene 1998;208(2):331–6.

83. Jung EY, Lee MN, Yang HY, et al. The repressive activity of hepatitis C virus core protein on the transcription of p21(waf1) is regulated by protein kinase A-mediated phosphorylation. Virus Res 2001;79(1–2):109–15.

84. Yoshida I, Oka K, Hidajat R, et al. Inhibition of p21/Waf1/Cip1/Sdi1 expression by hepatitis C virus core protein. Microbiol Immunol 2001;45(10):689–97.

85. Ghosh AK, Steele R, Meyer K, et al. Hepatitis C virus NS5A protein modulates cell cycle regulatory genes and promotes cell growth. J Gen Virol 1999;80(Pt 5):1179–83.

86. Honda M, Kaneko S, Shimazaki T, et al. Hepatitis C virus core protein induces apoptosis and impairs cell-cycle regulation in stably transformed Chinese hamster ovary cells. Hepatology 2000;31(6):1351–9.

87. Cho JW, Baek WK, Suh SI, et al. Hepatitis C virus core protein promotes cell proliferation through the upregulation of cyclin E expression levels. Liver 2001;21(2):137–42.

88. Street A, Macdonald A, McCormick C, et al. Hepatitis C virus NS5A-mediated activation of phosphoinositide 3-kinase results in stabilization of cellular beta-catenin and stimulation of beta-catenin-responsive transcription. J Virol 2005; 79(8):5006–16.

89. Milward A, Mankouri J, Harris M. Hepatitis C virus NS5A protein interacts with {beta}-catenin and stimulates its transcriptional activity in a phosphoinositide-3 kinase-dependent fashion. J Gen Virol 2010;91(2):373–81.

90. Ding Q, Xia W, Liu JC, et al. Erk associates with and primes GSK-3beta for its inactivation resulting in upregulation of beta-catenin. Mol Cell 2005;19(2):159–70.

91. Longato L, de la Monte S, Kuzushita N, et al. Overexpression of insulin receptor substrate-1 and hepatitis Bx genes causes premalignant alterations in the liver. Hepatology 2009;49(6):1935–43.

92. Shih WL, Kuo ML, Chuang SE, et al. Hepatitis B virus X protein inhibits transforming growth factor-beta -induced apoptosis through the activation of phosphatidylinositol 3-kinase pathway. J Biol Chem 2000;275(33):25858–64.

93. Lee YI, Kang-Park S, Do SI. The hepatitis B virus-X protein activates a phosphatidylinositol 3-kinase-dependent survival signaling cascade. J Biol Chem 2001; 276(20):16969–77.

94. Ueda H, Ullrich SJ, Gangemi JD, et al. Functional inactivation but not structural mutation of p53 causes liver cancer. Nat Genet 1995;9(1):41–7.

95. Wang XW, Gibson MK, Vermeulen W, et al. Abrogation of p53-induced apoptosis by the hepatitis B virus X gene. Cancer Res 1995;55(24):6012–6.

96. Clippinger AJ, Bouchard MJ. Hepatitis B virus HBx protein localizes to mitochondria in primary rat hepatocytes and modulates mitochondrial membrane potential. J Virol 2008;82(14):6798–811.

97. Su F, Theodosis CN, Schneider RJ. Role of NF-kappaB and myc proteins in apoptosis induced by hepatitis B virus HBx protein. J Virol 2001;75(1):215–25.

98. Yun C, Um HR, Jin YH, et al. NF-kappaB activation by hepatitis B virus X (HBx) protein shifts the cellular fate toward survival. Cancer Lett 2002;184(1):97–104.

99. Tanimoto H, Yan Y, Clarke J, et al. Hepsin, a cell surface serine protease identified in hepatoma cells, is overexpressed in ovarian cancer. Cancer Res 1997; 57(14):2884–7.

100. Magee JA, Araki T, Patil S, et al. Expression profiling reveals hepsin overexpression in prostate cancer. Cancer Res 2001;61(15):5692–6.

101. Zhang JL, Zhao WG, Wu KL, et al. Human hepatitis B virus X protein promotes cell proliferation and inhibits cell apoptosis through interacting with a serine protease Hepsin. Arch Virol 2005;150(4):721–41.

102. Zhang X, Dong N, Yin L, et al. Hepatitis B virus X protein upregulates survivin expression in hepatoma tissues. J Med Virol 2005;77(3):374–81.

103. Beresford PJ, Zhang D, Oh DY, et al. Granzyme A activates an endoplasmic reticulum-associated caspase-independent nuclease to induce single-stranded DNA nicks. J Biol Chem 2001;276(46):43285–93.

104. Lamontagne J, Pinkerton M, Block TM, et al. Hepatitis B and hepatitis C virus replication upregulates serine protease inhibitor Kazal, resulting in cellular resistance to serine protease-dependent apoptosis. J Virol 2010;84(2):907–17.

105. Kamegaya Y, Hiasa Y, Zukerberg L, et al. Hepatitis C virus acts as a tumor accelerator by blocking apoptosis in a mouse model of hepatocarcinogenesis. Hepatology 2005;41(3):660–7.

106. Machida K, Tsukiyama-Kohara K, Seike E, et al. Inhibition of cytochrome c release in Fas-mediated signaling pathway in transgenic mice induced to express hepatitis C viral proteins. J Biol Chem 2001;276(15):12140–6.

107. Majumder M, Ghosh AK, Steele R, et al. Hepatitis C virus NS5A protein impairs TNF-mediated hepatic apoptosis, but not by an anti-FAS antibody, in transgenic mice. Virology 2002;294(1):94–105.

108. Ghosh AK, Majumder M, Steele R, et al. Hepatitis C virus NS5A protein protects against TNF-alpha mediated apoptotic cell death. Virus Res 2000;67(2):173–8.

109. Lan KH, Sheu ML, Hwang SJ, et al. HCV NS5A interacts with p53 and inhibits p53-mediated apoptosis. Oncogene 2002;21(31):4801–11.

110. Nanda SK, Herion D, Liang TJ. The SH3 binding motif of HCV [corrected] NS5A protein interacts with Bin1 and is important for apoptosis and infectivity. Gastroenterology 2006;130(3):794–809.

111. He Y, Nakao H, Tan SL, et al. Subversion of cell signaling pathways by hepatitis C virus nonstructural 5A protein via interaction with Grb2 and P85 phosphatidylinositol 3-kinase. J Virol 2002;76(18):9207–17.

112. Peng L, Liang D, Tong W, et al. Hepatitis C Virus NS5A activates the mammalian target of rapamycin (mTOR) pathway, contributing to cell survival by disrupting the interaction between FK506-binding protein 38 (FKBP38) and mTOR. J Biol Chem 2010;285(27):20870–81.

113. Wang J, Tong W, Zhang X, et al. Hepatitis C virus non-structural protein NS5A interacts with FKBP38 and inhibits apoptosis in Huh7 hepatoma cells. FEBS Lett 2006;580(18):4392–400.
114. Saito K, Meyer K, Warner R, et al. Hepatitis C virus core protein inhibits tumor necrosis factor alpha-mediated apoptosis by a protective effect involving cellular FLICE inhibitory protein. J Virol 2006;80(9):4372–9.
115. Hara Y, Hino K, Okuda M, et al. Hepatitis C virus core protein inhibits deoxycholic acid-mediated apoptosis despite generating mitochondrial reactive oxygen species. J Gastroenterol 2006;41(3):257–68.
116. Ray RB, Steele R, Meyer K, et al. Transcriptional repression of p53 promoter by hepatitis C virus core protein. J Biol Chem 1997;272(17):10983–6.
117. Herzer K, Weyer S, Krammer PH, et al. Hepatitis C virus core protein inhibits tumor suppressor protein promyelocytic leukemia function in human hepatoma cells. Cancer Res 2005;65(23):10830–7.
118. Lee SH, Kim YK, Kim CS, et al. E2 of hepatitis C virus inhibits apoptosis. J Immunol 2005;175(12):8226–35.
119. Tahara H, Nakanishi T, Kitamoto M, et al. Telomerase activity in human liver tissues: comparison between chronic liver disease and hepatocellular carcinomas. Cancer Res 1995;55(13):2734–6.
120. Miura N, Horikawa I, Nishimoto A, et al. Progressive telomere shortening and telomerase reactivation during hepatocellular carcinogenesis. Cancer Genet Cytogenet 1997;93(1):56–62.
121. Yokota T, Suda T, Igarashi M, et al. Telomere length variation and maintenance in hepatocarcinogenesis. Cancer 2003;98(1):110–8.
122. Zhang X, Dong N, Zhang H, et al. Effects of hepatitis B virus X protein on human telomerase reverse transcriptase expression and activity in hepatoma cells. J Lab Clin Med 2005;145(2):98–104.
123. Liu H, Luan F, Ju Y, et al. In vitro transfection of the hepatitis B virus PreS2 gene into the human hepatocarcinoma cell line HepG2 induces upregulation of human telomerase reverse transcriptase. Biochem Biophys Res Commun 2007;355(2):379–84.
124. Zhu Z, Wilson AT, Gopalakrishna K, et al. Hepatitis C virus core protein enhances Telomerase activity in Huh7 cells. J Med Virol 2010;82(2):239–48.
125. Ray RB, Meyer K, Ray R. Hepatitis C virus core protein promotes immortalization of primary human hepatocytes. Virology 2000;271(1):197–204.
126. Majano PL, Garcia-Monzon C, Lopez-Cabrera M, et al. Inducible nitric oxide synthase expression in chronic viral hepatitis. Evidence for a virus-induced gene upregulation. J Clin Invest 1998;101(7):1343–52.
127. Moon EJ, Jeong CH, Jeong JW, et al. Hepatitis B virus X protein induces angiogenesis by stabilizing hypoxia-inducible factor-1alpha. FASEB J 2004;18(2):382–4.
128. Sanz-Cameno P, Martin-Vilchez S, Lara-Pezzi E, et al. Hepatitis B virus promotes angiopoietin-2 expression in liver tissue: role of HBV x protein. Am J Pathol 2006;169(4):1215–22.
129. Lee SW, Lee YM, Bae SK, et al. Human hepatitis B virus X protein is a possible mediator of hypoxia-induced angiogenesis in hepatocarcinogenesis. Biochem Biophys Res Commun 2000;268(2):456–61.
130. Yang JC, Teng CF, Wu HC, et al. Enhanced expression of vascular endothelial growth factor-A in ground glass hepatocytes and its implication in hepatitis B virus hepatocarcinogenesis. Hepatology 2009;49(6):1962–71.

131. Zhang J, Niu D, Sui J, et al. Protein profile in hepatitis B virus replicating rat primary hepatocytes and HepG2 cells by iTRAQ-coupled 2-D LC-MS/MS analysis: insights on liver angiogenesis. Proteomics 2009;9(10):2836–45.

132. Hassan M, Selimovic D, Ghozlan H, et al. Hepatitis C virus core protein triggers hepatic angiogenesis by a mechanism including multiple pathways. Hepatology 2009;49(5):1469–82.

133. Nasimuzzaman M, Waris G, Mikolon D, et al. Hepatitis C virus stabilizes hypoxia-inducible factor 1alpha and stimulates the synthesis of vascular endothelial growth factor. J Virol 2007;81(19):10249–57.

134. Kanda T, Steele R, Ray R, et al. Hepatitis C virus core protein augments androgen receptor-mediated signaling. J Virol 2008;82(22):11066–72.

135. Chung TW, Lee YC, Kim CH. Hepatitis B viral HBx induces matrix metalloproteinase-9 gene expression through activation of ERK and PI-3K/AKT pathways: involvement of invasive potential. FASEB J 2004;18(10):1123–5.

136. Lara-Pezzi E, Gomez-Gaviro MV, Galvez BG, et al. The hepatitis B virus X protein promotes tumor cell invasion by inducing membrane-type matrix metalloproteinase-1 and cyclooxygenase-2 expression. J Clin Invest 2002; 110(12):1831–8.

137. Liu LP, Liang HF, Chen XP, et al. The role of NF-kappaB in Hepatitis b virus X protein-mediated upregulation of VEGF and MMPs. Cancer Invest 2010;28(5): 443–51.

138. Yu FL, Liu HJ, Lee JW, et al. Hepatitis B virus X protein promotes cell migration by inducing matrix metalloproteinase-3. J Hepatol 2005;42(4):520–7.

139. Matsuzaki K, Murata M, Yoshida K, et al. Chronic inflammation associated with hepatitis C virus infection perturbs hepatic transforming growth factor beta signaling, promoting cirrhosis and hepatocellular carcinoma. Hepatology 2007;46(1):48–57.

140. Battaglia S, Benzoubir N, Nobilet S, et al. Liver cancer-derived hepatitis C virus core proteins shift TGF-beta responses from tumor suppression to epithelial-mesenchymal transition. PLoS One 2009;4(2):e4355.

141. Wright TL. Antiviral therapy and primary and secondary prevention of hepatocellular carcinoma. Hepatol Res 2007;37(Suppl 2):S294–8.

142. Lanier AP, Holck P, Ehrsam Day G, et al. Childhood cancer among Alaska Natives. Pediatrics 2003;112(5):e396.

143. Wichajarn K, Kosalaraksa P, Wiangnon S. Incidence of hepatocellular carcinoma in children in Khon Kaen before and after national hepatitis B vaccine program. Asian Pac J Cancer Prev 2008;9(3):507–9.

144. Lin SM, Yu ML, Lee CM, et al. Interferon therapy in HBeAg positive chronic hepatitis reduces progression to cirrhosis and hepatocellular carcinoma. J Hepatol 2007;46(1):45–52.

145. Camma C, Giunta M, Andreone P, et al. Interferon and prevention of hepatocellular carcinoma in viral cirrhosis: an evidence-based approach. J Hepatol 2001; 34(4):593–602.

146. Yang YF, Zhao W, Zhong YD, et al. Interferon therapy in chronic hepatitis B reduces progression to cirrhosis and hepatocellular carcinoma: a meta-analysis. J Viral Hepat 2009;16(4):265–71.

147. Ohata K, Hamasaki K, Toriyama K, et al. High viral load is a risk factor for hepatocellular carcinoma in patients with chronic hepatitis B virus infection. J Gastroenterol Hepatol 2004;19(6):670–5.

148. Ikeda K, Arase Y, Kobayashi M, et al. Consistently low hepatitis B virus DNA saves patients from hepatocellular carcinogenesis in HBV-related cirrhosis.

A nested case-control study using 96 untreated patients. Intervirology 2003; 46(2):96–104.

149. Sung JJ, Tsoi KK, Wong VW, et al. Meta-analysis: treatment of hepatitis B infection reduces risk of hepatocellular carcinoma. Aliment Pharmacol Ther 2008; 28(9):1067–77.

150. Liaw YF, Sung JJ, Chow WC, et al. Lamivudine for patients with chronic hepatitis B and advanced liver disease. N Engl J Med 2004;351(15):1521–31.

151. Yuen MF, Seto WK, Chow DH, et al. Long-term lamivudine therapy reduces the risk of long-term complications of chronic hepatitis B infection even in patients without advanced disease. Antivir Ther 2007;12(8):1295–303.

152. Yoshida H, Shiratori Y, Moriyama M, et al. Interferon therapy reduces the risk for hepatocellular carcinoma: national surveillance program of cirrhotic and noncirrhotic patients with chronic hepatitis C in Japan. IHIT Study Group. Inhibition of Hepatocarcinogenesis by Interferon Therapy. Ann Intern Med 1999;131(3): 174–81.

153. Azzaroli F, Accogli E, Nigro G, et al. Interferon plus ribavirin and interferon alone in preventing hepatocellular carcinoma: a prospective study on patients with HCV related cirrhosis. World J Gastroenterol 2004;10(21):3099–102.

154. Lee WM, Dienstag JL, Lindsay KL, et al. Evolution of the HALT-C Trial: pegylated interferon as maintenance therapy for chronic hepatitis C in previous interferon nonresponders. Control Clin Trials 2004;25(5):472–92.

155. Afdhal NH, Brown R, Freilich B, et al. Colchicine versus PEG interferon alfa-2b long-term therapy: results of the 4-year copilot trial. J Hepatol 2008; 48(Suppl 2):S4.

156. Bruix J, Poynard T, Colombo M, et al. Pegintron maintenance therapy in cirrhotic (Metavir F4) HCV patients, who failed to respond to interferon/ribavirin therapy: final results of the EPIC[3] cirrhosis maintenance trial (Co-Pilot abstract). J Hepatol 2009;50(Suppl 1):S22.

Insulin Resistance and Other Metabolic Risk Factors in the Pathogenesis of Hepatocellular Carcinoma

Asma Siddique, MD, Kris V. Kowdley, MD*

KEYWORDS

- Insulin resistance • Nonalcoholic steatohepatitis
- Hepatocellular carcinoma • Diabetes mellitus type 2

Coinciding with the increased incidence of hepatocellular carcinoma (HCC), world-wide and in the United States,[1–3] there has been a significant increase in the global incidence of obesity and diabetes, the two major risk factors for nonalcoholic steato-hepatitis (NASH). In this context, 15% to 50% of patients with HCC have no specific identifiable risk factors, such as hepatitis B virus (HBV) or hepatitis C virus (HCV) infection, and are labeled as having "cryptogenic cirrhosis."[4] A recent study of 105 patients with HCC of whom 29% carried a diagnosis of cryptogenic cirrhosis, found that 50% had nonalcoholic fatty liver disease (NAFLD)-related cirrhosis.[5]

OBESITY AND HCC

Overweight (body mass index [BMI; calculated as the weight in kilograms divided by height in meters squared, ie, kg/m^2] between 25 and 30) and obesity (BMI of 30 or higher) have been identified as independent risk factors for various cancers including postmenopausal breast cancer, endometrial cancer, colorectal cancer, renal cell cancer, and adenocarcinoma of the esophagus.[6] There is also a possible association between obesity and gallbladder, pancreas, thyroid, and hematologic malignancies.[6] With regard to HCC, data suggest that there is a 1.5- to 4-fold increased risk among obese individuals.[6–8] In a large prospective study involving 900,000 United States

Supported in part by K24 grant DK02957 to KVK.

Center for Liver Disease, Virginia Mason Medical Center, Digestive Disease Institute, 1100 Ninth Avenue, PO Box 900, Seattle, WA 98111, USA

* Corresponding author.

E-mail address: kris.kowdley@vmmc.org

adults initially free from cancer and followed for 16 years, obese men and obese women, respectively, had a 14% and 20% increased incidence of cancer-related death, after controlling for other risk factors.[6] In the morbidly obese (BMI >40), the death rate from cancer was 52% higher in men and 62% higher in women, respectively, compared with those of normal weight.[6] The relative risk of liver cancer among obese individuals in this population was 2.0- to 4.0-fold, as seen in other studies. A large Danish study of 43,965 obese individuals found an overall 16% increased incidence of cancers in general and a relative risk of 1.9 for liver cancer, compared with nonobese individuals.[7] Similarly, in a study in Sweden of more than 28,000 obese individuals, Wolk and colleagues[8] found an almost threefold increased risk of HCC as in slim counterparts. Regimbeau and colleagues,[9] analyzed 19,271 explanted liver specimens for HCC; after controlling for confounding variables such as age and gender, there was a slightly higher prevalence of HCC in obese than in nonobese patients. Furthermore, obesity was also an independent risk factor for HCC in patients with alcoholic and cryptogenic cirrhosis, but not among those with viral hepatitis, primary biliary cirrhosis, or metabolic liver diseases. A meta-analysis of 11 cohort studies confirmed that overweight and obese individuals had a 17% and 89% increased risk of liver cancer, respectively, compared with those with normal weight; moreover, the relative risk was significantly higher for men than for women.[10] The investigators estimated that overweight or obesity was a risk factor for HCC in 28% of men and 27% of women, respectively.[10]

The mechanism that links obesity and cancer is not clear. It is hypothesized that dysregulation of adipokines and insulin resistance may both contribute to tumorigenesis.[11] Both adipose tissue excess and adipose tissue deficiency (ie, lipodystrophy) are associated with features of the metabolic syndrome.[12] Adipose tissue is no longer considered a passive reservoir for energy storage but is currently viewed as an essential and active endocrine organ, as it secretes adipocyte-specific proteins called adipocytokines and other hormones that exert a wide range of physiologic effects, and may also contribute to obesity-related complications.[13] The adipocytokines, which include tumor necrosis factor (TNF)-α, resistin, leptin, and adiponectin among others, act at both the local (autocrine/paracrine) and systemic (endocrine) levels to create a milieu that results in inhibition of apoptosis, increased cellular proliferation, angiogenesis, and worsened insulin resistance.[12,14] Adipose tissue also expresses molecules such as vascular endothelial growth factor (VEGF), which exert a direct effect on cellular metabolism and proinflammatory prooncogenic proteins such as TNF-α, interleukin (IL)-6, and IL-1.[15]

DIABETES MELLITUS AND HCC

Patients with cirrhosis frequently develop impaired glucose tolerance or overt diabetes mellitus (DM), making it difficult to assess whether a direct relationship exists between DM and HCC. Results of several studies have convincingly shown that DM is an independent risk factor for the development of HCC.[16–19] In a large prospective study among United States veterans, which included 173,643 patients with and 650,620 patients without DM, a twofold increase in the relative risk of HCC was reported in DM patients,[16] after adjustment for confounding factors such as HBV, HCV, and alcoholic cirrhosis. Adami and colleagues[17] reported an overall fourfold increase in primary liver cancer in a cohort of 153,852 diabetics in Sweden who were followed for 1 to 24 years; after excluding patients with concomitant diseases such as cirrhosis, alcoholism, and hepatitis, the increased HCC risk persisted and was approximately threefold. Similarly, in a study from Denmark, standardized incidence ratios (SIRs) were estimated for primary liver cancer at 4.0 in males and 2.1

in women, in a cohort of 109,581 diabetics.[18] Finally, investigators using Surveillance, Epidemiology and End-Results (SEER) registries identified and compared 2061 patients with HCC with noncancer controls.[19] DM was reported in 43% and 19% of subjects with HCC and controls, respectively; after adjusting for other HCC risk factors (HBV, HCV, alcoholic liver disease, and hemochromatosis), DM was associated with a threefold increase risk of HCC.

NAFLD has now emerged as the most common chronic liver disease in Western countries, with approximately 20% to 30% of the general population affected. Furthermore, the prevalence of NAFLD is likely to increase given the rising incidence of obesity and DM.[20,21] NAFLD is closely linked to the metabolic syndrome, which includes obesity, DM, hyperlipidemia, and insulin resistance.[22,23] Approximately 10% of patients with NAFLD are likely to progress to NASH and 8% to 26% of individuals with NASH progress to cirrhosis, which is an independent risk factor for HCC.[24,25] Although the exact factors that influence the progression of NAFLD to the more severe NASH are not clear, BMI and DM are independent risk factors for progression of fibrosis.[26] Moreover, the association of NASH with other components of the metabolic syndrome increases the risk for developing chronic liver disease and cirrhosis, and subsequently HCC.[27]

In a recent review of 4406 HCC patients who were identified from a claims database, 59% had NAFLD/NASH as the underlying etiology followed by DM (36%) and HCV infection (22%).[28] In another study of 195 patients with NASH cirrhosis and 315 patients with HCV cirrhosis, who were followed for a mean period of 3.2 years, HCC was identified in 12.8% and 20.3% of NASH and HCV patients, respectively. The yearly cumulative incidence of HCC was 2.6% in NASH cirrhosis compared with 4.0% in HCV cirrhosis, respectively. NASH-cirrhotic individuals who drank alcohol were at higher risk of developing HCC than nondrinkers.[29] Similarly, comparing NASH-associated cirrhosis to HCV-associated cirrhosis in Japanese subjects during a 5-year follow-up period, the incidence of HCC was 11.3% versus 30.5% in these 2 respective groups.[30] In contrast to these many positive associations, it is not clear why Hui and colleagues,[31] in Australia, found that HCC did not develop in patients with NASH cirrhosis compared with a 17% prevalence in age-matched and gender-matched HCV-cirrhosis controls.

Although the mechanism of carcinogenesis in patients With NAFLD/ NASH remains uncertain, it is plausible that insulin resistance and oxidative stress are contributing factors, as is now discussed.

OXIDATIVE STRESS, REACTIVE OXYGEN SPECIES, AND HCC

Insulin resistance leads to increased hepatocyte lipogenesis, decreased hepatic secretion of very-low-density lipoproteins, and increased hepatic uptake of circulating free fatty acids (FFA) that come from peripheral lipolysis.[23,32] The resulting liver phenotype is characterized by increased hepatic triglyceride accumulation and macrovesicular steatosis, with varying degrees of necroinflammation and fibrosis.[33]

Increased production of TNF-α from adipose tissue and oxidative stress results in an upregulation of suppressors of cytokines signaling (SOCS 1 and 3), which bind to tyrosine Janus kinases (JAK) and inhibit phosphorylation of signal transducer and activator of transcription (STAT) proteins, resulting in inhibition of insulin signaling pathways that leads to hepatic insulin resistance.[34,35] Oxidative stress also stimulates production of reactive oxygen species (ROS) in the liver,[36] which increases the expression of the cytokines, transforming growth factor (TGF)-β. and IL-8, and generates lipid peroxidation products, such as 4-hydroxynonenal (4-HNE). These molecules are chemoattractants for neutrophils, and likely contribute to the neutrophil infiltration and inflammation in the fatty liver.[37] ROS activate fibrogenesis by stimulating hepatic stellate cells.[36,38] ROS also impair mitochondrial respiration, deplete mitochondrial cytochrome *c*, and cause oxidative damage to the mitochondrial genome, thereby activating the apoptosis cascade.[39] Furthermore, other products of lipid peroxidation (such as malondialdehyde) can cause DNA mutations. *trans*-4-Hydroxy-2-nonenal, another major by-product of lipid peroxidation, likely plays a major role in the pathogenesis of HCC, due to mutations induced in the tumor protein *p53* gene.[40] Downstream targets of p53 include p21/Wafl, and growth arrest DNA damage gene (GADD) 45 and 14-3-3, which mediate G2/M arrest.[41] p53 protein also has apoptotic properties due to its action on Bax.[42] Furthermore, activation of activating protein (AP)-1 and nuclear factor kappa B (NF-κB) by oxidative stress causes either cellular proliferation or apoptosis depending on the cellular redox state. Oxidative stress has also been shown to cause decreased expression of the nuclear respiratory factor (*Nrf*)1 gene; Nrf1L knock-out mice show increased susceptibility to oxidative stress, increases in intracellular ROS, development of fatty liver with inflammation, hepatic cell death, fibrosis, and ultimately liver cancer.[43]

INSULIN RESISTANCE AND HCC

Insulin resistance is characterized by reduced sensitivity to insulin and, as a result, impaired ability of insulin to suppress glucose production and stimulate peripheral glucose elimination. To overcome insulin resistance and maintain normal metabolic functions, insulin secretion is increased, leading to a state of compensatory hyperinsulinemia.[44] The liver also secretes insulin-like growth factor (IGF)-1. IGF-1 is one of the most potent activators of cellular proliferation via the Akt (also called protein kinase B [PKB]) signaling pathway, and is an inhibitor of apoptosis (**Fig. 1**).[45] Chronic hyperinsulinemia has been associated with a variety of cancers. Changes in the expression of the IGF axis, which consists of IGF-1 and IGF-2, its receptors IGF1R and IGF2R, and IGF-binding proteins (IGFB1–6), have been observed in rodent models of HCC and in human HCC cell lines.[46,47]

Insulin resistance and compensatory hyperinsulinemia promote increased phosphorylation and activation of downstream pathways, resulting in inhibition of apoptosis and increased mitogenesis, which thereby promotes tumorigenesis. Insulin resistance may also directly accelerate hepatocarcinogenesis via the stimulation of hepatic neovascularization.[48] Insulin causes upregulation of hepatic growth hormone (GH) receptors, and GH is the principal stimulus for IGF-1 activation. IGF-1, like insulin, promotes cell proliferation, upregulates endothelial growth factor, and inhibits apoptosis.[49] Hyperinsulinemia further reduces liver synthesis and blood levels of IGFBP1 and IGFBP2, which lead to increased bioavailability of IGF-1.[50] IGF signaling in HCC has been shown to increase production of IGFs, IGFBPs, IGFBP proteases, and IGF receptor expression.[50] IGF-1 also has mitogenic effects on a variety of cancer cell lines and activates mitogen-activated protein kinase (MAPK), and increases expression of the c-fos and c-jun protooncogenes in cultured HCC cells.[51,52] IGF-2 may also be overexpressed as result of a reduced expression of IGFBP in cirrhotic patients.[50] IGF-2 promotes proliferation, survival, and migration in HCC cells through binding to its IGF type 1 receptor. This receptor, as well as its main substrates insulin receptor substrate (IRS)-1 and IRS-2, are overexpressed in HCC and in experimental models of liver carcinogenesis.[53]

Hyperinsulinemia and the activated insulin receptors cause phosphorylation of IRS-1, a key protein involved in cellular proliferation that transmits insulin signals through two main pathways: phosphatase and tensin homolog (PTEN)/P13K/Akt and MAPK kinase

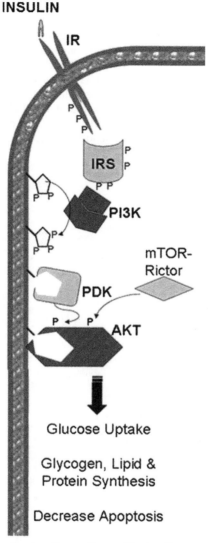

Fig. 1. The canonical insulin signaling pathway. The insulin receptor (IR) phosphorylates itself as well as insulin receptor substrate (IRS). PI3 kinase (PI3K) phosphorylates 3-phosphoinositides, which produce binding sites for PIP3-dependent kinase (PDK) and Akt via their PH domains. Akt is phosphorylated by PDK and mammalian target of rapamycin (mTOR)-Rictor, which lead to active Akt kinase activity and its pleiotropic effects. P denotes key phosphorylation events. (*From* Holland WL, Summers SA. Sphingolipids, insulin resistance, and metabolic disease: new insights from in vivo manipulation of sphingolipid metabolism. Endocr Rev 2008;29(4):381–402; © The Endocrine Society; with permission.)

(MAPKK),[54] which is also referred to as MEK (MAP kinase or extracellullar signal-related kinase [ERK] kinase). PTEN/P13K/Akt, an important pathway in cellular proliferation and apoptosis, also plays an important role in the pathogenesis of HCC.[55] PTEN is a tumor suppressor gene, and its activity is reduced by mutations or deletions in several malignancies.[56,57] Loss of PTEN results in activation of the downstream effector

Akt.[58] Akt is also activated by insulin and IGF-1. Activated Akt promotes cell survival by inhibiting proapoptotic protein Bcl-2 family member BAD.[59] Under normal circumstances BAD interacts with Bcl-XL and causes apoptosis. Phosphorylation of BAD by Akt prevents its binding to Bcl-XL and thereby suppresses apoptosis. Activated Akt thereby plays an important role in promoting cell growth and survival, and also inhibits apoptosis. The central role of Akt in insulin signaling is shown in **Fig. 2**.

However, despite these compelling circumstantial data linking hyperinsulinemia to cancer, a 10-year prospective study from Korea of 1,298,385 patients showed that cancer risk was influenced by fasting blood glucose in a dose-dependent manner rather than insulin resistance, which challenges a supposed direct action of insulin on promotion of cancers.[60]

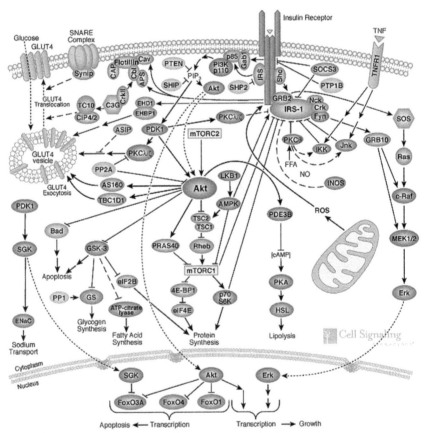

Fig. 2. Insulin is the major hormone controlling critical energy functions such as glucose and lipid metabolism. Insulin activates the insulin receptor tyrosine kinase (IR), which phosphorylates and recruits different substrate adaptors such as the IRS family of proteins. Tyrosine-phosphorylated IRS then displays binding sites for numerous signaling partners. Among them, PI3K has a major role in insulin function, mainly via the activation of the Akt/PKB and the protein kinase Cζ cascades. Activated Akt induces glycogen synthesis, through inhibition of GSK-3; protein synthesis via mTOR and downstream elements; and cell survival, through inhibition of several proapoptotic agents (Bad, Forkhead family transcription factors, GSK-3). (Pathway diagram reproduced *courtesy of* Cell Signaling Technology Inc. www.cellsignal.com.)

LEPTIN AND HCC

Hyperleptinemia is noted in both obesity and type 2 diabetes. The link between hepatic fibrosis and leptin, and its profibrogenic and angiogenic properties, suggests that this protein may be a risk factor for the development of HCC.[6] Male mice treated with simultaneous carbon tetrachloride and/or leptin had significant leptin-enhanced hepatic necroinflammatory and fibrotic changes.[61] The *db/db* mouse—a model of obesity, diabetes, and dyslipidemia that caused by homozygous genetic hepatic leptin receptor deficiency—when fed a diet deficient in methionine and choline (MCD diet) develops insulin resistance and hyperleptinemia, and a picture that mimics severe human NASH[62] with liver fibrosis. By comparison, leptin-deficient obese, diabetic, and genetically leptin-deficient ob/ob mice fed an MCD diet do not develop liver fibrosis, suggesting that leptin has an important role in hepatic fibrogenesis. Furthermore, in a NASH rat model Kitade and colleagues[63] were able to demonstrate increased leptin-mediated neovascularization in the liver with progression of NASH, while leptin inhibition mitigated both fibrogenesis and hepatocarcinogenesis.

Leptin, the product of the obese (Ob) gene, is an adipokine predominant in adipose tissue. Leptin acts centrally in the hypothalamus and decreases appetite, regulates food intake, and increases energy expenditure.[64] Of the 6 isoforms of leptin receptors (ObRa through ObRf), ObRb is the most important mediator of the biologic effects of leptin.[64] Obesity in humans is frequently associated with elevated leptin levels, suggesting that leptin resistance may be present.[65] Failure of elevated leptin to mediate weight loss in this setting is likely caused by mechanisms that attenuate leptin signaling, including inhibition of SOCS3 by adenosine monophosphate (AMP)-activated protein kinase (AMPK) due to leptin resistance.[64,66]

In liver disease, serum leptin levels are substantially elevated; patients with alcohol and viral cirrhosis may have a twofold increase in leptin as compared with controls.[67] Leptin is upregulated by cytokines such as IL-1, TNFα, and insulin, which are often elevated in patients with cirrhosis.[68–70] Circulating free leptin levels are also significantly higher in NASH patients and in HCC patients than in healthy controls.[71,72] Wang and colleagues[72] evaluated 36 HCC specimens and corresponding adjacent nontumorous liver tissue, and found that adjacent liver cells expressed higher levels of leptin and its receptor than adjacent HCC cells, suggesting that leptin acts as a growth factor to hepatocytes and may have a role in initiation and progression of HCC.

Leptin binds to its receptors, and causes phosphorylation of JAK2 and the downstream STAT3. The JAK/STAT signaling pathway then triggers a signaling cascade involving activations of PI3K/Akt and MEK 1/2 (**Fig. 3**).[73] These signal pathways increase cyclin D1 protein expression, resulting in proliferation of hepatocytes and HCC cells.[74] Inhibition of any of these signal pathways blocks the action of leptin. Leptin also inhibits TGF-β1-induced apoptosis by downregulating proapoptotic Bax expression.[74] Therefore, by increasing cellular proliferation and decreasing apoptosis, leptin may function as a growth factor for HCC cells. Activation of these pathways also results in an increase in methionine adenosyl transferase (MAT)2A and MAT2β gene expression, markers of liver cell growth, and differentiation.

Leptin may also contribute to hepatic fibrogenesis via TGF-β and activation of hepatic stellate cells (HSCs).[75] HSCs are liver specific, and are involved in wound healing and development of fibrosis in the setting of chronic liver disease.[76] HSCs regulate inflammation and promote angiogenesis via secretion of various cytokines, including chemokines, by acting through several pathways including ERK/Akt, nuclear factor kappa D (NF-κD), and hypoxia-inducible factor 1 (HIF-1).[77] Activated HSCs proliferate

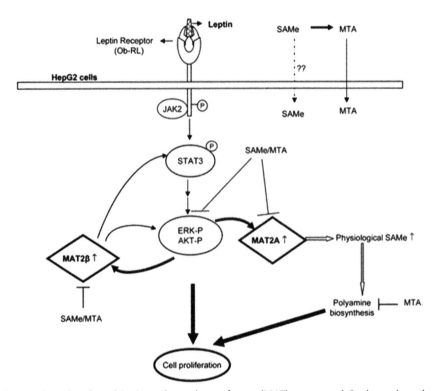

Fig. 3. The role of methionine adenosyl transferase (MAT) genes and S-adenosyl methyltransferase (SAMe) in leptin-induced mitogenic response in HepG2 cells. Upon leptin interaction with its receptor, Ob-RL, activation of Janus kinase 2 (JAK2) occurs via transphosphorylation of the receptor as well as subsequent phosphorylation of the signal transducer and activator of transcription (STAT) proteins. This process leads to a series of downstream events including activation of extracellular signal-related kinase (ERK)/mitogen-activated protein kinase (MAPK) and PI3-K/Akt survival pathways in HepG2 cells. Leptin signaling induces MAT2A and MAT2β genes via activation of these survival pathways, which further leads to enhanced cell proliferation. The MAT2A-encoded protein induces leptin's mitogenic response by raising intracellular SAMe levels, leading to polyamine biosynthesis and growth. The MAT2β gene interacts with leptin signaling components and modulates cell growth. Pharmacologic doses of SAMe and metastasis-associated (MTA) proteins act as inhibitors of leptin signaling and growth in HepG2 cells. (*From* Ramani K, Yang H, Xia M, et al. Leptin's mitogenic effect in human liver cancer cells requires induction of both methionine adenosyltransferase 2A and 2beta. Hepatology 2008;47(2):521–31; Copyright © 2007 American Association for the Study of Liver Diseases. Wiley and Sons; with permission.)

and secrete collagen and other extracellular matrix components, which ultimately results in liver fibrogenesis.[76] Increased expression of has been observed in the areas surrounding HCC and hepatic metastases secondary to activation of HSCs via cyclo-oxygenase (COX)-2 dependent prostaglandin (PG)E$_2$.[78] VEGF upregulation creates a proangiogenic microenvironment, which leads to progression of liver fibrogenesis and possibly cancer.[78] The role of leptin in carcinogenesis may be more complex. As mentioned earlier, because leptin expression was shown to be increased in adjacent noncancerous liver tissues but markedly decreased in the cancerous lesions, it is possible that leptin may be associated with angiogenesis but not with the proliferation of HCC cells.[72]

Furthermore, Ellinav and colleagues[79] reported that administration of leptin in a murine model of HCC resulted in a significant reduction in tumor size and improved survival.

In summary, leptin remains a reasonable candidate for promotion of cancer via effects on angiogenesis and other pathways; the presence of leptin resistance in obesity suggests a possible relation between altered regulation of this pathway and liver cancer.

ADIPOCYTOKINES AND HCC

The plasma concentration of adiponectin, a hormone exclusively secreted by adipose tissue, is markedly decreased in obesity, type 2 DM, and atherosclerosis.[80] Obesity is associated with a state of low-grade chronic inflammation characterized by upregulation of TNF-α, IL-6, and other proinflammatory cytokines, which inhibit expression of adiponectin.[81] Maeda and colleagues[82] have shown that adiponectin knock-out mice had high levels of plasma TNF-α, and TNF-α mRNA in adipose tissue. These mice developed severe insulin resistance, had increased atherogenesis, and significant endothelial dysfunction in response to vascular injury. Administration of adiponectin to these mice resulted in improvement of insulin resistance. Similarly, a rhesus monkey model of obesity and type 2 DM is characterized by low levels of adiponectin.[83]

Adiponectin has several beneficial effects. The anti-inflammatory effects of adiponectin can be linked to stimulation of the anti-inflammatory cytokines and inhibition of proinflammatory markers, including TNF-α and IL-6, the NF-κB pathway, and chemokines.[81] Adiponectin exerts atheroprotective properties by inhibition of monocyte adhesion to endothelial cells, macrophage cytokine production, lipid accumulation in macrophages, and phagocytosis.[84] There are convincing data showing an inverse relationship between serum adiponectin concentration and inflammatory markers such as C-reactive protein, and development of features of the metabolic syndrome.[85] Low adiponectin levels have also been strongly implicated in the development of insulin resistance.[86] Adiponectin-induced AMPK upregulates glucose transporter (GLUT)-4 gene expression and inhibits transcription of phosphoenolpyruvate carboxykinase (PEPCK) and glucose-6-phosphatase, which regulate hepatic gluconeogenesis.[87] Insulin resistance and chronic hyperinsulinemia result in reduced synthesis of IGFBP1 and IGFBP2, and increased bioavailability of IGF1, which promotes cellular proliferation, upregulates EGF, and inhibits apoptosis, thereby promoting carcinogenesis.[88] Insulin reduces the expression of AdipoR1 and AdipoR2 via a PI3K/Forkhead boxO1-dependent pathway in cultured hepatocytes.[89] Patients with insulin resistance and type 2 DM have significantly reduced adiponectin levels, which increase on administration of insulin-sensitizing drugs, such as the thiazolidinediones (TZDs).[85] Missense mutations in adiponectin genes have been identified in subjects with type 2 DM and hypoadiponectinemia.[90] These data suggest that hyperinsulinemia may negatively regulate adiponectin.

Low levels of adiponectin have been implicated in many common cancers including breast, colorectal, and prostate in men, and breast and endometrial cancer in women.[91–94] Mouse NASH models that have low levels of adiponectin demonstrate increased progression of hepatic fibrosis, whereas administration of adiponectin reduces inflammation and steatosis. Moreover, these animals also had accelerated tumorigenesis, suggesting that adiponectin probably contributes to NASH cirrhosis and HCC.[95] Similarly, patients with HCC had lower levels of plasma adiponectin as well as an inverse relationship between adiponectin expression and tumor size.[96] Saxena and colleagues[97] showed that HCC cells overexpress AdipoR1 and AdipoR2, leading to increased adiponectin-binding capacity, while adiponectin treatment inhibited HCC tumorigenesis in vivo by inhibition of cellular proliferation and induction of apoptosis.

AdipoR1 is expressed mainly in skeletal muscle but is also present in endothelial cells and other tissues, whereas AdipoR2 is predominantly expressed in the liver.[98] These receptors mediate the cellular function of adiponectin by activating two main downstream signaling pathways: AMPK and peroxisome proliferator-activated receptor (PPAR)-α. AMPK activation by novel small molecules appears to show promise for the treatment of diabetes and metabolic syndrome via effects on glucose and lipid metabolism.[99]

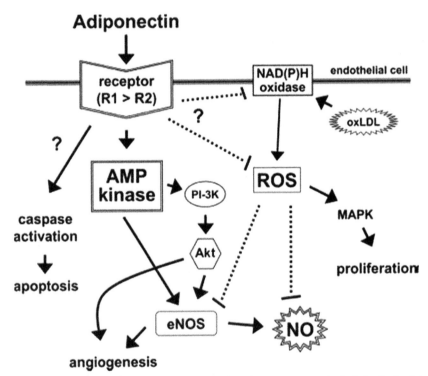

Fig. 4. Many potential signaling pathways exist for adiponectin in endothelial cells. Both iso-forms of the adiponectin receptor (AdipoR1 and AdipoR2) are expressed in endothelial cells, but mRNA for the AdipoR1 receptor, with a higher affinity for globular adiponectin (gAd), is more abundant. As in metabolically responsive tissues, one of the major signaling effects of adiponectin in endothelial cells is activation of AMP kinase. AMP kinase, in turn, activates endothelial nitric oxide synthase (eNOS) via a pathway that also appears to be dependent on Akt activation, which is linked upstream to phosphatidylinositol 3-kinase (PI-3K) signaling. Both eNOS activation and Akt activation contribute to the effects of adiponectin on angiogenesis. Adiponectin also inhibits oxidized low-density lipoprotein (oxLDL)–induced superoxide production, possibly through inhibition of cellular NAD(P)H oxidase activity. Reduced reactive oxygen species (ROS) generation may enhance NO production and diminish cell proliferation by adiponectin by ameliorating the suppression of eNOS activity and NO quenching by ROS and by blocking oxLDL-induced MAPK activation, respectively. Adiponectin can also lead to endothelial apoptosis via upstream caspase activation. The solid arrows and dotted lines reflect stimulatory and inhibitory effects, respectively. (*From* Goldstein BJ, Scalia R. Adiponectin: A novel adipokine linking adipocytes and vascular function. J Clin Endocrinol Metab 2004;89(6):2563–68; © The Endocrine Society; with permission.)

The antiproliferative and proapoptotic effect of adiponectin is mediated by AMPK, which has been shown to cause cell-cycle arrest in HepG2 cells via p53 phosphorylation of tuberous sclerosis protein (TSC) 2, phosphorylation and inhibition of translation elongation factor (TEF) 2 (EF2), and/or suppression of mammalian target of rapamycin (mTOR), thereby decreasing protein synthesis and cell growth.[100] mTOR pathway activation via phosphatidylinositol (PI) 3-kinase and PKB/Akt signaling plays an important role in activation of cell growth and proliferation (**Fig. 4**). mTOR stimulates cell growth by activating ribosomal protein S6 kinase (S6K1) and by increasing phosphorylation of elongation factor-4E binding protein 1 (4E-BP1), resulting in protein synthesis.[101] In addition, activated AMPK positively regulates 2 important proteins for the control of growth arrest and apoptosis, namely p53 and p21.[102] In addition, c-Jun N-terminal kinase (JNK) and STAT3 are important downstream effectors of adiponectin. JNK regulates cell proliferation and apoptosis while STAT3 stimulates cell proliferation and prevents apoptosis.[103] Adiponectin has been shown to stimulate JNK and suppress STAT3 in HepG2 cells. Thus, adiponectin may play a pivotal role in the pathogenesis of HCC via the JNK/STAT3 signal pathway (see **Fig. 4**).

In summary, the beneficial effect of adiponectin on tumorigenesis is probably multifactorial and likely involves the effect of adiponectin on insulin resistance, a direct effect on tumor cells, and suppression of endothelial cell proliferation, migration, and survival, thereby inhibiting neovascularization.

SUMMARY

There are many causes of HCC, and NAFLD/NASH is now emerging as a leading risk factor owing to the epidemic of obesity and type 2 DM. The mechanisms leading to HCC in obesity and type 2 DM likely involve interactions between several signaling pathways, including oxidative stress, inflammation, oncogenes, adiponectins, and insulin resistance associated with visceral adiposity and diabetes. Understanding the molecular signaling pathways involved in the pathogenesis of HCC will aid in the development of molecular therapies targeting specific receptors and/or signaling proteins for the prevention and treatment of HCC. In addition, a better understanding of the role of insulin and leptin resistance and adiponectin deficiency in these pathways may provide greater awareness of dietary, lifestyle, and pharmacologic interventions.

REFERENCES

1. Ferlay J, Autier P, Boniol M, et al. Estimates of the cancer incidence and mortality in Europe in 2006. Ann Oncol 2007;18(3):581–92.
2. Parkin DM. Global cancer statistics in the year 2000. Lancet Oncol 2001;2(9): 533–43.
3. Altekruse SF, McGlynn KA, Reichman ME. Hepatocellular carcinoma incidence, mortality, and survival trends in the United States from 1975 to 2005. J Clin Oncol 2009;27(9):1485–91.
4. Di Bisceglie AM, Order SE, Klein JL, et al. The role of chronic viral hepatitis in hepatocellular carcinoma in the United States. Am J Gastroenterol 1991;86(3): 335–8.
5. Marrero JA, Fontana RJ, Su GL, et al. NAFLD may be a common underlying liver disease in patients with hepatocellular carcinoma in the United States. Hepatology 2002;36:1349–54.

6. Calle EE, Rodriguez C, Walker-Thurmond K, et al. Overweight, obesity, and mortality from cancer in a prospectively studied cohort of U.S. Adults. N Engl J Med 2003;348:1625–38.

7. Møller H, Mellemgaard A, Lindvig K, et al. Obesity and cancer risk: a Danish record-linkage study. Eur J Cancer 1994;30(3):344–50.

8. Wolk A, Gridley G, Svensson M, et al. A prospective study of obesity and cancer risk (Sweden). Cancer Causes Control 2001;12(1):13–21.

9. Regimbeau JM, Colombat M, Mognol P, et al. Obesity and diabetes as a risk factor for hepatocellular carcinoma. Liver Transpl 2004;10(2 Suppl 1):S69–73.

10. Larsson SC, Wolk A. Overweight, obesity and risk of liver cancer: a meta-analysis of cohort studies. Br J Cancer 2007;97(7):1005–8.

11. Castagnetta L, Granata OM, Cocciadiferro L, et al. Sex steroids, carcinogenesis, and cancer progression. Ann N Y Acad Sci 2004;1028:233–46.

12. Grundy SM, Brewer HB Jr, Cleeman JI, et al. Definition of metabolic syndrome: report of the National Heart, Lung, and Blood Institute/American Heart Association conference on scientific issues related to definition. American Heart Association; National Heart, Lung, and Blood Institute. Circulation 2004;109(3):433–8.

13. Rajala MW, Scherer PE. Minireview: the adipocyte—at the crossroads of energy homeostasis, inflammation, and atherosclerosis. Endocrinology 2003;144:3765–73.

14. Harrison SA. Liver disease in patients with diabetes mellitus. J Clin Gastroenterol 2006;40:68–76.

15. Weisberg SP, McCann D, Desai M, et al. Obesity is associated with macrophage accumulation in adipose tissue. J Clin Invest 2003;112:1796–808.

16. El-Serag HB, Tran T, Everhart JE. Diabetes increases the risk of chronic liver disease and hepatocellular carcinoma. Gastroenterology 2004;126(2):460–8.

17. Adami HO, Chow WH, Nyrén O, et al. Excess risk of primary liver cancer in patients with diabetes mellitus. J Natl Cancer Inst 1996;88(20):1472–7.

18. Wideroff L, Gridley G, Mellemkjaer L, et al. Cancer incidence in a population-based cohort of patients hospitalized with diabetes mellitus in Denmark. J Natl Cancer Inst 1997;89(18):1360–5.

19. Davila JA, Morgan RO, Shaib Y, et al. Diabetes increases the risk of hepatocellular carcinoma in the United States: a population based case control study. Gut 2005;54(4):533–9.

20. Browning JD, Szczepaniak LS, Dobbins R, et al. Prevalence of hepatic steatosis in an urban population in the United States: impact of ethnicity. Hepatology 2004;40:1387–95.

21. Zelber-Sagi S, Nitzan-Kaluski D, Halpern Z, et al. Prevalence of primary nonalcoholic fatty liver disease in a population-based study and its association with biochemical and anthropometric measures. Liver Int 2006;26:856–63.

22. Marchesini G, Bugianesi E, Forlani G, et al. Nonalcoholic fatty liver, steatohepatitis, and the metabolic syndrome. Hepatology 2003;37:917–23.

23. Chitturi S, Abeygunasekera S, Farrell GC, et al. NASH and insulin resistance: Insulin hyper-hypersecretion and specific association with the insulin resistance syndrome. Hepatology 2002;35:373–9.

24. Matteoni CA, Younossi ZM, Gramlich T, et al. Nonalcoholic fatty liver disease: a spectrum of clinical and pathological severity. Gastroenterology 1999;116:1413–9.

25. Ong JP, Younossi ZM. Epidemiology and natural history of NAFLD and NASH. Clin Liver Dis 2007;11:1–16.

26. Adams LA, Sanderson S, Lindor KD, et al. The histological course of nonalcoholic fatty liver disease: a longitudinal study of 103 patients with sequential liver biopsies. J Hepatol 2005;42:132–8.

27. Siegel AB, Zhu AX. Metabolic syndrome and hepatocellular carcinoma: two growing epidemics with a potential link. Cancer 2009;115:5651–61.
28. Sanyal A, Poklepovic A, Moyneur E, et al. Population-based risk factors and resource utilization for HCC: US perspective. Curr Med Res Opin 2010;26(9): 2183–91.
29. Ascha MS, Hanouneh IA, Lopez R, et al. The incidence and risk factors of hepatocellular carcinoma in patients with nonalcoholic steatohepatitis. Hepatology 2010;51(6):1972–8.
30. Tokushige K, Hashimoto E, Yatsuji S, et al. Prospective study of hepatocellular carcinoma in nonalcoholic steatohepatitis in comparison with hepatocellular carcinoma caused by chronic hepatitis C. J Gastroenterol 2010;45(9):960–7.
31. Hui JM, Kench JG, Chitturi S, et al. Long-term outcomes of cirrhosis in nonalcoholic steatohepatitis compared with hepatitis C. Hepatology 2003;38(2):420–7.
32. Malhi H, Gores GJ. Molecular mechanisms of lipotoxicity in nonalcoholic fatty liver disease. Semin Liver Dis 2008;28(4):360–9.
33. Tiniakos DG, Vos MB, Brunt EM. Nonalcoholic fatty liver disease: pathology and pathogenesis. Annu Rev Pathol 2010;5:145–71.
34. Ueki K, Kondo T, Kahn CR. Suppressor of cytokine signaling 1 (SOCS-1) and SOCS-3 cause insulin resistance through inhibition of tyrosine phosphorylation of insulin receptor substrate proteins by discrete mechanisms. Mol Cell Biol 2004;24:5434–46.
35. Hotamisligil GS, Peraldi A, Budavari A, et al. IRS-1 mediated kinase activity in TNF-a and obesity induced insulin resistance. Science 1996;272:665–8.
36. Poli G. Pathogenesis of liver fibrosis: the role of oxidative stress. Mol Aspects Med 2000;21:49–98.
37. Pessayre D, Fromenty B. NASH: a mitochondrial disease. J Hepatol 2005;42(6): 928–40.
38. Canbay A, Friedman S, Gores GJ. Apoptosis: the nexus of liver injury and fibrosis. Hepatology 2004;39:273–8.
39. Tafani M, Schneider TG, Pastorino JG, et al. Cytochrome dependent activation of caspase 3 by tumor necrosis factor requires induction of the mitochondrial permeability transition. Am J Pathol 2000;156:2111–21.
40. Hu W, Feng Z, Eveleigh J, et al. The major lipid peroxidation product, trans-4 hydroxy-2-nonenal, preferentially forms DNA adducts at codon 249 of human p53 gene, a unique mutational hotspot in hepatocellular carcinoma. Carcinogenesis 2002;23:1781–9.
41. Taylor WR, Stark GR. Regulation of the G2/M transition by p53. Oncogene 2001; 20(15):1803–15.
42. Levine AJ. p53, the cellular gatekeeper for growth and division. Cell 1997;88(3): 323–31.
43. Xu Z, Chen L, Leung L, et al. Liver-specific inactivation of the Nrf1 gene in adult mouse leads to nonalcoholic steatohepatitis and hepatic neoplasia. Proc Natl Acad Sci U S A 2005;102:4120–5.
44. Bugianesi E, McCullough AJ, Marchesini G. Insulin resistance: a metabolic pathway to chronic liver disease. Hepatology 2005;42:987–1000.
45. Kaaks R, Lukanova A. Energy balance and cancer: the role of insulin and insulin-like growth factor-I. Proc Nutr Soc 2001;60(1):91–106.
46. Stoll BA. Western nutrition and the insulin resistance syndrome: a link to breast cancer. Eur J Clin Nutr 1999;53:83–7.
47. Alexia C, Fallot G, Lasfer M, et al. An evaluation of the role of insulin-like growth factors (IGF) and of type-I IGF receptor signalling in hepatocarcinogenesis and

in the resistance of hepatocarcinoma cells against drug-induced apoptosis. Biochem Pharmacol 2004;68:1003–15.

48. Kaji K, Yoshiji H, Kitade M, et al. Impact of insulin resistance on the progression of chronic liver diseases. Int J Mol Med 2008;22:801–8.

49. Prisco M, Romano G, Peruzzi F, et al. Insulin and IGF-I receptors signaling in protection from apoptosis. Horm Metab Res 1999;31(2-3):80–9.

50. Scharf JG, Braulke T. The role of the IGF axis in hepatocarcinogenesis. Horm Metab Res 2003;35:685–93.

51. Price JA, Kovach SJ, Johnson T. Insulin-like growth factor I is a comitogen for hepatocyte growth factor in a rat model of hepatocellular carcinoma. Hepatology 2002;36(5):1089–97.

52. Stumpo DJ, Blackshear PJ. Insulin and growth factor effects on c-fos expression in normal and protein kinase C-deficient 3T3-L1 fibroblasts and adipocytes. Proc Natl Acad Sci U S A 1986;83(24):9453–7.

53. Boissan M, Beurel E, Wendum D, et al. Overexpression of insulin receptor substrate-2 in human and murine hepatocellular carcinoma. Am J Pathol 2005;167:869–77.

54. Malaguarnera M, Di Rosa M, Nicoletti F, et al. Molecular mechanisms involved in NAFLD progression. J Mol Med 2009;87(7):679–95.

55. Chen JS, Wang Q, Fu XH, et al. Involvement of PI3K/PTEN/AKT/mTOR pathway in invasion and metastasis in hepatocellular carcinoma: Association with MMP-9. Hepatol Res 2009;39(2):177–86.

56. Salmena L, Carracedo A, Pandolfi PP. Tenets of PTEN tumor suppression. Cell 2008;133:403–14.

57. Carnero A, Blanco-Aparicio C, Renner O, et al. The PTEN/PI3K/AKT signalling pathway in cancer, therapeutic implications. Curr Cancer Drug Targets 2008; 8:187–98.

58. Kandel ES, Hay N. The regulation and activities of the multifunctional serine/threonine kinase Akt/PKB. Exp Cell Res 1999;253(1):210–29.

59. Lawlor MA, Alessi DR. PKB/Akt: a key mediator of cell proliferation, survival and insulin responses? J Cell Sci 2001;114(Pt 16):2903–10.

60. Jee SH, Ohrr H, Sull JW, et al. Fasting serum glucose level and cancer risk in Korean men and women. JAMA 2005;293:194–202.

61. Ikejima K, Honda H, Yoshikawa M, et al. Leptin augments inflammatory and profibrogenic responses in the murine liver induced by hepatotoxic chemicals. Hepatology 2001;34:288–97.

62. Sahai A, Malladi P, Pan X, et al. Obese and diabetic db/db mice develop marked liver fibrosis in a model of nonalcoholic steatohepatitis: role of short-form leptin receptors and osteopontin. Am J Physiol Gastrointest Liver Physiol 2004;287(5):G1035–43.

63. Kitade M, Yoshiji H, Kojima H, et al. Leptin-mediated neovascularization is a prerequisite for progression of nonalcoholic steatohepatitis in rats. Hepatology 2006 Oct;44(4):983–91.

64. Myers MG, Cowley MA, Münzberg H. Mechanisms of leptin action and leptin resistance. Annu Rev Physiol 2008;70:537–56.

65. Considine RV, Sinha MK, Heiman ML, et al. Serum immunoreactive-leptin concentrations in normal weight and obese humans. N Engl J Med 1996;334:292–5.

66. Vilà L, Roglans N, Alegret M, et al. Suppressor of cytokine signaling-3 (SOCS-3) and a deficit of serine/threonine (Ser/Thr) phosphoproteins involved in leptin transduction mediate the effect of fructose on rat liver lipid metabolism. Hepatology 2008;48(5):1506–16.

67. Henriksen JH, Holst JJ, Møller S, et al. Increased circulating leptin in alcoholic cirrhosis: relation to release and disposal. Hepatology 1999;29(6):1818–24.
68. Saxena NK, Titus MA, Ding X, et al. Leptin as a novel profibrogenic cytokine in hepatic stellate cells: mitogenesis and inhibition of apoptosis mediated by extracellular regulated kinase (Erk) and Akt phosphorylation. FASEB J 2004;18(13): 1612–4.
69. Grunfeld C, Zhao C, Fuller J, et al. Endotoxin and cytokines induce expression of leptin, the OB gene product, in hamsters. A role for leptin in the anorexia of infection. J Clin Invest 1996;97:2152–7.
70. Kolacynski JW, Nyce MR, Considine RV, et al. Acute and chronic effects of insulin on leptin production in humans in vivo and in vitro. Diabetes 1996;45:699–701.
71. Hafner SM, Miettinen H, Karhapaa, et al. Leptin concentrations, sex hormones, and cortisol in non-diabetic men. J Clin Endocrinol Metab 1997;82:1807–9.
72. Wang XJ, Yuan SL, Lu Q, et al. Potential involvement of leptin in carcinogenesis of hepatocellular carcinoma. World J Gastroenterol 2004;10(17):2478–81.
73. Frühbeck G. Intracellular signalling pathways activated by leptin. Biochem J 2006;393(Pt 1):7–20.
74. Ramani K, Yang H, Xia M, et al. Leptin's mitogenic effect in human liver cancer cells requires induction of both methionine adenosyltransferase 2A and 2beta. Hepatology 2008;47(2):521–31.
75. Ikejima K, Takei Y, Honda H, et al. Leptin receptor-mediated signaling regulates hepatic fibrogenesis and remodeling of extracellular matrix in the rat. Gastroenterology 2002;122(5):1399–410.
76. Moreira RK. Hepatic stellate cells and liver fibrosis. Arch Pathol Lab Med 2007; 131(11):1728–34.
77. Friedman SL. Molecular regulation of hepatic fibrosis, an integrated cellular response to tissue injury. J Biol Chem 2000;275(4):2247–50.
78. Yoshiji H, Kuriyama S, Yoshii J, et al. Vascular endothelial growth factor and receptor interaction is a prerequisite for murine hepatic fibrogenesis. Gut 2003; 52:1347–54.
79. Elinav E, Abd-Elnabi A, Pappo O, et al. Suppression of hepatocellular carcinoma growth in mice via leptin, is associated with inhibition of tumor cell growth and natural killer cell activation. J Hepatol 2006;44(3):529–36.
80. Hu E, Liang P, Spiegelman BM. AdipoQ is a novel adipose-specific gene dysregulated in obesity. J Biol Chem 1996;271:10697–703.
81. Tilg H, Moschen AR. Adipocytokines: mediators linking adipose tissue, inflammation and immunity. Nat Rev Immunol 2006;6(10):772–83.
82. Maeda N, Shimomura I, Kishida K, et al. Diet-induced insulin resistance in mice lacking adiponectin/ACRP30. Nat Med 2002;8(7):731–7.
83. Hotta K, Funahashi T, Bodkin NL, et al. Circulating concentrations of the adipocyte protein adiponectin are decreased in parallel with reduced insulin sensitivity during the progression to type 2 diabetes in rhesus monkeys. Diabetes 2001;50(5):1126–33.
84. Zhang H, Cui J, Zhang C. Emerging role of adipokines as mediators in atherosclerosis. World J Cardiol 2010;2(11):370–6.
85. Hirose H, Kawai T, Yamamoto Y, et al. Effects of pioglitazone on metabolic parameters, body fat distribution and serum adiponectin levels in Japanese male patients with type 2 diabetes. Metabolism 2002;51:314–7.
86. Weyer C, Funahashi T, Tanaka S, et al. Hypoadiponectimia in obesity and type 2 diabetes: close association with insulin resistance and hyperinsulinemia. J Clin Endocrinol Metab 2001;86:1930–5.

87. Gruzman A, Babai G, Sasson S. Adenosine monophosphate-activated protein kinase (AMPK) as a new target for antidiabetic drugs: a review on metabolic, pharmacological and chemical considerations. Rev Diabet Stud 2009;6(1): 13–36.

88. Sandhu MS, Dunger DB, Giovannucci EL. Insulin, insulin-like growth factor-I (IGF-I), IGF binding proteins, their biologic interactions, and colorectal cancer. J Natl Cancer Inst 2002;94(13):972–80.

89. Tsuchida A, Yamauchi T, Ito Y, et al. Insulin/Foxo1 pathway regulates expression levels of adiponectin receptors and adiponectin sensitivity. J Biol Chem 2004; 279:30817–22.

90. Kondo H, Shimomura I, Matsukawa Y, et al. Association of adiponectin mutation with type 2 diabetes: a candidate gene for the insulin resistance syndrome. Diabetes 2002;51(7):2325–8.

91. Chen X, Wang Y. Adiponectin and breast cancer. Med Oncol 2010. [Epub ahead of print].

92. Wei EK, Giovannucci E, Fuchs CS, et al. Low plasma adiponectin levels and risk of colorectal cancer in men: a prospective study. J Natl Cancer Inst 2005;97(22): 1688–94.

93. Michalakis K, Williams CJ, Mitsiades N, et al. Serum adiponectin concentrations and tissue expression of adiponectin receptors are reduced in patients with prostate cancer: a case control study. Cancer Epidemiol Biomarkers Prev 2007;16(2):308–13.

94. Rzepka-Górska I, Bedner R, Cymbaluk-Płoska A, et al. Serum adiponectin in relation to endometrial cancer and endometrial hyperplasia with atypia in obese women. Eur J Gynaecol Oncol 2008;29(6):594–7.

95. Kamada Y, Matsumoto H, Tamura S, et al. Hypoadiponectinemia accelerates hepatic tumor formation in a nonalcoholic steatohepatitis mouse model. J Hepatol 2007;47(4):556–64.

96. Wree A, Kahraman A, Gerken G, et al. Obesity affects the liver—the link between adipocytes and hepatocytes. Digestion 2011;83(1–2):124–33.

97. Saxena NK, Fu PP, Nagalingam A, et al. Adiponectin modulates C-jun N-terminal kinase and mammalian target of rapamycin and inhibits hepatocellular carcinoma. Gastroenterology 2010;139(5):1762–73, 1773.e1–5.

98. Kadowaki T, Yamauchi T. Adiponectin and adiponectin receptors. Endocr Rev 2005;26(3):439–51.

99. Cool B, Zinker B, Chiou W, et al. Identification and characterization of a small molecule AMPK activator that treats key components of type 2 diabetes and the metabolic syndrome. Cell Metabolism 2006;3:403–16.

100. Motoshima H, Goldstein BJ, Igata M, et al. AMPK and cell proliferation–AMPK as a therapeutic target for atherosclerosis and cancer. J Physiol 2006;574(Pt 1): 63–71.

101. Wang X, Proud CG. The mTOR pathway in the control of protein synthesis. Physiology (Bethesda) 2006;21:362–9.

102. Feng Z, Zhang H, Levine AJ, et al. The coordinate regulation of the p53 and mTOR pathways in cells. Proc Natl Acad Sci U S A 2005;102(23):8204–9.

103. Miyazaki T, Bub JD, Uzuki M, et al. Adiponectin activates c-Jun NH2 terminal kinase and inhibits signal transducer and activator of transcription 3. Biochem Biophys Res Commun 2005;333(1):79–87.

Diagnosis of Hepatocellular Carcinoma: Role of Tumor Markers and Liver Biopsy

Stevan A. Gonzalez, MD, MS[a], Emmet B. Keeffe, MD[b],*

KEYWORDS

- Hepatocellular carcinoma • Cirrhosis • α-Fetoprotein
- Des-γ-carboxyprothrombin • Glypican-3
- Immunohistochemistry • Proteomics

The ability to establish a diagnosis of HCC in patients with chronic liver disease at an early time point is critical to providing effective treatment, including surgical resection, locoregional ablative therapy, and liver transplantation. Consequently, surveillance strategies with the goal of increasing the rate of early detection of HCC, primarily through serum α-fetoprotein (AFP) assessment and hepatic imaging, have led to increased survival in high-risk populations.[1,2] Once a hepatic lesion is identified through surveillance, the diagnosis of HCC can be achieved through the use of dynamic contrast-enhanced cross-sectional imaging, tumor markers, and/or liver biopsy. These topics are dealt with in depth in the articles elsewhere in this issue by Anis and Irshad, Frenette and Gish, and Roskams, respectively. Although imaging modalities have become the primary means of establishing the diagnosis of HCC as a result of their increased sensitivity and specificity, serum tumor markers and liver biopsy continue to have an important role, particularly in the setting of small or atypical hepatic lesions. Advances in the development of novel serum tumor markers with higher sensitivity and specificity, as well as the use of immunohistochemical techniques to identify molecular markers on biopsy specimens, may contribute greatly to early recognition of HCC in cases that would otherwise remain undiagnosed.

Disclosures: Drs Gonzalez and Keeffe have nothing to disclose.
[a] Division of General and Transplant Hepatology, Baylor Regional Transplant Institute, Baylor All Saints Medical Center at Fort Worth, Baylor University Medical Center at Dallas, 1250 8th Avenue, Suite 515, Fort Worth, TX 76104, USA
[b] Division of Gastroenterology and Hepatology, Department of Medicine, Stanford University Medical Center, 750 Welch Road, Suite 210, Palo Alto, CA 94304-1509, USA
* Corresponding author.
E-mail address: ekeeffe@stanford.edu

Clin Liver Dis 15 (2011) 297–306
doi:10.1016/j.cld.2011.03.012
1089-3261/11/$ – see front matter © 2011 Elsevier Inc. All rights reserved.

DIAGNOSIS OF HCC

The diagnosis of HCC has primarily relied on the presence of typical features seen on contrast-enhanced imaging studies, histopathological assessment, and serum AFP levels. Prior guidelines incorporated serum AFP into the diagnostic algorithm, in which elevated AFP levels in conjunction with a contrast-enhanced imaging study were sufficient in the diagnosis of lesions larger than 2 cm.[3,4] In light of data revealing poor sensitivity of AFP in the diagnosis of HCC, the most recent guideline of the American Association for the Study of Liver Diseases (AASLD) no longer includes measurement of serum AFP in the diagnostic algorithm for hepatic nodules found on surveillance imaging[5] (see also the article elsewhere in this issue by Sherman). However, AFP remains the tumor marker most commonly used in clinical practice, both in surveillance strategies and for the diagnosis of HCC. Whether AFP will remain the preferred tumor marker in conjunction with imaging studies or be combined with other more sensitive tests in the future remains to be seen.

The current AASLD guideline provides strategies for achieving the diagnosis of HCC based on the size of hepatic nodules seen on surveillance imaging (**Table 1**). For lesions less than 1 cm in size, follow-up surveillance imaging is recommended at 3-month intervals to assess for an increase in size. Lesions larger than 1 cm require definitive contrast-enhanced imaging with either dynamic 4-phase computed tomography (CT) or magnetic resonance imaging (MRI). The presence of typical features on these imaging studies, including intense uptake of contrast during arterial phases followed by decreased enhancement (washout) during portal venous phases, have a very high sensitivity and specificity for the diagnosis of HCC.[6–9] In cases of atypical enhancement of the suspected lesion, an additional contrast-enhanced imaging study can be performed. Although interpretation of liver biopsy specimens for a definitive histopathological diagnosis of HCC is not used as frequently, it has an important role in the setting of lesions with atypical features on imaging studies.

TUMOR MARKERS
AFP

AFP is a glycoprotein produced during embryologic development by the fetal liver and yolk sac. AFP shares primary and secondary structural features with albumin and is a member of the albumin multigene family.[10,11] Serum AFP levels decline during the course of normal gestation, but maternal levels may increase in association with fetal

Table 1
Diagnostic approach for hepatic nodules based on current guidelines

Nodule Size	Primary Imaging Assessment and Strategy	Secondary Assessment for Atypical Features
<1 cm	Repeat imaging every 3 months until >1 cm	Role of liver biopsy not established
>1 cm	Contrast-enhanced cross-sectional imaging study (CT or MRI) to assess for typical features[a]	Contrast-enhanced cross-sectional imaging study with alternative modality (CT or MRI) (or) liver biopsy if atypical features on first or second imaging study

[a] Dynamic 4-phase computed tomography (CT) or magnetic resonance imaging (MRI).

Data from Bruix J, Sherman M. Management of hepatocellular carcinoma: an update. Hepatology 2010:000;1–35. Available at: http://publish.aasld.org/practiceguidelines/Documents/Bookmarked%2520Practice%2520Guidelines/HCCUpdate2010.pdf. Accessed November 20, 2010.

disorders. In adulthood, elevations in serum AFP can be seen in the setting of various malignancies in addition to HCC, including germ cell tumors, gastric cancer, and intra-hepatic cholangiocarcinoma.[11–13] Elevations in serum AFP can also occur in patients with cirrhosis in the absence of malignancy; in these circumstances, the elevated AFP level may correlate with elevations in serum aminotransferase levels or grade of nec-roinflammatory activity on liver biopsy.[14]

AFP has long been recognized as a tumor marker for HCC, and has played a prom-inent role in the diagnosis of HCC according to previous guidelines.[3,4] However, the utility of serum AFP as a diagnostic tool may be increasingly limited as imaging modal-ities have become more advanced and evidence has emerged demonstrating a low sensitivity of AFP in the diagnosis of HCC. One large prospective cohort study of more than 1000 patients diagnosed with HCC revealed that 46% of patients had normal serum AFP levels (<20 ng/mL).[15] Data derived predominantly from case-control and prospective cohort studies, involving mostly patients with cirrhosis secondary to chronic hepatitis C virus (HCV) infection, have shown sensitivities of 41% to 65% and specificities of 80% to 94% for serum AFP levels greater than 20 ng/mL (**Table 2**).[15–18] As AFP levels increase to more than 200 ng/mL, the specificity approaches 100%; however, the sensitivity is reduced to as low as 20%.[17,18] AFP levels greater than 400 ng/mL have been considered to be virtually diagnostic of HCC, but sensitivity is then decreased further, to less than 20%.[16,18] The low sensi-tivity associated with serum AFP levels, elevated false-negative rate, and poor discriminatory ability in the diagnosis of HCC have all significantly limited reliance on AFP as a diagnostic test.[15]

Several factors may influence the diagnostic accuracy of serum AFP levels, including the etiology of chronic liver disease, patient ethnicity, prevalence of HCC within certain populations, and the size of nodules identified during surveillance imaging studies. Although some reports have suggested that serum AFP levels may be more effective as a surveillance and diagnostic tool in patients with chronic hepa-titis B virus (HBV) infection,[19] others have not demonstrated a difference when comparing patients with chronic HBV versus HCV infection.[20] The use of AFP in patients of certain ethnic backgrounds, particularly African Americans, seems to be associated with a much lower sensitivity than is apparent in non-African Americans.[21] The prevalence of HCC within a population can have a major impact on the positive predictive value (PPV) of AFP, as demonstrated in a large case-control study in which

Table 2
Performance characteristics of serum tumor markers in the diagnosis of hepatocellular carcinoma

Tumor Marker	Sensitivity (%)	Specificity (%)
α-Fetoprotein (AFP)[15–18]		
>20 ng/mL	41–65	80–94
>200 ng/mL	20–45	99–100
>400 ng/mL	<20	99–100
Lens culinaris agglutinin-reactive α-fetoprotein (AFP-L3)[24–27,a]	39–75	83–90
Des-γ-carboxyprothrombin (DCP)[29–31,b]	41–74	70–100
Glypican-3 (GPC-3)[36–39]	40–53	90–100
Proteomic profiling[40–43]	61–92	76–91

[a] Proportion of AFP-L3 used as cutoff ranges from 10% to 35%.[24–27]
[b] Cutoff values for DCP were 60 mAU/mL[29] and 150 mAU/mL.[30,31]

an 85% PPV associated with AFP levels of greater than 20 ng/mL decreased to 25% when the prevalence of HCC decreased from 50% to 5%.[20] In addition, the efficacy of AFP in establishing the diagnosis of HCC may be diminished as the size of hepatic nodules seen during surveillance imaging decreases. A retrospective series of consecutive patients diagnosed with a single HCC mass smaller than 2 cm reported low sensitivities associated with serum AFP, in which fewer than 20% of patients had a serum AFP level greater than 100 ng/mL and only 11% had a level greater than 200 ng/mL.[22]

Despite the poor reliability and low sensitivity of serum AFP in the diagnosis of HCC, AFP levels appear to have prognostic value, as elevations in AFP are significantly associated with increased tumor size and stage, extrahepatic metastases, portal vein thrombosis, and decreased survival.[15] Recent data have also pointed out that progression of AFP levels in patients with HCC before liver transplantation may be associated with an increased risk of tumor recurrence and decreased survival following transplantation.[23]

Lens culinaris Agglutinin-Reactive AFP

AFP is characterized by molecular microheterogeneity, in which different isoforms of AFP can be identified through electrophoretic techniques based on reactivity to specific lectins.[10] Of 3 major isoforms of AFP, a fucosylated variant reactive to *Lens culinaris* agglutinin has been associated with HCC. The relative proportion of the *Lens culinaris* agglutinin-reactive AFP (AFP-L3) to total serum AFP is significantly increased in patients with HCC, in contrast to those with elevated AFP in the absence of HCC.[24] Several prospective studies have reported a higher sensitivity and specificity associated with AFP-L3 in the diagnosis of HCC relative to total serum AFP in patients with elevated baseline AFP levels (see **Table 2**)[24–27]; however, data demonstrating a significant advantage of AFP-L3 over total AFP are limited. One recent prospective study noted a significantly higher specificity of AFP-L3 when compared with total AFP levels.[27] In this study, both sensitivity and specificity of AFP-L3 improved as AFP levels increased and the negative predictive value (NPV) of AFP-L3 was greater than 80%, suggesting that it may have a role as a secondary test in conjunction with total serum AFP.

Des-γ-Carboxyprothrombin

Des-γ-carboxyprothrombin (DCP), also known as Prothrombin Induced by Vitamin K Absence II (PIVKA II), is an abnormal prothrombin molecule resulting from the absence of vitamin K–dependent activity of γ-glutamyl carboxylase on the prothrombin precursor molecule. Serum DCP levels are increased in patients with HCC, possibly due to decreased activity of the γ-glutamyl carboxylase enzyme or altered vitamin K metabolism.[28] Although prospective data using DCP as a diagnostic tool for detection of HCC are limited, one large prospective cohort study found DCP to have greater specificity in comparison with AFP (91% vs 78%, respectively); however the sensitivity of DCP was low, at 41% (see **Table 2**).[29] Recent case-control studies have reported mixed results, in which there is no clear advantage to the use of DCP,[30,31] although the low sensitivity associated with DCP may be offset when used in conjunction with AFP.[29] An additional concern regarding the utility of DCP is the emergence of data suggesting that DCP is inferior to AFP in the detection of small or early HCC nodules based on receiver-operating characteristic analysis.[32] DCP levels are also raised by warfarin and other 4-hydroxcoumarin–containing anticoagulants, which interfere with vitamin K–mediated carboxylation of prothrombin and other blood coagulation proteins. Warfarin prevents vitamin K epoxide reductase from recycling oxidized vitamin K to its reduced form that participates in γ-glutamyl protein carboxylation. DCP is elevated in proportion to the degree of warfarin-induced anticoagulation, which may be used in patients with portal vein thrombosis, Budd-Chiari syndrome, and other hypercoagulable states.

Glypican-3

Glypican-3 (GPC-3) is a cell-surface heparin sulfate proteoglycan that is overexpressed in HCC cells and may be involved in promoting tumor growth.[33–35] GPC-3 can be identified histologically through immunohistochemistry as well as in the serum of individuals with HCC. Several studies have reported a very high specificity (90%–100%) associated with serum GPC-3 in patients with HCC (see **Table 2**).[36–39] Similar to serum AFP, the sensitivity of serum GPC-3 in patients with HCC remains relatively low; however, when GPC-3 is measured in conjunction with AFP, the reported sensitivity appears to improve.

Proteomic Profiling

Proteomic techniques involving surface-enhanced laser desorption/ionization time-of-flight mass spectrometry have been used to provide reproducible profiles of protein expression associated with HCC. The use of proteomic array technology also can be used to identify expression of specific serum protein fragments that may function as new biomarkers for HCC. Although prospective longitudinal data are limited, early studies have demonstrated high sensitivity and specificity in the detection of established HCC in comparison with non-HCC cohorts (see **Table 2**).[40–43]

Other Serum Tumor Markers

Additional potential serum biomarkers have been identified in association with early diagnosis of HCC, including α1-fucosidase, human telomerase reverse transcriptase, squamous cell carcinoma antigen, Golgi protein 73, and transforming growth factor β1. Although these are promising candidates in the effort to develop novel tumor markers for HCC with sufficient sensitivity and specificity to perform as diagnostic tools, further studies in larger cohorts will be required to more accurately determine whether these markers will be useful.

LIVER BIOPSY
Histopathology and Role in Diagnosis

As early diagnosis of HCC has an impact on survival, efforts to achieve a definitive diagnosis in small lesions, particularly those less than 2 cm in size, are important considerations. Recent prospective studies have reported that up to 67% of new nodules smaller than 2 cm identified during surveillance imaging in patients with cirrhosis are indeed HCC.[7,8] In lesions found to have atypical imaging characteristics, a percutaneous biopsy should be considered in order to achieve a definitive diagnosis.[5] Histopathologic assessment can differentiate between premalignant lesions, known as low-grade or high-grade dysplastic nodules, and early HCC. Small lesions found to be HCC may be further classified as distinctly nodular type, which are predominantly moderately differentiated, or indistinctly nodular type, which are more likely to be well differentiated.[44] An unresolved question is whether imaging studies alone are sufficient to diagnose small lesions, or if a definitive assessment through liver biopsy is required for most lesions.

Recent data have suggested that a single dynamic contrast-enhanced imaging study such as CT or MRI with typical enhancement patterns has sufficient specificity for the diagnosis of small HCC of 1 to 2 cm size in the absence of histopathologic evaluation.[8] Consequently, updated guidelines no longer require 2 positive imaging studies for lesions of this size, and liver biopsy now enters the algorithm as an alternative strategy to a second dynamic imaging study if atypical imaging features are encountered on initial imaging (see **Table 1**).[5] Although the specificity of contrast-enhanced MRI has been reported as high as 96% for hepatic nodules of 1 to 2 cm in size,[7,9] a significant proportion of small HCC may appear hypovascular or have atypical features, resulting in a false-negative rate of 20% to 38%.[9,45] In cases of small nodules with atypical enhancement a biopsy should be considered, as it may significantly improve the likelihood of correctly achieving a diagnosis of HCC. As the ability to diagnose small lesions improves with more advanced imaging capability, the need for biopsy and its importance in the diagnosis of HCC may likely be diminished.

In the setting of small hepatic nodules of less than 2 cm in size, obtaining a reliable tissue specimen for the diagnosis of HCC can be challenging and the potential for false-negative results, that is, failure to sample the lesion, must be taken into consideration. In one prospective study of patients with cirrhosis who presented with solitary nodules smaller than 2 cm, the false-negative rate was reported to be 30%. A second biopsy was then performed that established the diagnosis of HCC in over half of the patients who had an initial false-negative result.[7] Although the overall sensitivity, specificity, and PPV of biopsy for the diagnosis of HCC are reported to be as high as 90% to 100%, the NPV remains remarkably low, at 14%.[46–48] Thus, a negative result on biopsy, particularly in small nodules, does not exclude HCC, and a second attempt at achieving a histopathologic diagnosis of HCC should be considered. Some data suggest that almost 70% of hepatic nodules of less than 1 cm in size may indeed be HCC in patients with cirrhosis[47]; however, others have reported a much lower proportion of less than 25%.[7] The use of biopsy for lesions this small has not been fully endorsed because of the technical challenge of obtaining a reliable specimen and the increased potential for false negatives.

Safety and Risk of Needle Tract Seeding

Overall, percutaneous liver biopsy for assessment of hepatic nodules is well tolerated and safe. In addition to obtaining diagnostic information, a biopsy may be useful in determining tumor grade before treatment or transplantation.[49] A concern frequently raised when considering percutaneous biopsy of a hepatic nodule is the potential risk of needle tract seeding of the tumor and the associated increased risk of recurrence, particularly in patients who are liver transplant candidates. Although needle tract seeding does happen, it seems to occur very rarely. In the largest series to date, the incidence of needle tract seeding in more than 1000 patients with HCC who underwent ultrasound-guided percutaneous biopsy was 0.76%.[50] Other studies with more than 100 patients have reported the incidence of tumor seeding following percutaneous biopsy to be in the range of 1.6% to 3.4%.[48] Despite concerns of a potential risk of HCC recurrence with immunosuppression therapy following liver transplantation, there is no clear evidence demonstrating an increased risk of needle tract seeding and recurrent HCC in this setting; therefore, previous biopsy of HCC should not be a barrier to transplant candidacy.[48]

Immunohistochemical Analysis

Several molecular tumor markers found in association with HCC have been identified and can be detected through the use of immunohistochemistry.[44,51] The use of these techniques in the assessment of biopsy specimens may be increasingly important in establishing the diagnosis of HCC, particularly in the setting of early tumors that may demonstrate features of both high-grade dysplasia and HCC. GPC-3, as well as other markers including heat-shock protein 70 (HSP70) and glutamine synthase, can be effectively detected in HCC biopsy tissue through immunohistochemistry.[52] Several studies have demonstrated high sensitivity and specificity associated with GPC-3 immunostaining in particular.[36–39,52–56] Immunohistochemistry for the presence of GPC-3 may be an effective diagnostic tool in identifying HCC in early lesions and in discriminating between high-grade dysplastic nodules and well-differentiated HCC with high specificity[52,55,56]; however, its sensitivity may be diminished as the size of hepatic nodules decreases.[57] This topic is covered in depth in the article elsewhere in this issue by Roskams, who insists that biopsies for HCC should be done universally in clinical trials of HCC therapy, as an adjunct to decisions concerning all modes of therapy in individual cases, and for prognosis.

SUMMARY

Serum tumor markers and histopathologic assessment of hepatic nodules by liver biopsy continue to play an important selective role in the diagnosis of HCC, particularly in settings where imaging modalities cannot achieve a definitive diagnosis. The ability to discriminate between dysplastic nodules and early HCC has become increasingly important, as the efficacy of treatments for HCC, including liver transplantation, depends on recognition at an early phase. Although tumor markers for HCC such as AFP are characterized by low sensitivity, the emergence of new highly sensitive and specific biomarkers through the use of microarray technology, proteomics, and other techniques may significantly improve noninvasive methods of diagnosing HCC. Likewise, the use of novel molecular markers in the interpretation of liver biopsy specimens may more accurately recognize the transition from high-grade dysplasia to HCC.

REFERENCES

1. Zhang BH, Yang BH, Tang ZY. Randomized controlled trial of screening for hepatocellular carcinoma. J Cancer Res Clin Oncol 2004;130:417–22.
2. Sangiovanni A, Del Ninno E, Fasani P, et al. Increased survival of cirrhotic patients with a hepatocellular carcinoma detected during surveillance. Gastroenterology 2004;126:1005–14.
3. Bruix J, Sherman M, Llovet JM, et al. Clinical management of hepatocellular carcinoma. Conclusions of the Barcelona-2000 EASL conference. European Association for the Study of the Liver. J Hepatol 2001;35:421–30.
4. Bruix J, Sherman M. Management of hepatocellular carcinoma. Hepatology 2005; 42:1208–36.
5. Bruix J, Sherman M. Management of hepatocellular carcinoma: an update. Hepatology 2010;000:1–35. Available at: http://publish.aasld.org/practiceguidelines/Documents/Bookmarked%20Practice%20Guidelines/HCCUpdate2010.pdf. Accessed November 20, 2010.
6. Burrel M, Llovet JM, Ayuso C, et al. MRI angiography is superior to helical CT for detection of HCC prior to liver transplantation: an explant correlation. Hepatology 2003;38:1034–42.
7. Forner A, Vilana R, Ayuso C, et al. Diagnosis of hepatic nodules 20 mm or smaller in cirrhosis: prospective validation of the noninvasive diagnostic criteria for hepatocellular carcinoma. Hepatology 2008;47:97–104.
8. Sangiovanni A, Manini MA, Iavarone M, et al. The diagnostic and economic impact of contrast imaging techniques in the diagnosis of small hepatocellular carcinoma in cirrhosis. Gut 2010;59:638–44.

9. Leoni S, Piscaglia F, Golfieri R, et al. The impact of vascular and nonvascular findings on the noninvasive diagnosis of small hepatocellular carcinoma based on the EASL and AASLD criteria. Am J Gastroenterol 2010;105:599–609.

10. Mizejewski GJ. Alpha-fetoprotein structure and function: relevance to isoforms, epitopes, and conformational variants. Exp Biol Med (Maywood) 2001;226: 377–408.

11. Terentiev AA, Moldogazieva NT. Structural and functional mapping of alpha-fetoprotein. Biochemistry (Mosc) 2006;71:120–32.

12. Adachi Y, Tsuchihashi J, Shiraishi N, et al. AFP-producing gastric carcinoma: multivariate analysis of prognostic factors in 270 patients. Oncology 2003;65: 95–101.

13. Shen WF, Zhong W, Xu F, et al. Clinicopathological and prognostic analysis of 429 patients with intrahepatic cholangiocarcinoma. World J Gastroenterol 2009;15: 5976–82.

14. Di Bisceglie AM, Sterling RK, Chung RT, et al. Serum alpha-fetoprotein levels in patients with advanced hepatitis C: results from the HALT-C Trial. J Hepatol 2005;43:434–41.

15. Farinati F, Marino D, De Giorgio M, et al. Diagnostic and prognostic role of alpha-fetoprotein in hepatocellular carcinoma: both or neither? Am J Gastroenterol 2006;101:524–32.

16. Gebo KA, Chander G, Jenckes MW, et al. Screening tests for hepatocellular carcinoma in patients with chronic hepatitis C: a systematic review. Hepatology 2002;36:S84–92.

17. Gupta S, Bent S, Kohlwes J. Test characteristics of alpha-fetoprotein for detecting hepatocellular carcinoma in patients with hepatitis C. A systematic review and critical analysis. Ann Intern Med 2003;139:46–50.

18. Daniele B, Bencivenga A, Megna AS, et al. Alpha-fetoprotein and ultrasonography screening for hepatocellular carcinoma. Gastroenterology 2004;127: S108–12.

19. McMahon BJ, Bulkow L, Harpster A, et al. Screening for hepatocellular carcinoma in Alaska natives infected with chronic hepatitis B: a 16-year population-based study. Hepatology 2000;32:842–6.

20. Trevisani F, D'Intino PE, Morselli-Labate AM, et al. Serum alpha-fetoprotein for diagnosis of hepatocellular carcinoma in patients with chronic liver disease: influence of HBsAg and anti-HCV status. J Hepatol 2001;34:570–5.

21. Nguyen MH, Garcia RT, Simpson PW, et al. Racial differences in effectiveness of alpha-fetoprotein for diagnosis of hepatocellular carcinoma in hepatitis C virus cirrhosis. Hepatology 2002;36:410–7.

22. Rapaccini GL, Pompili M, Caturelli E, et al. Hepatocellular carcinomas <2 cm in diameter complicating cirrhosis: ultrasound and clinical features in 153 consecutive patients. Liver Int 2004;24:124–30.

23. Vibert E, Azoulay D, Hoti E, et al. Progression of alpha-fetoprotein before liver transplantation for hepatocellular carcinoma in cirrhotic patients: a critical factor. Am J Transplant 2010;10:129–37.

24. Sato Y, Nakata K, Kato Y, et al. Early recognition of hepatocellular carcinoma based on altered profiles of alpha-fetoprotein. N Engl J Med 1993;328:1802–6.

25. Shiraki K, Takase K, Tameda Y, et al. A clinical study of lectin-reactive alpha-fetoprotein as an early indicator of hepatocellular carcinoma in the follow-up of cirrhotic patients. Hepatology 1995;22:802–7.

26. Wang SS, Lu RH, Lee FY, et al. Utility of lentil lectin affinity of alpha-fetoprotein in the diagnosis of hepatocellular carcinoma. J Hepatol 1996;25:166–71.

27. Sterling RK, Jeffers L, Gordon F, et al. Clinical utility of AFP-L3% measurement in North American patients with HCV-related cirrhosis. Am J Gastroenterol 2007; 102:2196–205.

28. Inagaki Y, Tang W, Makuuchi M, et al. Clinical and molecular insights into the hepatocellular carcinoma tumour marker des-gamma-carboxyprothrombin. Liver Int 2011;31(1):22–35.

29. Ishii M, Gama H, Chida N, et al. Simultaneous measurements of serum alpha-fetoprotein and protein induced by vitamin K absence for detecting hepatocellular carcinoma. South Tohoku District Study Group. Am J Gastroenterol 2000; 95:1036–40.

30. Marrero JA, Feng Z, Wang Y, et al. Alpha-fetoprotein, des-gamma carboxyprothrombin, and lectin-bound alpha-fetoprotein in early hepatocellular carcinoma. Gastroenterology 2009;137:110–8.

31. Lok AS, Sterling RK, Everhart JE, et al. Des-gamma-carboxy prothrombin and alpha-fetoprotein as biomarkers for the early detection of hepatocellular carcinoma. Gastroenterology 2010;138:493–502.

32. Nakamura S, Nouso K, Sakaguchi K, et al. Sensitivity and specificity of des-gamma-carboxy prothrombin for diagnosis of patients with hepatocellular carcinomas varies according to tumor size. Am J Gastroenterol 2006;101:2038–43.

33. Sung YK, Hwang SY, Park MK, et al. Glypican-3 is overexpressed in human hepatocellular carcinoma. Cancer Sci 2003;94:259–62.

34. Zhu ZW, Friess H, Wang L, et al. Enhanced glypican-3 expression differentiates the majority of hepatocellular carcinomas from benign hepatic disorders. Gut 2001;48:558–64.

35. Capurro MI, Xiang YY, Lobe C, et al. Glypican-3 promotes the growth of hepatocellular carcinoma by stimulating canonical Wnt signaling. Cancer Res 2005;65: 6245–54.

36. Hippo Y, Watanabe K, Watanabe A, et al. Identification of soluble NH2-terminal fragment of glypican-3 as a serological marker for early-stage hepatocellular carcinoma. Cancer Res 2004;64:2418–23.

37. Nakatsura T, Yoshitake Y, Senju S, et al. Glypican-3, overexpressed specifically in human hepatocellular carcinoma, is a novel tumor marker. Biochem Biophys Res Commun 2003;306:16–25.

38. Capurro M, Wanless IR, Sherman M, et al. Glypican-3: a novel serum and histochemical marker for hepatocellular carcinoma. Gastroenterology 2003;125: 89–97.

39. Liu H, Li P, Zhai Y, et al. Diagnostic value of glypican-3 in serum and liver for primary hepatocellular carcinoma. World J Gastroenterol 2010;16:4410–5.

40. Poon TC, Yip TT, Chan AT, et al. Comprehensive proteomic profiling identifies serum proteomic signatures for detection of hepatocellular carcinoma and its subtypes. Clin Chem 2003;49:752–60.

41. Paradis V, Degos F, Dargere D, et al. Identification of a new marker of hepatocellular carcinoma by serum protein profiling of patients with chronic liver diseases. Hepatology 2005;41:40–7.

42. Schwegler EE, Cazares L, Steel LF, et al. SELDI-TOF MS profiling of serum for detection of the progression of chronic hepatitis C to hepatocellular carcinoma. Hepatology 2005;41:634–42.

43. Zinkin NT, Grall F, Bhaskar K, et al. Serum proteomics and biomarkers in hepatocellular carcinoma and chronic liver disease. Clin Cancer Res 2008;14:470–7.

44. Roskams T, Kojiro M. Pathology of early hepatocellular carcinoma: conventional and molecular diagnosis. Semin Liver Dis 2010;30:17–25.

45. Bolondi L, Gaiani S, Celli N, et al. Characterization of small nodules in cirrhosis by assessment of vascularity: the problem of hypovascular hepatocellular carcinoma. Hepatology 2005;42:27–34.

46. Durand F, Regimbeau JM, Belghiti J, et al. Assessment of the benefits and risks of percutaneous biopsy before surgical resection of hepatocellular carcinoma. J Hepatol 2001;35:254–8.

47. Caturelli E, Solmi L, Anti M, et al. Ultrasound guided fine needle biopsy of early hepatocellular carcinoma complicating liver cirrhosis: a multicentre study. Gut 2004;53:1356–62.

48. Durand F, Belghiti J, Paradis V. Liver transplantation for hepatocellular carcinoma: role of biopsy. Liver Transpl 2007;13:S17–23.

49. Colecchia A, Scaioli E, Montrone L, et al. Pre-operative liver biopsy in cirrhotic patients with early hepatocellular carcinoma represents a safe and accurate diagnostic tool for tumour grading assessment. J Hepatol 2011;54(2):300–5.

50. Chang S, Kim SH, Lim HK, et al. Needle tract implantation after sonographically guided percutaneous biopsy of hepatocellular carcinoma: evaluation of doubling time, frequency, and features on CT. AJR Am J Roentgenol 2005;185:400–5.

51. Chan ES, Yeh MM. The use of immunohistochemistry in liver tumors. Clin Liver Dis 2010;14:687–703.

52. Di Tommaso L, Destro A, Seok JY, et al. The application of markers (HSP70 GPC3 and GS) in liver biopsies is useful for detection of hepatocellular carcinoma. J Hepatol 2009;50:746–54.

53. Wang XY, Degos F, Dubois S, et al. Glypican-3 expression in hepatocellular tumors: diagnostic value for preneoplastic lesions and hepatocellular carcinomas. Hum Pathol 2006;37:1435–41.

54. Wang FH, Yip YC, Zhang M, et al. Diagnostic utility of glypican-3 for hepatocellular carcinoma on liver needle biopsy. J Clin Pathol 2010;63:599–603.

55. Libbrecht L, Severi T, Cassiman D, et al. Glypican-3 expression distinguishes small hepatocellular carcinomas from cirrhosis, dysplastic nodules, and focal nodular hyperplasia-like nodules. Am J Surg Pathol 2006;30:1405–11.

56. Llovet JM, Chen Y, Wurmbach E, et al. A molecular signature to discriminate dysplastic nodules from early hepatocellular carcinoma in HCV cirrhosis. Gastroenterology 2006;131:1758–67.

57. Shafizadeh N, Ferrell LD, Kakar S. Utility and limitations of glypican-3 expression for the diagnosis of hepatocellular carcinoma at both ends of the differentiation spectrum. Mod Pathol 2008;21:1011–8.

Hepatocellular Carcinoma: Molecular and Genomic Guideline for the Clinician

Catherine Frenette, MD[a],*, Robert G. Gish, MD[b]

KEYWORDS

- Hepatocellular carcinoma • Multikinase inhibitors
- Targeted therapy • Molecular classification

Conventional approaches to prognostic classification and treatment recommendations for the worldwide burden that is hepatocellular carcinoma (HCC)[1] have largely relied on clinicopathological characteristics, such as tumor size, Child-Turcotte-Pugh score, serum levels of α-fetoprotein (AFP), number of nodules, functional performance estimates (such as the Eastern Cooperative Oncology [ECOG] performance status), vascular invasion, distant metastases, and tumor grade. With improved DNA-microarray methods, defining the genomic and molecular changes that occur during the development of HCC should improve the classification and prognostication of liver tumors. Additional testing with RNA and proteomics will further add to the profiling of HCC. The development of sorafenib and other new targeted therapies in development has been made possible by the discovery and understanding of the molecular and genetic pathogenesis of hepatocellular carcinoma, and the signaling pathways that are important in the progression of the disease from dysplastic lesions to cancer and further progression of disease clinically. The understanding of these pathways will in the future enable the clinician to focus the treatment patients with HCC and customize single or combination therapy and allow refinement of treatment sequencing. Furthermore, investigators will be able to understand the basis of newer therapies that need to enter investigational trials. The discussion that follows complements the information in articles elsewhere in this issue, all in relation to HCC, by

There is no funding support for this article.

Disclosures: Dr Frenette serves on the Speakers Board for Onyx Pharmaceuticals. Dr Gish serves on the Speakers Board for Onyx Pharmaceuticals, is a paid consultant for Bristol Meyers Squibb, and is an unpaid consultant for OSI Pharmaceuticals.

[a] The Methodist Center for Liver Disease, J.C. Walter Transplant Center, Department of Medicine, The Methodist Hospital, 6550 Fannin Street, SM 1001, Houston, TX 77098, USA

[b] Center for Hepatobiliary Disease and Abdominal Transplantation, University of California, 200 West Arbor Drive, MC 8413, San Diego, CA 92103-8413, USA

* Corresponding author.

E-mail address: ctfrenette@tmhs.org

Clin Liver Dis 15 (2011) 307–321
doi:10.1016/j.cld.2011.03.010
1089-3261/11/$ – see front matter © 2011 Elsevier Inc. All rights reserved.

Roskams on Anatomic Pathology, Siddique and Kowdley on Insulin Resistance and Other Metabolic Risk Factors, the Diagnostic Role of Tumor Markers and Liver Biopsy by Gonzalez and Keeffe, the Role of Oncogenic Viruses by Zemel, Isaschar, and Tur-Kaspa, and Systemic Therapy by Wrzenski, Taddei, and Strazzabosco.

PATHOGENESIS OF HCC

Development of hepatocellular carcinoma involves a complex, multistep pathway where normal hepatocytes proliferate in the setting of chronic inflammation and altered intracellular signaling, and subsequently develop into regenerative nodules, with evolution to dysplastic nodules and cancer.[2] Most often, this occurs in a chronically diseased liver caused by hepatitis B virus (HBV) or hepatitis C virus (HCV). The most important molecular event that occurs in cancer development is aberrant gene expression. Genetic and epigenetic changes may occur, such as direct integration into the cellular DNA and "injury" with genetic mutations and translocations; or epigenetic modulations of genes such as DNA methylation, which results in altered gene expression without any changes in the base sequence of DNA, can occur.[3] Modifications of DNA sequences that do not directly encode mRNA and proteins can modify the generation of micro-RNA (miRNA); this can then result in dysregulation of primary gene signaling.[4] Cancer cells do not invent new pathways of signaling, but instead use preexisting pathways that are dormant or less active in normal cells. The changes in genetics, epigenetics, or miRNA allow these pathways to become overactive in cancer cells, increasing cell proliferation and signaling and decreasing cell apoptosis, with escape from the normal growth inhibition and regulation of growth from the extracellular matrix.

The pathogenesis of hepatocellular carcinoma is incredibly complex, since the development of a malignant signature can occur with several different mechanisms. This process results in different subtypes of HCC that are similar on pathologic examination, but clinically behave in different manners. For example, HCC related to HBV infection can have the HBV DNA (full or partial sequences) incorporated into many different areas in the host DNA, whereas the HCV virus does not incorporate into the host DNA and the development of HCC is related to decades of liver cell damage and regeneration.[3] HCV, through oxidative injury, can also result in cellular DNA modification.

Elevated expression of transforming growth factor (TGF)-α and insulin-like growth factor (IGF)-2 are both responsible for accelerated hepatocyte proliferation.[5–7] This increased expression reflects the expression of several genes that are upregulated by epigenetic mechanisms during the preneoplastic stage, resulting from the combined actions of cytokines produced by chronic inflammation, viral transactivation, and the regenerative response of the liver to cell loss. As hepatocytes repeatedly proliferate in response to these signals, monoclonal hepatocyte populations develop with progressive telomere shortening that predisposes to the development of dysplasia.

GENETIC ALTERATIONS

Nearly all liver cancer cells contain many genes and genetic loci that have structural alterations, but specific genetic or allelic alterations studies rarely affect more than half of liver cancers studied. The amount of variation among these genetic alterations has prompted the development of genetic and molecular subclassifications of HCC.

Many different genetic alterations have been discovered in HCC, including gains in chromosomes 1q, 6p, 8q, 17q, and 20q, and losses in 4q, 8p, 13q, 16q, and 17p.[8]

Mutations in the tumor suppressor gene p53 occur frequently in human cancer development, but are only found in 29% of HCC. In addition, HBV-induced HCC is also closely linked to p53 alterations.[9] Expression of HBV viral protein HBX inactivates p53-dependent activities, a tumor suppressor gene, which includes p53-mediated apoptosis.[10,11] Activation of oncogenes such as k-Ras seems to occur at a lower rate than in other human cancers, only occurring in 3% to 10% of liver cancers.[12] Other oncogenes are thought to be more important, such as c-met, which was shown to be expressed in 40% of HCC.[13]

Knowing what genetic alterations have occurred can help to assess the prognosis of disease. In tumors with a p53 mutation, loss of heterozygosity (LOH) of 17p was found in 95% of liver cancers.[9] These tumors are more often poorly differentiated and at a more advanced stage of disease at diagnosis.[9] Many tumor suppressor genes on several different chromosomes have been found to have LOH, including 17p (p53), 13q (RB1, retinoblastoma 1), 16p (AXIN1, axis inhibition protein 1), 9p (CDKN2A, cyclin-dependent kinase inhibitor 2A), and 6q (IGFR2R, insulin-like growth factor 2 receptor).[3] These changes can result in further inactivation of tumor suppressor genes, and signal the development of malignant cell development.

Another tumor suppressor gene, retinoblastoma gene Rb, which is located on chromosome 13q14, also appears to be involved in HCC development, with 43% of tumors showing alteration in this gene.[14] Inactivation of Rb contributes to tumor progression and metastasis in many patients rather than tumor initiation, and therefore tends to occur at more advanced stages of disease.[15]

LOH on chromosome 16, corresponding to tumor suppressor gene AXIN1, occurs in more than 50% of cases of HCC, and occurs more frequently in large, poorly differentiated, and metastatic liver cancers, but not early liver cancers.[3] This LOH also plays a role in tumor aggressiveness rather than tumor initiation.

DNA methylation is a key process in the epigenetic control of gene expression. Hypermethylation can lead to the inactivation of tumor suppressor genes and invasion-suppressor genes, and predisposes for allelic loss.[16,17] Hypomethylation of DNA increases the expression of oncogenes.[18] The level of DNA methylation is controlled by DNA methyltransferase, which transfers a methyl group from S-adenosylmethionine (SAMe) to the 5-position of cytidine. Increased expression of DNA methyltransferase is another step involved in human carcinogenesis.[19] Of interest, DNA methyltransferase mRNA levels are significantly higher in liver tissue showing chronic hepatitis or cirrhosis than in normal liver tissue, and are even higher in HCC cells.[20,21] This finding suggests that increased DNA methyltransferase expression is also a step that is responsible for hepatocarcinogenesis, especially in the early stages of disease.

Changes in DNA methylation are reversible, and correcting this aberrant process seems to be more feasible than correcting genetic alterations such as gene mutations. Reducing DNA methyltransferase activity has been shown, in experimental models, to inhibit tumor development, and thus may be a potential target for the prevention and subsequent treatment of HCC.[22,23]

Microsatellite instability also occurs in hepatocytes as a preneoplastic lesion. In the early preneoplastic stage, structural alterations in DNA occur slowly, but as dysplasia and neoplasia develop the rate of development of structural alterations and amount of alterations increase sharply.[24] Individual liver cancers often contain multiple allelic deletions and chromosomal losses and gains concurrently, which emphasize the complexity of HCC development. Through the progression of HCC from small, well-differentiated tumors to large, poorly differentiated, and metastatic tumors, further chromosomal alterations occur, resulting in a tumor with areas of diverse mixtures of genomic aberrations.[25]

GENETIC CLASSIFICATION OF HCC

Many genetic alterations accumulate during HCC development and may involve more than 20 different genes, with at least 3 and probably more different signaling pathways affected, as follows:

1. The Wnt pathway, a term derived from the genetic mutation in *Drosophila melanogaster* fruit fly, which produces a wingless phenotype. The *wingless* gene is a homolog to the *int-1* gene of vertebrates, which was originally identified near insertion sites for mammillary tumor virus in mice where virus integration causes amplification of *Wnt* genes. Wnt is a catenation of *wingless* and *int*.
2. The extracellular signal-related kinase, or ERK, pathway
3. The mammalian target of rapamycin, or mTOR, pathway.

The goal of discovering particular genetic and molecular alterations is to apply the knowledge to clinical management and treatment of HCC. As such, several different groups have attempted to first classify HCC into different groups based on the etiology, clinical characteristics, and aggressiveness, and then to identify the associated genetic alterations. For instance, Laurent-Puig and colleagues[26] analyzed a large number of genetic alterations in the same series of tumors, which enabled the definition of two mechanisms of HCC development.[26] These investigators found that LOH was the most frequent genetic alteration, and half the tumors exhibited LOH on more than 5 chromosome arms (Pathway I). In the other half of HCCs, tumors were chromosome stable, and the β-catenin mutation was the one most frequently observed (Pathway II). The tumors in Pathway I were predominantly from HBV-infected patients, were poorly differentiated, and had a poor prognosis. Pathway II tumors were generally non-HBV–infected, and were large and well differentiated.

Another genetic classification system was developed by Katoh and colleagues.[27] These researchers analyzed chromosomal alteration profiles, named cluster A and cluster B, that were associated with viral infection status, serum AFP levels, and presence of intrahepatic metastasis, as well as patient survival. All liver cancers had chromosomal alterations to varying degrees, but more frequent and pronounced alterations were observed in cluster A, which had a worse prognosis and poorer survival than cluster B (**Fig. 1**). In addition, subclusters were noted that may respond

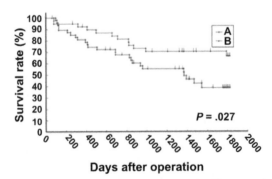

Fig. 1. Kaplan-Meier survival curve demonstrating survival difference after partial hepatectomy in patients with hepatocellular carcinoma, with stratification based on chromosomal alteration profiles. (*From* Katoh H, Ojima H, Kokubu A, et al. Genetically distinct and clinically relevant classification of hepatocellular carcinoma: putative therapeutic targets. Gastroenterology 2007;133:1480; with permission.)

well to different treatments, such as a subcluster A1 that was characterized by amplification on 1q and/or 6p, and which may respond to molecular inhibitors available for vascular endothelial growth factor (VEGF). A subcluster A3 showed a higher rate of 17q gain/amplification, and results of in vitro experiments show that these cell lines respond well to rapamycin, an mTOR inhibitor that directly inhibits the activity of S6 kinases.[28] These data suggest that molecular stratification of individual liver cancers into genetically homogeneous subclasses could provide an opportunity for developing optimal tailor-made therapeutic agents.

A third genetic classification system has been developed by Boyault and colleagues.[29] This classification also found 6 main subgroups based on genetic alterations in the tumors, The primary clinical determinant of class membership in this scheme is HBV infection, with other main determinants being genetic and epigenetic alterations, including chromosomal instability, β-catenin and p53 mutations, and parental imprinting.

More than 6 different groups have attempted to develop HCC classification systems based on genetic alteration of the tumor cells.[27–34] The fact that so many different groups have attempted to classify HCC highlights the importance and difficulty of understanding the genetic basis of hepatocellular carcinoma. All of the genetic classification systems have similar findings, notably that HBV infection, chromosomal instability, and changes in β-catenin and p53 seem to be the most important factors in tumor behavior. The classification systems can identify tumors that are at high risk for being poorly differentiated histologically, having vascular invasion, and having poor patient survival. With further investigation, these classification systems may be used to determine the targeted therapies that would be best suited to particular patients in each unique subclass of HCC.

NONTUMOR TISSUE AND PROGRESSION OF HCC

In addition to the genetic alterations in tumor tissue, when HCC is resected the genetic alterations in the tissue adjacent to the tumor also seems to affect survival. Hoshida and colleagues[35] analyzed 186 gene signatures, 113 of which were associated with a good prognosis and 73 with a poor prognosis. Early recurrence of tumor is associated with clinical and histopathological factors associated with the resected tumor, but late recurrence (more than 2 years after resection) is associated with the gene-expression signature of the nontumoral liver tissue. This finding indicates that late occurrences are likely to be new primary tumors rather than actual recurrences. The poor-prognosis signature contained gene sets that are associated with inflammation, such as interferon signaling, activation of nuclear factor kappa B (NF-κB), and signaling by TNF-α.

The impact of inflammation on the risk of metastasis remains unclear. Budhu and colleagues[36] investigated the impact of inflammatory changes on the risk of metastasis in HCC. Using two gene clusters, patients with metastatic disease were found to have a significantly different microenvironment in nontumor tissue compared with patients without metastatic disease. Unlike the findings of Hoshida and colleagues, where inflammation conferred a poor prognosis, the gene set investigated by Budhu showed that patients without metastasis seemed to have an increase in inflammatory cytokines compared with patients with metastatic disease. In fact, patients with metastatic disease had a global decrease in proinflammatory cytokines.

The use of nontumoral gene expression profiling may be used to identify patients at the highest risk of recurrence in order to target intensive follow-up or use of adjuvant therapies. However, there remain many unanswered questions as to the true genetic changes that will offer the best profiling available, and further research is needed before clinical tests that can be applied to patient care can be embraced.

MICRORNAS

miRNAs are small, noncoding RNA gene products that play key regulatory roles in mRNA translation and degradation.[37,38] In addition, each miRNA has the capability to regulate the expression of hundreds of coding genes and modulate multiple cellular pathways including those for proliferation, apoptosis, and stress response.[39] miRNAs are frequently produced from "fragile" DNA sites, common break points, or regions of amplification or LOH. Research has clearly shown that miRNAs play a significant role in human hepatocarcinogenesis.[40] Mature miRNAs are relatively stable; this characteristic may make miRNAs excellent molecular markers that may be used as a tool for further cancer diagnosis and prognosis. Budhu and colleagues[4] analyzed a 20-miRNA signature that could significantly predict metastatic (M) from nonmetastatic (NM) status with an accuracy of 76%. In this cohort of patients with early-stage HCC, the patients with M status had a 500-day survival rate of 38%, compared with 73% 500-day survival in patients with NM status. This outcome was related to the presence of metastatic disease and higher recurrence rate in patients with miRNA profiles consistent with M status. Ji and colleagues[41] investigated miRNA patterns in 455 resected HCC specimens, and found that overexpression of miRNA-26 was associated with overall survival, while lower expression was associated with response to interferon in the adjuvant setting. Other important miRNAs are miR-122 and miR-221, both of which are associated with a poor prognosis as well.[42,43] Many other miRNAs are being studied to elucidate their roles in liver cancer. The ability to understand the alterations in miRNA expression in liver cancer may be used in the future to accurately predict prognosis and potentially offer adjuvant therapy.

MOLECULAR PATHWAYS

HCC has traditionally been considered a chemotherapy-resistant tumor. However, in 2007, with the approval of sorafenib, for the first time a systemic targeted therapy was accepted as standard of care in the treatment of HCC.[44] In many cancers, specific drugs are indicated for specific subtypes of cancer. For instance, trastuzumab (Herceptin) is only effective in patients with breast cancer who express the erythroblastic leukemia virus oncogene homolog 2 (ERBB2), also known as the human epidermal growth factor (HER)-2 gene, as is imatinib (Gleevec) for patients with chronic myeloid leukemia resulting from the breakpoint cluster region (BCR)-Abelson leukemia virus (ABL) gene fusion.[45,46] With improved knowledge of specific pathways that are upregulated in HCC, targeted therapies for the subtypes of HCC will also be able to be employed in the future.

The Wnt/β-catenin signaling pathway, many other receptor tyrosine kinases activating downstream of Ras/Raf/MAPK or ERK kinase (MEK)/ERK signaling, and the Akt/mTOR signaling pathways have all been identified to be important in liver cancer, and would serve as markers of cancer activation and targets of therapy.[7,47–49] Other molecular signals are important in stimulating tumor signaling pathways, including epidermal growth factor (EGF), VEGF, IGF, fibroblast growth factor (FGF), and others (**Fig. 2**). These molecular signals are current targets of therapy that are in development for cancer treatment not only in liver cancer but in many other cancers as well (**Table 1**).

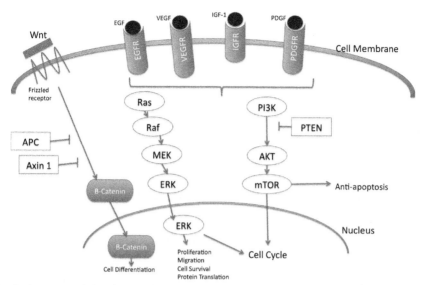

Fig. 2. Summary of signaling pathways and stimulating growth factors important in hepatocellular carcinoma. Cell membrane receptors: EGF, epidermal growth factor; IGF, insulin-like growth factor; PDGF, platelet-derived growth factor; VEGF, vascular endothelial growth factor. See text for explanation of the remaining acronyms.

Table 1
Current targeted therapies in clinical use or under investigation

Drug	Molecular Target	Cancer
Sorafenib	VEGFR, PDGFR, raf	Liver, renal
Brivinib	VEGFR2, FGFR	Liver, solid organ, colon
Erlotinib	EGFR	Liver, lung, pancreatic
Linifanib	VEGFR, PDGFR	Lung, liver
Sirolimus	mTOR	Liver, Kaposi's, renal
Sunitinib	VEGFR, PDGFR, cKIT	Renal, GIST
PI-88	FGF, VEGF	Lung, liver
Trastuzumab	HER2	Breast
Rituximab	CD20	Lymphoma
Imatinib	BCR-ABL, cKIT	CML, GIST
Cetuximab	EGFR	Colon, head/neck
Bevacizumab	VEGF	Colon, lung, breast
Dasatinib	BCR-ABL, src	CML
Lapatinib	HER2, EGFR	Breast

Abbreviations: BCR-ABL, breakpoint cluster region-Abelson leukemia virus; CML, chronic myelocytic leukemia; EGFR, epidermal growth factor receptor; FGF, fibroblast growth factor; FGFR, fibroblast growth factor receptor; GIST, gastrointestinal stromal tumor; HER2, human epidermal growth factor 2; mTOR, mammalian target of rapamycin; PDGFR, platelet-derived growth factor receptor; VEGF, vascular endothelial growth factor; VEGFR, vascular endothelial growth factor receptor.

RAt Sarcoma (Ras) Pathway

The Ras pathway is a dominant signaling pathway promoting cell proliferation and survival. The binding of growth factors (EGF, IGF-1, and platelet-derived growth factor [PDGF]) to their receptors activates Ras, which in turn activates Raf, MEK, and ERK. The phosphorylated ERK in the nucleus activates transcription factors such as c-Jun, which regulate the expression of genes involved in proliferation and survival.[50] Aberrant activation of the Ras/Raf pathway can occur at multiple different levels, and has been shown to be upregulated in multiple solid tumors. Newell and colleagues[51] performed extensive genomic analysis in a cohort of 351 tumor samples, and found several different methods of Ras signaling in HCC. Overexpression with H-Ras, DNA copy number gains with B-Raf, and aberrant methylation of key genes in this pathway are all different ways in which the Ras pathway may be upregulated in HCC. In addition, these investigators identified MAP2K4, which is a negative regulator of Ras signaling and may be a new candidate tumor suppressor gene in HCC.

Sorafenib is the first multikinase inhibitor approved for the treatment of nonresectable HCC. Sorafenib blocks the Ras/Raf pathway at multiple levels, and has been shown to improve survival in patients.[52] It is the first drug to follow the proof of concept that blocking upregulated pathways in hepatocellular carcinoma may improve tumor response to systemic therapy. The ability of sorafenib to increase survival of patients with liver cancer seems to be related to its ability to block the Ras/Raf pathway. In patients with liver cancer, ERK tissue concentrations are upregulated, and the level of upregulation seems to be related to the response of sorafenib.[53]

Wnt/β-Catenin Pathway

β-Catenin has a dual function in adhesion and Wnt signaling. It can acquire oncogenic activity as the result of mutations within its N-terminus.[54] These mutations result in loss of negative regulation of β-catenin, resulting in high cytoplasmic and nuclear levels, which then activate the transcription of Wnt target. In HCC, β-catenin mutations are found in 13% to 43% of tumors, and are mutated in some adenomas with a higher risk of malignant potential.[20,55–58] In addition, HCV has been shown to act as a Wnt ligand to upregulate cell signaling pathways, and causes mutations in β-catenin.[59,60]

The Wnt pathway may also be activated by several other methods. Inactivation of the tumor suppressor gene adenomatous polyposis coli or upregulation of the frizzled-7 receptor also causes activation of the pathway.[61,62] The AXIN1 gene noted earlier is also important in the Wnt pathway. It codes for a protein of a complex that inhibits the Wnt pathway, and mutation with subsequent inactivation of this gene results in activation of Wnt target genes.[63]

Activation of the Wnt signaling pathway has many carcinogenic properties, such as increased gene products responsible for proliferation (myc), activation of oncogenes (such as c-myc and cyclin D), antiapoptosis (survivin), invasion (matrix metalloproteinases [MMPs]), and angiogenesis (VEGF).[63] Thus, activation of Wnt not only regulates tissue development but also influences tumor growth and progression.

At present there are no therapies available that target this pathway; however, there are some molecules in preclinical trials that interfere with various locations in this pathway.[64,65]

Akt/mTOR Signaling

Another important signaling pathway in HCC is the Akt/mTOR signaling pathway. This pathway is frequently amplified and overexpressed in various cancers, and is activated in approximately half of patients with liver cancer.[66] Akt is a serine/threonine kinase that acts as a cytoplasmic regulator of numerous signals related to cell cycling (cyclin D1), cell survival (Mdm2/p53), cardiovascular homeostasis (endothelial nitric oxide synthase), and cell growth (mTOR).[63] The tumor suppressor phosphatase and tensin homolog (PTEN) is a negative regulator of the pathway, and its loss activates Akt.

mTOR complex 1 (mTORC1) is a downstream target of Akt that acts as a central regulator of cell growth and proliferation by activating S6 kinase, which regulates protein synthesis and allows progression from the G1 to the S phase of the cell cycle. Rather than activation through somatic mutations of the pathway components, aberrant pathway signaling is associated with activation of IGF and/or EGF.[67]

Gene expression studies in human HCC tissue have found dysregulation of this pathway to be important in tumor progression.[67] EGF was upregulated, particularly in advanced HCC, and the tumor suppressor PTEN was downregulated in advanced HCC. Also, a subgroup of patients had very high upregulation of IGF-2. In addition, there is a clear shift of mTOR localization in cirrhotic tissue and HCC. In cirrhosis, staining of mTOR is predominantly membranous, whereas in HCC it is typically located in the cytoplasm. Lastly, mTOR positivity is a negative prognostic factor in HCC, with these patients having increased tumor multinodularity and decreased time to recurrence after treatment.

Blocking the mTOR cascade is thought to be a therapeutic option in HCC. mTOR inhibitors, such as sirolimus or everolimus, may decrease tumor growth and expand survival. Potentially combining these drugs with epidermal growth factor receptor (EGFR) inhibitors may allow blockade of the signaling pathway at many levels, which could potentially offer synergy in treatments. Such has been shown in mouse models to be effective in vivo, and has been confirmed in small trials in humans.[68] Larger human trials are under way.[67] In addition, the combination of sorafenib to block the Ras/Raf pathway, and sirolimus to block the mTOR pathway, may be another effective way to treat liver cancer.[51,69] mTOR may also interact with other pathways in complex ways. Recently it was found that mTOR inhibition may result in MAPK activation[70]; this suggests that tumors are finding "escape mechanisms" for pathway blockades, which may form the mechanism for tumor resistance to treatments. The understanding of the pathway interactions may allow planning for treatment regimens with combination therapies similar to treatment of resistant-prone viruses.

IGF

IGF is increasingly being recognized as playing a key role in liver cancer signaling. IGF has a major role in fetal development, cell proliferation, differentiation, growth, and apoptosis, and has been implicated in multiple malignancies. IGF-1 stimulates growth through cellular proliferation and inhibition of apoptosis.[71] IGF-2 is overexpressed up to tenfold above normal in 20% to 30% of human liver cancers.[6] IGFR-2 receptor is a tumor suppressor, and is downregulated in a subset of liver cancers.

The importance of IGF-1 and IGF-2 is highlighted by the rising incidence of liver cancer in patients with insulin resistance, diabetes mellitus, and nonalcoholic steatohepatitis,[72] as discussed in detail in the article by Siddique and Kowdley elsewhere in this issue. Hyperinsulinemia upregulates the production of IGF-1 and activated insulin receptor substrate (IRS)-1, which is upregulated in liver cancer and is involved in cytokine signaling pathways. In addition, IGF-1 activates the Akt/mTOR pathway which, as discussed earlier, is important in liver cancer.[73]

EGFR

EGFR is an active target for several oncogenic chemotherapeutics. It may be attacked extracellularly through the use of antibodies that block its receptor, or intracellularly with binding of the receptor's tyrosine kinase domain.[74] Targeting EGFR has been used in many solid tumor treatments, including cancer of the colon and rectum, head and neck, lung, and pancreas. EGFR is overexpressed in 40% to 70% of liver cancers, and activation of the receptor has been implicated in pathogenesis of HCC.[75,76] EGFR activation results in signaling through both the Ras pathway and mTOR pathways already discussed, and is an important targeting receptor in HCC.

Angiogenesis/VEGF Pathway

HCC is a highly vascular tumor, and development of new blood vessels is key to allowing progression of disease. Avascular tumors only grow to a certain size and then undergo regression if their metabolic demands are not met. Angiogenesis depends on activation, proliferation, and migration of endothelial cells to create a functional system of blood vessels.[77] The main factors that stimulate angiogenesis are hypoxia and inflammation. Hypoxia induces expression of hypoxia-inducible factor 1 (HIF1) and IGF-2, both of which stimulate expression of VEGF and other growth factors such as FGF, hepatocyte growth factor, and TGF.[78] Endothelial cells proliferate in response to growth factors secreted by themselves (autocrine stimulation) or by surrounding cells (paracrine stimulation). In the development of pathologic angiogenesis such as happens in tumor formation in the liver, capillarized vascular structures develop instead of the sinusoidal vascular pattern that occurs in normal tissue. This process hampers the physiologic interchange of oxygen and metabolic factors, which further stimulates hypoxia and tissue injury. It also impairs the effective delivery of therapeutic drugs to the tumor.[79] Therefore, development of pharmaceutical interventions may be directed at inhibiting progression of angiogenesis as well as facilitating the transcellular route of delivery.

The importance of angiogenesis in tumor development is highlighted by the knowledge that VEGF levels correlate with vascular invasion and metastasis.[80,81] In addition, FGF levels seem to correlate with advanced tumor stage, vascular invasion, and postoperative relapse.[82] In patients undergoing transarterial chemoembolization (TACE), VEGF levels also correlate with response rate.[83] Patients who have VEGF levels above the mean have a high rate of nonresponse to TACE, with residual tumor activity of greater than 30%. In addition, it has been found that VEGF levels significantly increase in the 24 hours after TACE and decrease after 48 to 72 hours. Therefore, VEGF could be used in monitoring response to treatment, and potentially could be a target for adjuvant treatments such as sorafenib, in patients undergoing transarterial therapy when used as a neoadjuvant medication.

TGF-β

TGF-β is a cytokine that controls many aspects of cell biology, including proliferation, migration, adhesion, differentiation, and modification of the cellular microenvironment.[7] Genetic alterations of TGF-β have been reported in cancer, but the implications are complex, as TGF-β can exhibit both tumor-suppressive and oncogenic properties.[84–86] TGF-β acts as a tumor suppressor at the early stages of tumor development by inhibiting proliferation and inducing apoptosis, but as carcinogenesis progresses TGF-β action changes and can contribute to tumor progression. When cell lines exhibit the late TGF-β signature, they possess a more invasive phenotype and have worse prognosis with a shorter patient survivals.[7]

Because TGF-β activity changes as cancer progresses, it may be possible to develop a gene-expression signature that can help offer prognosis and staging for patients with liver cancer.

FUTURE THERAPIES

In understanding the complex molecular and genetic changes that occur in hepatocellular carcinoma development and progression, it may help to develop future therapies for HCC. At diagnosis, most patients are not candidates for curative therapies, and would benefit from individualized analysis of their tumor genotype and phenotype. With further research, one can envision using therapy that targets an individual's specific tumor type by focusing narrowly on the dominant or codominant tumor-signaling pathway. The hope is that combination therapy will provide greater survival and potentially long-term remission. Thus, new drugs need to be developed that target the single or multiply-activated pathways. Safely performed liver and tumor biopsies can identify a patient's particular tumor fingerprint. Pathways may be blocked vertically, and at more than one location in a particular pathway in this future scenario, which may lead to high-level blockade and prevent tumor resistance via use of alternative "escape" pathways. By contrast, horizontal blockade refers to the use of different drugs targeting different parallel pathways, which may limit the tumor cell's ability to develop resistance to therapy. Horizontal blockade may also limit overlapping toxicities. All of these treatment strategies need to be investigated further to determine the best efficacy and least toxicity of the regimens.

In this article the authors review in detail the molecular and genomic changes that occur in liver cancer. This topic remains a complex one, and discoveries thus far have only scratched the surface. Understanding the molecular and genomic changes that are active in HCC has already allowed targeted therapies to be developed and studied, and will further advance the treatment of liver cancer, allowing for more personalized medicine that may translate into increased survival for patients.

REFERENCES

1. Parkin DM, Bray F, Ferlay J, et al. Estimating the world cancer burden: Globocan 2000. Int J Cancer 2001;94:153–6.
2. Hui AM, Makuuchi M. Molecular basis of multistep hepatocarcinogenesis: genetic and epigenetic events. Scand J Gastroenterol 1999;8:737–42.
3. Laurent-Puig P, Zucman-Rossi J. Genetics of hepatocellular tumors. Oncogene 2006;25:3778–86.
4. Budhu A, Jia HL, Forgues M, et al. Identification of metastasis-related micro-RNAs in hepatocellular carcinoma. Hepatology 2008;47:897–907.
5. Thorgeirsson SS, Grisham JW. Molecular pathogenesis of human hepatocellular carcinoma. Nat Genet 2002;31:339–46.
6. Tovar V, Alsinet C, Villanueva A, et al. IGF activation in a molecular subclass of hepatocellular carcinoma and pre-clinical efficacy of IGF-1R blockage. J Hepatol 2010;52:550–9.
7. Coulouarn C, Factor VM, Thorgeirsson SS. Transforming growth factor-beta gene expression signature in mouse hepatocytes predicts clinical outcome in human cancer. Hepatology 2008;47:2059–67.
8. Hoshida Y, Toffanin S, Lackenmayer A, et al. Molecular classification and novel targets in hepatocellular carcinoma: recent advancements. Semin Liver Dis 2010;30:35–51.

9. Oda T, Tsuda H, Scarpa A, et al. p53 gene mutation spectrum in hepatocellular carcinoma. Cancer Res 1992;52(22):6358–64.

10. Feitelson MA, Zhu M, Duan LX, et al. Hepatitis Bx antigen and p53 are associated in vitro and in liver tissues from patients with primary hepatocellular carcinoma. Oncogene 1993;8:1109–17.

11. Tanaka S, Toh Y, Adachi E, et al. Tumor progression in hepatocellular carcinoma may be mediated by p53 mutation. Cancer Res 1993;53:2884–7.

12. Tsuda H, Hirohashi S, Shimosato Y, et al. Low incidence of point mutation of c-Ki-ras and N-ras oncogenes in human hepatocellular carcinoma. Jpn J Cancer Res 1989;80(3):196–9.

13. Boix L, Rosa JL, Ventura F, et al. c-met mRNA expression in human hepatocellular carcinoma. Hepatology 1994;19(1):88–91.

14. Zhang X, Xu HJ, Murakami Y, et al. Deletions of chromosome 13q, mutations in retinoblastoma 1, and retinoblastoma protein state in human hepatocellular carcinoma. Cancer Res 1994;54:4177–82.

15. Weinberg RA. The retinoblastoma protein and cell cycle control. Cell 1995;81:323–30.

16. Herman JG, Merlo A, Mao L, et al. Inactivation of the CDKN2/p16/MTS1 gene is frequently associated with aberrant DNA methylation in all common human cancers. Cancer Res 1995;55:4525–30.

17. Yoshiura K, Kanai Y, Ochiai A, et al. Silencing of the E-cadherin invasion-suppressor gene by CpG methylation in human carcinomas. Proc Natl Acad Sci U S A 1995;92:7416–9.

18. Cheah MS, Wallace CD, Hoffman RM. Hypomethylation of DNA in human cancer cells: a site-specific change in the c-myc oncogene. J Natl Cancer Inst 1984;73:1057–65.

19. El-Deiry WS, Nelkin BD, Celano P, et al. High expression of the DNA methyltransferase gene characterizes human neoplastic cells and progression stages of colon cancer. Proc Natl Acad Sci U S A 1991;88:3470–4.

20. Sun L, Hui AM, Kanai Y, et al. Increased DNA methyltransferase expression is associated with an early stage of human hepatocarcinogenesis. Jpn J Cancer Res 1998;88:1165–70.

21. Kanai Y, Hui AM, Sun L, et al. DNA hypermethylation at the D17S5 locus and reduced HIC-1 mRNA expression are associated with hepatocarcinogenesis. Hepatology 1999;29:703–9.

22. MacLeod AR, Szyf M. Expression of antisense to DNA methyltransferase mRNA induces DNA methylation and inhibits tumorigenesis. J Biol Chem 1995;270:8037–43.

23. Ramchandani S, MacLeod AR, Pinard M, et al. Inhibition of tumorigenesis by a cytosine DNA, methyltransferase, antisense oligodeoxynucleotide. Proc Natl Acad Sci U S A 1997;94:684–9.

24. Salvucci M, Lemoine A, Saffroy R, et al. Microsatellite instability in European hepatocellular carcinoma. Oncogene 1999;18(1):181–7.

25. Kazachkov Y, Yoffe B, Khaoustov VI, et al. Microsatellite instability in human hepatocellular carcinoma: relationship to p53 abnormalities. Liver 1998;18(3):156–61.

26. Laurent-Puig P, Legoix P, Bluteau O, et al. Genetic alterations associated with hepatocellular carcinomas define distinct pathways of hepatocarcinogenesis. Gastroenterology 2001;120(7):1763–73.

27. Katoh H, Ojima H, Kokubu A, et al. Genetically distinct and clinically relevant classification of hepatocellular carcinoma: putative therapeutic targets. Gastroenterology 2007;133:1475–86.

28. Sabatini DM. mTOR and cancer: insights into a complex relationship. Nat Rev Cancer 2006;6:729–34.
29. Boyault S, Richman DS, de Reynies A, et al. Transcriptome classification of HCC is related to gene alterations and to new therapeutic targets. Hepatology 2007; 45:42–52.
30. Lee J-S, Chu I-S, Heo J, et al. Classification and prediction of survival in hepato-cellular carcinoma by gene expression profiling. Hepatology 2004;40:667–76.
31. Thorgeirsson SS, Lee J-S, Grisham JW. Functional genomics of hepatocellular carcinoma. Hepatology 2006;43:S145–50.
32. Lee JS, Thorgeirsson SS. Comparative and integrative functional genomics of HCC. Oncogene 2006;25:3801–9.
33. Katoh H, Shibata T, Kokubu A, et al. Epigenetic instability and chromosomal insta-bility in hepatocellular carcinoma. Am J Pathol 2006;168:1375–84.
34. Cillo U, Bassanello M, Vitale A, et al. The critical issue of hepatocellular carci-noma prognostic classification: which is the best tool available? J Hepatol 2004;40:124–31.
35. Hoshida Y, Villanueva A, Kobayashi M, et al. Gene expression in fixed tissues and outcome in hepatocellular carcinoma. N Engl J Med 2008;359(19):1995–2004.
36. Budhu A, Forgues M, Ye Q-H, et al. Prediction of venous metastases, recurrence, and prognosis in hepatocellular carcinoma based on a unique immune response signature of the liver microenvironment. Cancer Cell 2006;10:99–111.
37. Lagos-Quintana M, Rauhut R, Lendeckel W, et al. Identification of novel genes encoding for small expressed RNAs. Science 2001;294:853–8.
38. Lau NC, Lim LP, Weinstein EG, et al. An abundant class of tiny RNAs with prob-ably regulatory roles in *Caenorhabditis elegans*. Science 2001;294:858–62.
39. Ambros V. MicroRNA pathways in flies and worms: growth, death, fat, stress, and timing. Cell 2003;113:673–6.
40. Gregory RJ, Shiekhattar R. MicroRNA biogenesis and cancer. Cancer Res 2005; 65:3509–12.
41. Ji J, Shi J, Budhu A, et al. MicroRNA expression, survival, and response to inter-feron in liver cancer. N Engl J Med 2009;361(15):1437–47.
42. Coulouarn C, Factor VM, Anderon JB, et al. Loss of miRNA-122 expression in liver cancer correlates with suppression of the hepatic phenotype and gain of meta-static properties. Oncogene 2009;28(40):3526–36.
43. Gramantieri L, Ferracin M, Fornari F, et al. Cyclin G1 is a target of miRNA-122a, a microRNA frequently down-regulated in human hepatocellular carcinoma. Cancer Res 2007;67(13):6092–9.
44. National Comprehensive Cancer Network, Inc. The NCCN Clinical Practice Guidelines in Oncology. Hepatobiliary Cancers (Version 2.2010). Available at: http://www.nccn.org. Accessed November 28, 2010.
45. Vogel CL, Cobleigh MA, Tripathy D, et al. Efficacy and safety of trastuzumab as a single agent in first-line treatment of HER2-overexpressing metastatic breast cancer. J Clin Oncol 2002;20:719–26.
46. le Coutre P, Mologni L, Cleris L, et al. In vivo eradication of human BCR/ABL posi-tive leukemia cells with an ABL kinase inhibitor. J Natl Cancer Inst 1999;91(2): 163–8.
47. Branda M, Wands JR. Signal transduction cascades and hepatitis B and C related hepatocellular carcinoma. Hepatology 2006;43:891–902.
48. Lee JS, Heo J, Libbrecht L, et al. A novel prognostic subtype of human hepato-cellular carcinoma derived from hepatic progenitor cells. Nat Med 2006;12: 410–6.

49. Chiang DY, Villanueva A, Hoshida Y, et al. Focal gains of VEGFA and molecular classification of hepatocellular carcinoma. Cancer Res 2008;68(16):6779–88.

50. Dhillon AS, Hagan S, Rath O, et al. MAP kinase signaling pathways in cancer. Oncogene 2007;26:3279–90.

51. Newell P, Toffanin S, Villanueva A, et al. Ras pathway activation in hepatocellular carcinoma and anti-tumoral effect of combined sorafenib and rapamycin in vivo. J Hepatol 2009;51:725–33.

52. Llovet JM, Ricci S, Mazzaferro V, et al. Sorafenib in advanced hepatocellular carcinoma. N Engl J Med 2008;359(4):378–90.

53. Abou-Alfa GK, Schwartz L, Ricci S, et al. Phase II study of sorafenib in patients with advanced hepatocellular carcinoma. J Clin Oncol 2006;24(26):4293–300.

54. Morin PJ, Sparks AB, Korinek V, et al. Activation of beta-catenin-Tcf signaling in colon cancer by mutations in beta-catenin or APC. Science 1997;275(5307):1787–90.

55. de la Coste A, Romagnolo B, Billuart P, et al. Somatic mutations of the beta-catenin gene are frequent in mouse and human hepatocellular carcinomas. Proc Natl Acad Sci U S A 1998;95:8847–51.

56. Hsu HC, Jeng YM, Mao TL, et al. Beta-catenin mutations are associated with a subset of low-stage hepatocellular carcinoma negative for hepatitis B virus and with favorable prognosis. Am J Pathol 2000;157:763–70.

57. Huang H, Fujii H, Sankila A, et al. Beta-catenin mutations are frequent in human hepatocellular carcinomas associated with hepatitis C infection. Am J Pathol 1999;155:1795–801.

58. Legoix P, Bluteau O, Bayer J, et al. Beta-catenin mutations in hepatocellular carcinoma correlate with a low rate of loss of heterozygosity. Oncogene 1999;18:4044–6.

59. Fukutomi T, Zhou Y, Kawai S, et al. Hepatitis C virus core protein stimulates hepatocyte growth: correlation with upregulation of wnt-1 expression. Hepatology 2005;41(5):1096–105.

60. Devereux TR, Stern MC, Flake GP, et al. CTNNB1 mutations and beta-catenin protein accumulation in human hepatocellular carcinomas associated with high exposure to aflatoxin B1. Mol Carcinog 2001;31(2):68–73.

61. Breuhahn K, Longerich T, Schirmacher P. Dysregulation of growth factor signaling in human hepatocellular carcinoma. Oncogene 2006;25:3787–800.

62. Villanueva A, Newell P, Chiang DY, et al. Genomics and signaling pathways in hepatocellular carcinoma. Semin Liver Dis 2007;27:55–76.

63. Roberts LR, Gores GJ. Hepatocellular carcinoma: molecular pathways and new therapeutic targets. Semin Liver Dis 2005;25:212–25.

64. Dihlmann S, von Knebel Doeberitz M. Wnt/beta-catenin pathway as a molecular target for future anti-cancer therapeutics. Int J Cancer 2005;113:515–24.

65. Emami KH, Nguyen C, Ma H, et al. A small molecule inhibitor of beta-catenin/CREB-binding protein transcription. Proc Natl Acad Sci U S A 2004;101:12682–7.

66. Llovet JM, Bruix J. Novel advancements in the management of hepatocellular carcinoma in 2008. J Hepatol 2008;48:S20–37.

67. Villanueva A, Chiang DK, Newell P, et al. Pivotal role of mTOR signaling in hepatocellular carcinoma. Gastroenterology 2008;135:1972–83.

68. Rizell M, Andersson M, Cahlin C, et al. Effects of the mTOR inhibitor sirolimus in patients with hepatocellular and cholangiocellular cancer. Int J Clin Oncol 2008;13(1):66–70.

69. Wang Z, Zhou J, Fan J, et al. Effect of rapamycin alone and in combination with sorafenib in an orthotopic model of human hepatocellular carcinoma. Clin Cancer Res 2008;14(16):5124–30.

70. Carracedo A, Ma L, Teruya-Feldstein J, et al. Inhibition of mTORC1 leads to MAPK pathway activation through a PI3K-dependent feedback loop in human cancer. J Clin Invest 2008;118:3065–74.
71. Starley BQ, Calcagno CJ, Harrison SA. Nonalcoholic fatty liver disease and hepatocellular carcinoma: a weighty connection. Hepatology 2010;51:1820–32.
72. El Serag HB, Rudolph KL. Hepatocellular carcinoma: epidemiology and molecular carcinogenesis. Gastroenterology 2007;132:2557–76.
73. Stickel F, Hellerbrand C. Non-alcoholic fatty liver disease as a risk factor for hepatocellular carcinoma: mechanisms and implications. Gut 2010;59:1303–7.
74. Llovet JM, Bruix J. Molecular targeted therapies in hepatocellular carcinoma. Hepatology 2008;48:1312–27.
75. Buckley AF, Burgart LJ, Sahai V, et al. Epidermal growth factor receptor expression and gene copy number in conventional hepatocellular carcinoma. Am J Clin Pathol 2008;129:245–51.
76. Schiffer E, Housset C, Cacheux W, et al. Gefitinib, an EGFR inhibitor, prevents hepatocellular carcinoma development in the rat liver with cirrhosis. Hepatology 2005;41:307–14.
77. Semela D, Dufour JF. Angiogenesis and hepatocellular carcinoma. J Hepatol 2004;41(5):864–80.
78. Kim KR, Moon HE, Kim KW. Hypoxia-induced angiogenesis in human hepatocellular carcinoma. J Mol Med 2002;80(11):703–14.
79. Sanz-Cameno O, Trapero-Marugan M, Chaparro M, et al. Angiogenesis: from chronic liver inflammation to hepatocellular carcinoma. J Oncol 2010;2010: 272170.
80. Yamaguchi R, Yano H, Iemura A, et al. Expression of vascular endothelial growth factor in human hepatocellular carcinoma. Hepatology 1998;28:68–77.
81. Nyun Park Y, Park C. Increased expression of vascular endothelial growth factors and angiogenesis in the early stage of multistep hepatocarcinogenesis. Arch Pathol Lab Med 2000;124:1061–5.
82. Poon RT, Ng IO, Lau C, et al. Correlation of serum basic fibroblastic growth factor levels with clinicopathologic features and postoperative recurrence in hepatocellular carcinoma. Am J Surg 2001;182:298–304.
83. Sergio A, Cristofori C, Cardin R, et al. Transcatheter arterial chemoembolization (TACE) in hepatocellular carcinoma (HCC): the role of angiogenesis and invasiveness. Am J Gastroenterol 2008;103:914–21.
84. Derynck R, Akhurst RJ, Balmain A. TGF-beta signaling in tumor suppression and cancer progression. Nat Genet 2001;29:117–29.
85. Pardali K, Moustakas A. Actions of TGF-beta as tumor suppressor and prometastatic factor in human cancer. Biochim Biophys Acta 2007;1775:21–62.
86. Siegel PM, Massague J. Cytostatic and apoptotic actions of TGF-beta in homeostasis and cancer. Nat Rev Cancer 2003;3:807–21.

Hepatocellular Carcinoma: Screening and Staging

Morris Sherman, MB BCh, PhD, FRCP(C)

KEYWORDS

- Hepatocellular carcinoma • Screening for HCC
- Staging of HCC • BCLC staging system

The incidence of hepatocellular carcinoma (HCC) is increasing in Western countries, and remains high in the East, making HCC one of the most common cancers. The tools are now available to diagnose this cancer early, stage it in a uniform manner, and apply treatments that are appropriate to each stage. In addition, with early detection a high rate of cure is possible, whereas in the past, with the ability to find small tumors, cure rates were very low. Thus is it important to manage patients at risk for HCC appropriately so that early detection is possible, and that stage-appropriate treatment can be offered when HCC develops.

SCREENING FOR HEPATOCELLULAR CARCINOMA
Objectives, Requirements, and Pitfalls

Conventionally, the term "screening" refers to a single test to identify a disease that is asymptomatic at the time of performing the test (eg, urine testing all newborns for phenylketonuria). In oncology, the term is used in connection with tests to detect preclinical cancer (eg, breast cancer screening, or precancerous lesions that have a high probability to develop into cancer, such as cervical dysplasia). The term "surveillance" in oncology is used to refer to tests done to detect residual or recurrent cancer after initial treatment. The terms have been used slightly differently with regard to hepatocellular carcinoma. Surveillance is the term that has been applied to the provision of recurrent testing to detect preclinical cancer. In this article, the more usual term, "screening," will be used.

Screening is much more than the application of a test to detect preclinical cancer. To be done properly and to have any possibility of reducing overall mortality from the disease, screening for HCC must include proper identification of the at-risk population and application of the most sensitive and specific tests to that population at the appropriate intervals. These tests must be able to detect HCCs at a stage when treatment is

Department of Medicine, University of Toronto, Toronto General Hospital, 585 University Avenue, Toronto, ON M5G 2N2, Canada
E-mail address: morris.sherman@uhn.on.ca

Clin Liver Dis 15 (2011) 323–334
doi:10.1016/j.cld.2011.03.003
1089-3261/11/$ – see front matter © 2011 Elsevier Inc. All rights reserved.

highly likely to produce a cure. This requires that there is also a validated program of follow-up of abnormal findings that maximizes the likelihood of detecting a false-positive screening test before the institution of treatment, and minimizes the number of tests required to confirm the diagnosis if HCC is present. Finally, there must be appropriate treatment available that has a high likelihood of producing a cure. There is no point in providing HCC screening if treatment is ineffective.

The objective of a screening program for cancer must be to reduce mortality from that cancer. Strictly speaking, this can be conclusively demonstrated only in a randomized controlled trial in which a screening group is compared with an unscreened group. There is one such trial of HCC screening, which will be discussed later in this article.[1] Although it might seem self-evident that early detection would decrease mortality, there are a number of reasons why this might not be so, and these are related to the criteria for the establishment of a proper screening program, as described in the previous paragraph. First, if a population is screened that has a very low risk of cancer, it will be very difficult to show that overall mortality is decreased significantly compared with an unscreened group. Thus, in the context of HCC screening, this means excluding patients at low risk for HCC from screening. Second, if the screening test is inadequately sensitive and specific, or the test does not detect disease early enough, ie, at a stage when cure is highly likely, mortality will likely not be affected. Clearly, if treatment does not cure disease, or at least prolong survival, screening will be ineffective. Finally, overdiagnosis, that is, the identification of preclinical lesions that will never develop into life-threatening cancer, if prevalent, will also mean that the reduction in overall mortality might also be insignificant. We examine all of these issues in turn.

The literature on HCC screening is fraught with studies that do not adhere to these principles, and which therefore make claims to benefit from screening that are not supported by the data. To properly assess the benefit of screening, sources of bias must be excluded. These include lead-time bias, in which the apparent increase in survival time is simply attributable to earlier diagnosis and the intervention has no effect, and length bias, in which slow-growing tumors are more likely to be identified and successfully treated than more rapidly growing tumors. Another bias is ascertainment bias, in which the test used to confirm the presence of HCC is not sufficiently specific, with the result that some lesions are called cancer when they are not.

Definition of the At-Risk Population

The relationship between chronic liver disease and the development of HCC is well known and needs no elaboration. However, it is equally well recognized that not all patients who fall in the at-risk population will develop HCC, and in many patients HCC develops long after the onset of risk factor (eg, cirrhosis). The challenge is twofold. The first is to identify the at-risk population, and then to determine the incidence of HCC at which screening becomes effective in that population. This second criterion is important, because there is a spectrum of HCC risk generally across any population. Even people without liver disease have a small, but finite risk of developing HCC. The question is what level of risk is high enough to warrant screening, and how should this cutoff be determined. Conventionally, an intervention is thought to be effective if it enhances life in the population by at least 3 months. If this increased survival can be achieved at a cost of less than about $50,000/life year gained, the intervention is considered cost-effective. The role that this type of analysis plays in identifying the population that should undergo HCC screening will be discussed later.

The at-risk populations can be broadly defined as those who have liver diseases associated with the development of HCC. These include cirrhosis of any etiology, and precirrhotic hepatitis C, probably precirrhotic steatohepatitis, and precirrhotic chronic hepatitis B or hepatitis B with regressed cirrhosis.[2] Cost-efficacy analysis has been used to attempt to determine the cutoff HCC incidence that makes screening worthwhile. There are now about 10 cost-efficacy analyses of screening for HCC.[3–12] The different analyses differ in the starting populations. Some included only hepatitis C, others included all cirrhosis. There is a single analysis of screening in hepatitis B. The analyses differ in the structure of the model used, the intervention applied, and the assumptions about the sensitivity and specificity of the surveillance tests. However, they almost all find that some methods of providing screening are cost-effective (eg, ultrasonography), whereas others (computed tomography [CT] scan or magnetic resonance imaging [MRI]) are not. Analysis suggested that among those with hepatitis B, if the risk of HCC was greater than about 0.2% per year, screening was effective and cost-effective.[13] Among patients with cirrhosis of other etiologies, screening became effective and cost-effective once the HCC incidence exceeded 1.5% to 2.0% per year.[4,9] The causes of cirrhosis that are associated with an incidence of 1.5% to 2.0% or higher are listed in **Table 1**.[2] Hepatitis B is different from other causes of cirrhosis because patients with hepatitis B frequently have better liver function than those with other forms of cirrhosis when the HCC develops. This means patients with hepatitis B are more likely to be able to undergo curative therapy. Thus, the threshold incidence for providing surveillance is lower than in diseases where cirrhosis is more frequent. However, because risk increases with age, in the noncirrhotic hepatitis B population the recommendation is to start screening men at about age 40 and women at about age 50.

Table 1
Groups for whom HCC surveillance is recommended

Population Group	Threshold Incidence for Efficacy of Surveillance (>25 LYG) (%/year)	Incidence of HCC
Asian male hepatitis B carriers older than 40 y	0.2	0.4%–0.6%/y
Asian female hepatitis B carriers older than 50 y	0.2	0.3%–0.6%/y
Hepatitis B carrier with family history of HCC	0.2	Incidence higher than without family history
African/North American Blacks with chronic hepatitis B	0.2	HCC occurs at a younger age
Cirrhotic hepatitis B carriers	0.2–1.5	3%–8%/y
Hepatitis C cirrhosis	1.5	3%–5%/y
Stage 4 primary biliary cirrhosis	1.5	3%–5%/y
Alcoholic cirrhosis	1.5	Unknown, but probably >1.5%/y
NAFLD cirrhosis	1.5	Unknown, but probably >1.5%/y
Genetic hemochromatosis and cirrhosis	1.5	3%–4%/y
Alpha 1-antitrypsin deficiency and cirrhosis	1.5	Unknown, but probably >1.5%/y
Other cirrhosis	1.5	Unknown

Abbreviations: HCC, hepatocellular carcinoma; LYG, life years gained; NAFLD, non-alcoholic fatty liver disease.

Screening is not recommended for noncirrhotic patients with liver disease other than hepatitis B, in whom the HCC incidence is lower than 1.5% to 2.0%, such as pre-cirrhotic hepatitis C or noncirrhotic steatohepatitis.[2] This is because these are populations in which screening will likely not lead to an overall reduction in mortality. That does not mean that individual practitioners who wish to provide screening should not do so; however, they should be aware that the costs are not justified by standard criteria. Those practitioners who do not provide screening for these groups should not be legally liable should HCC develop.

Even within the groups for whom screening is recommended, it is recognized that only a minority will develop cancer. There have been studies that have provided tools to more accurately identify patients who are at risk for HCC than the broad definitions we currently use. On the one hand, the results of these studies have the potential to increase the size of the screened group by identifying patients who do not meet current criteria but who are nonetheless at risk. On the other hand, they decrease the size of the current pool of individuals needing screening by documenting that some members of the group are at much lower risk than initially thought.

The first study evaluated the incidence of cancer in a moderately large hepatitis B–infected cohort in Hong Kong and determined risk factors that were associated with the development of cancer,[13] namely male gender, increasing age, higher hepatitis B virus (HBV) DNA levels in (log copies/mL), core promoter mutations, and the presence of cirrhosis. These factors were combined to develop a 5-year and 10-year score for the risk of developing HCC. This risk score requires external validation. Furthermore, the formula is cumbersome, and includes factors that may not be readily available, such as presence of precore mutations. There are 2 other similar analyses, one in hepatitis B, using data from the REVEAL study,[14] and one in hepatitis C, using data from the HALT-C study.[15] The HALT-C study analysis demonstrated that older age, African American race, lower platelet count, higher alkaline phosphatase, and esophageal varices were significant risk factors for HCC. These were combined to identify 3 groups at low, medium, and high risk of HCC.[15] This also needs validation and is not ready for use. In contrast, the analysis from the REVEAL study,[14,16] which came from Taiwan, has been validated, at least in other similar populations in Asia (Japan, Hong Kong, and China), and is now applicable to similar populations in the United States and Canada. This study remains to be validated in white and in those infected with hepatitis B genotypes other than B and C. This analysis led to the development of 3 models. The simplest model included age, gender, alcohol consumption, a family history of HCC, HBeAg status, and alanine aminotransferase. A more complex model included all these variables plus HBV DNA concentration. Finally, the most complex model includes all the previous factors plus HBV genotype (either B or C).[14] These models perform well compared with actual risk of HCC. Furthermore, they have been depicted graphically in the form of a nomogram (**Fig. 1**) that resembles the Framingham heart attack risk nomogram, thus making it easy for family physicians to use.[14]

Screening Tests

The next important factor is the screening test. Here it is important to recognize what we are asking the screening test to do. The test must find HCC at a stage when treatment is likely to be curative. Essentially, for HCC this means that the lesion should be single and smaller than about 3 cm, ideally smaller than 2 cm. This is because whatever treatment is applied, the likelihood of cure starts to decrease once the tumors are multiple or get larger than about 2.0 to 2.5 cm. Sala and colleagues[17] have shown that the likelihood of cure when radiofrequency ablation is the treatment used is highest

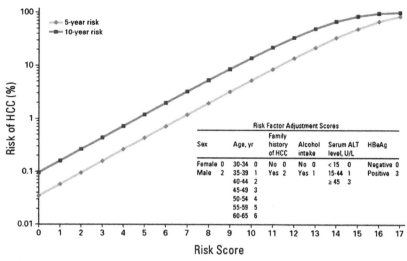

Fig. 1. Example of nomogram for assessing risk of hepatocellular carcinoma in patients with chronic hepatitis B. (*From* Yang HI, Sherman M, Su J, et al. Nomograms for risk of hepatocellular carcinoma in patients with chronic hepatitis B virus infection. J Clin Oncol 2010;28:2437–44; with permission.)

with lesions smaller than 2 cm, and treatment efficacy decreases substantially when there are multiple lesions or the lesion size exceeds 2 cm.[17] Similar data exist for the efficacy of resection. Thus, screening protocols that only identify patients with tumors larger than 3 cm are unlikely to decrease disease-related mortality. Many of the existing studies on screening have ignored this, particularly those that evaluate the use of serologic markers.

Studies that have attempted to evaluate the efficacy of screening tests have mostly been studied in patients who were known to have HCC. This is equivalent to determining the performance characteristics of the test as a diagnostic test. However, the performance characteristics of a screening test will be very different when the test is evaluated in preclinical cancer. First, smaller lesions are less likely to produce sufficient serologic markers to be detectable by even sensitive enzyme-linked immunosorbent assay (ELISA), let alone less sensitive biologic assays. Second, the use of the test in question to diagnose the HCC (eg, alpha fetoprotein [AFP]) in the first place introduces a bias.

Even when used as a test for diagnosis, the performance characteristics of serologic tests are not very good. The 3 serologic tests that have been evaluated are AFP, desgamma carboxy prothrombin (DCP, also known as the Protein Induced by Vitamin K Absence II [PIVKAII]), and the L3 fraction of AFP, which is more tumor specific than total AFP.

AFP has been best studied.[18–21] When evaluated as a diagnostic test, a value of about 20 ng/mL provides the optimal balance between sensitivity and specificity.[18] At this level, the sensitivity is only 60%. This is inadequately sensitive for general use. At higher AFP levels, sensitivity falls. For example, at a cutoff of 200 ng/mL the sensitivity is 22%. In this diagnostic study with an HCC prevalence of 50%, the positive predictive rate was 84%. However, in most clinics, the prevalence rates are closer to 5%, and possibly even less. At that level, the positive predictive value (PPV) of AFP drops to 42%, and even at a higher cutoff of 400 ng/mL, the PPV is only 60%.[18] These results indicate that AFP is a poor screening test. More recent data confirm the lack of efficacy of AFP as a screening test. In the HALT-C study,[22] a prospective study, patients with cirrhosis were screened with AFP and DCP. Measurements of DCP and AFP were taken at intervals. Both 12 months before diagnosis and at diagnosis, the performance characteristics of these tests were inadequate as screening tests. In another study, the performance characteristics of AFP, even as a diagnostic test, were inadequate, with a sensitivity of 66% and a specificity of 82%.[23] Therefore, AFP is no longer recommended as a screening test.

DCP is more sensitive than AFP for HCC screening, but is still not adequately sensitive.[22–27] Finally, there are reports that AFP, DCP, and AFP-L3 are all markers of advanced HCC. This automatically disqualifies them as effective screening tests, because the aim of a screening test is to find treatable disease, and advanced or poor prognosis tumors are too late for effective treatment.

Others have advocated the use of CT scanning for HCC screening. However, there are no data on the use of CT scanning as a screening test, rather than a diagnostic test. The performance characteristics are therefore unknown. A noncontrast CT scan does not have the sensitivity to detect small cancers. Arterial phase-only CT scans will identify a large number of false-positives, including cirrhotic nodules, dysplastic nodules, intrahepatic shunts, and transient attenuation defects, all of which will enhance in the arterial phase. Thus, a 3-phase or 4-phase CT will be required. This substantially increases the cost of surveillance, to the point that cost-efficacy analysis indicates that using CT scanning or MRI for HCC screening increases the cost by $100,000 to $300,000 per quality adjusted life year.[7]

This leaves ultrasonography as the screening test of choice. Ultrasonography is not ideal, but is better than any of the other tests used. A meta-analysis shows that ultrasound is more sensitive than AFP in detecting small HCCs.[28] A small HCC on ultrasound may take on one of several different appearances. The smallest lesions may be echogenic, because of the presence of fat in the cells. Other lesions may be hypoechoic, or show a "target lesion" appearance. None of these appearances is specific, and therefore an algorithm has been developed to improve the efficiency of investigation of lesions found on ultrasound. Ultrasound has been reported to have a sensitivity of between 65% and 80% and specificity greater than 90% when used as a screening test.[29] However, the performance characteristics have not been as well defined in nodular cirrhotic livers undergoing surveillance.[29–31] These performance characteristics, although not ideal, are superior to any of the serologic tests.

The most difficult ultrasounds are in obese individuals with fatty liver disease and cirrhosis. However, no alternative strategy for surveillance in such patients has been adequately tested.

Strategies such as alternating different surveillance modalities at intervals have no basis. The guiding principle should be that the best available screening test should be chosen, and it should be applied regularly. Combined use of AFP and ultrasonography increases detection rates, but also increases costs and false-positive rates.[32,33] Cost efficacy analysis suggests that adding AFP to ultrasonography increases costs substantially, without much increase in benefit.

Thus, the test of choice for HCC screening is ultrasonography.

Screening Interval

The ideal screening interval is 6 months. The only randomized controlled trial of HCC screening[1] used a 6-month interval, and showed enhanced survival. Data from a cohort study in Korea also suggested that survival was better after 6-monthly surveillance than 12-monthly surveillance.[34] In the United States, screening is poorly done, but even under these circumstances outcomes are better with screening than no screening,[35] and more frequent screening is better than less frequent screening. Screening does not need to be offered more frequently for those who are deemed to be at higher risk of HCC, because the frequency of screening is determined by the tumor growth rate and by the size of tumor that is associated with less than optimal outcomes. Neither of these is influenced by the degree of HCC risk.

With all these theoretical considerations in mind, it is important to ask whether there is any concrete evidence that screening decreases HCC mortality. There is indeed a single randomized controlled study in China[1] in which cluster randomization was used to compare survival in a screened and unscreened cohort of patients with chronic hepatitis B. In this study at 5 years, the mortality in the screened cohort was 37% less than in the unscreened cohort. Only resection was provided as therapy. It is possible that the results could be improved if some form of local ablation was available or if liver transplantation was available. Unfortunately, these results cannot be extrapolated to other causes of HCC. As discussed earlier, patients with cirrhosis are less likely to be able to undergo surgery, and in the hepatitis B cohort there are a relatively greater number of patients without cirrhosis who develop cancer.

A general problem with screening for cancer is the entity of overdiagnosis.[36] This is the identification of a lesion that is either precancer or even fully developed cancer that will not progress or grow. This may be because some premalignant lesions stabilize or regress and never become malignant, or because some cancers are very slow growing and do not cause ill health because of competing causes of death. Overdiagnosis can only really be identified in population studies. When the incidence of cancer increases, but the mortality from the disease stays stable, either treatment is progressively more effective (unlikely over a short term), or overdiagnosis is occurring. The increase in thyroid cancer in the recent past is not accompanied by an increase in mortality, indicating overdiagnosis. It is difficult to know whether overdiagnosis is an issue in liver cancer screening, but it is likely to be a factor. This is because the pathology of the small nodules identified by HCC screening has really only been defined in resected specimens, so that the behavior of these lesions cannot be followed. There are features on histology that suggest malignancy, such a stromal invasion, but this cannot be proven. The development of nodules that are clearly cancer within one of these nodules has been well described, suggesting that the first nodule was at least precancerous. However, the dysplasia/neoplasia sequence in liver tissue is hard to prove. So far, the data that exist are mainly based on histology.

STAGING OF HEPATOCELLULAR CARCINOMA

The purpose of developing a staging system for cancer is twofold. First, a staging system allows comparison between different clinical studies, and between results from clinical studies and what might be expected for an individual patient. Second, many staging systems are associated with stage-specific treatment regimens that are optimal for that stage.

There are a number of different methods of staging cancer. These can be clinical, surgical, radiological, or pathologic (eg, the Dukes staging for colon cancer).

Traditionally, clinical staging systems have been developed by cohort studies that have attempted to identify those factors most strongly associated with survival or lack thereof, and using those factors to develop a scoring system. This requires a fairly large cohort of untreated patients or at least uniformly treated patients, something that is seldom available today. Second, the scoring system has to be validated in external cohorts, ideally in other countries.

With HCC, there is an additional factor that has to be taken into account, and that is the underlying liver disease, which contributes to mortality. Thus, any staging system has to take liver function into account. The first clinical liver staging system was developed in Japan.[37] This was a relatively simple staging system that did take liver disease into account. It consisted of the size of the tumor (> or <50% of the liver volume), bilirubin, albumin, and ascites. This has since been superseded by several newer staging systems.[38–43] There are currently at least 8 separate staging systems. The classical TNM staging used in many other cancers has been applied to the liver; however, this staging system does not take liver function into account. Variants of this system that have attempted to include liver function are the sT or simplified TNM system,[43] and the staging system set up by the liver cancer study group of Japan.[39] The sT system does not include an assessment of liver function, but includes a measure of fibrosis as a surrogate of liver function. Both of these systems also suffer from the fact that they include features in the staging system that cannot be determined before surgery, such as the presence of microvascular invasion. Thus, nonsurgical patients cannot be staged, and surgical patients can be staged only after resection.

Of the several different staging systems, the one that seems to have been most widely accepted in the West is the Barcelona Cancer of the Liver Clinic staging (BCLC).[42] In Japan, the Japan Integrated Score is more widely used.[44] However, many of the major drug company trials that are currently under way or are being planned use the BCLC staging system (**Fig. 2**). For example, the SHARP trial, which was a randomized controlled trial that demonstrated survival benefit to the use of sorafenib, included only patients who were BCLC stage C.[45,46] Other trials (eg, STORM, a phase III randomized controlled trial of adjuvant therapy using sorafenib) are targeted at BCLC stage B.

The BCLC staging system has its problems. For example, it does not classify patients with single tumors larger than 5 cm in diameter. It does not classify recurrent disease after initial treatment. However, its main virtues are that it classifies patients

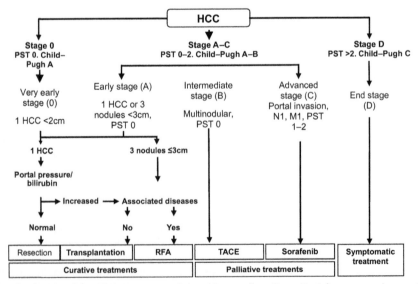

Fig. 2. The BCLC staging system and treatment allocation. Portal pressure is usually measured by the hepatic venous pressure gradient method. PST, performance status; RFA, radiofrequency ablation; TACE, transarterial chemoembolization.

who have different expectations of duration of survival, based on untreated patients, and it links staging with treatment. No other staging system does that. Until BCLC came along, most studies stratified patients as candidates for surgery or not, and all those who were not surgical candidates were lumped into a single category. The BCLC staging system stratifies unresectable HCC into 3 categories: BCLC B, C, and D, based on the extent of the tumor, the presence of vascular invasion, and the severity of the liver disease. Each of these factors separately is associated with reduced survival compared with patients in whom these factors are not present, and when more than one factor is present, survival is even worse.[47]

Therefore, all patients should be stage by the BCLC staging system, at least until something better comes along.

SUMMARY

Active screening of patients at risk for HCC has led to the identification of early HCCs that are amenable to treatment with a high rate of cure. This requires high-quality ultrasound examinations at 6-month intervals. However, if widely applied, screening has the potential to substantially reduce the mortality from this disease.

The application of the BCLC staging system should standardize assessment of prognosis and determination of the most effective treatments for each stage. With new molecular targeted agents coming, it is critical that studies are performed in patients stratified by stage into homogeneous groups. Because it is linked with therapy, the BCLC is ideally suited to this purpose.

REFERENCES

1. Zhang BH, Yang BH, Tang ZY. Randomized controlled trial of screening for hepatocellular carcinoma. J Cancer Res Clin Oncol 2004;130:417–22.
2. Bruix J, Sherman M; Practice Guidelines Committee, American Association for the Study of Liver Diseases. Management of hepatocellular carcinoma. Available at: http://www.aasld.org/practiceguidelines/documents/bookmarked%20practice%20guidelines/hccupdate2010.pdf. Accessed February 7, 2010.
3. Arguedas MR, Chen VK, Eloubeidi MA, et al. Screening for hepatocellular carcinoma in patients with hepatitis C cirrhosis: a cost-utility analysis. Am J Gastroenterol 2003;98:679–90.
4. Nouso K, Tanaka H, Uematsu S, et al. Cost-effectiveness of the surveillance program of hepatocellular carcinoma depends on the medical circumstances. J Gastroenterol Hepatol 2008;23:437–44.
5. Lin OS, Keeffe EB, Sanders GD, et al. Cost-effectiveness of screening for hepatocellular carcinoma in patients with cirrhosis due to chronic hepatitis C. Aliment Pharmacol Ther 2004;19:1159–72.
6. Thompson Coon J, Rogers G, Hewson P, et al. Surveillance of cirrhosis for hepatocellular carcinoma: systematic review and economic analysis. Health Technol Assess 2007;11:1–206.
7. Andersson KL, Salomon JA, Goldie SJ, et al. Cost effectiveness of alternative surveillance strategies for hepatocellular carcinoma in patients with cirrhosis. Clin Gastroenterol Hepatol 2008;6:1418–24.
8. Patel D, Terrault NA, Yao FY, et al. Cost-effectiveness of hepatocellular carcinoma surveillance in patients with hepatitis C virus-related cirrhosis. Clin Gastroenterol Hepatol 2005;3:75–84.

9. Sarasin FP, Giostra E, Hadengue A. Cost-effectiveness of screening for detection of small hepatocellular carcinoma in western patients with Child-Pugh class A cirrhosis. Am J Med 1996;101:422–34 Kang et al. J Gastro Hepatol 1992.

10. Saab S, Ly D, Nieto J, et al. Hepatocellular carcinoma screening in patients waiting for liver transplantation: a decision analytic model. Liver Transpl 2003;9: 672–81.

11. Shih ST, Crowley S, Sheu JC. Cost-effectiveness analysis of a two-stage screening intervention for hepatocellular carcinoma in Taiwan. J Formos Med Assoc 2010;109(1):39–55.

12. Collier J, Krahn M, Sherman M. A cost-benefit analysis of the benefit of screening for hepatocellular carcinoma. Hepatology 1999;30:481A.

13. Yuen MF, Tanaka Y, Fong DY, et al. Independent risk factors and predictive score for the development of hepatocellular carcinoma in chronic hepatitis B. J Hepatol 2009;50(1):80–8.

14. Yang HI, Sherman M, Su J, et al. Nomograms for risk of hepatocellular carcinoma in patients with chronic hepatitis B virus infection. J Clin Oncol 2010;28(14): 2437–44.

15. Lok AS, Seeff LB, Morgan TR, et al. Incidence of hepatocellular carcinoma and associated risk factors in hepatitis C-related advanced liver disease. Gastroenterology 2009;136(1):138–48.

16. Chen CJ, Yang HI, Su J, et al. Risk of hepatocellular carcinoma across a biological gradient of serum hepatitis B virus DNA level. JAMA 2006;295(1):65–73.

17. Sala M, Llovet JM, Vilana R, et al. Initial response to percutaneous ablation predicts survival in patients with hepatocellular carcinoma. Hepatology 2004; 40:1352–60.

18. Trevisani F, D'Intino PE, Morselli-Labate AM, et al. Serum alpha-fetoprotein for diagnosis of hepatocellular carcinoma in patients with chronic liver disease: influence of HBsAg and anti-HCV status. J Hepatol 2001;34(4):570–5.

19. Pateron D, Ganne N, Trinchet JC, et al. Prospective study of screening for hepatocellular carcinoma in Caucasian patients with cirrhosis [see comments]. J Hepatol 1994;20:65–71.

20. Zoli M, Magalotti D, Bianchi G, et al. Efficacy of a surveillance program for early detection of hepatocellular carcinoma. Cancer 1996;78:977–85.

21. Izuno K, Fujiyama S, Yamasaki K, et al. Early detection of hepatocellular carcinoma associated with cirrhosis by combined assay of des-gamma-carboxy prothrombin and alpha-fetoprotein: a prospective study. Hepatogastroenterology 1995;42:387–93.

22. Lok AS, Sterling RK, Everhart JE, et al. Des-gamma-carboxy prothrombin and alpha fetoprotein as biomarkers for the early detection of hepatocellular carcinoma. Gastroenterology 2010;138(2):493–502.

23. Marrero JA, Feng Z, Wang Y, et al. Alpha-fetoprotein, des-gamma carboxyprothrombin, and lectin-bound alpha-fetoprotein in early hepatocellular carcinoma. Gastroenterology 2009;137(1):110–8.

24. Grazi GL, Mazziotti A, Legnani C, et al. The role of tumor markers in the diagnosis of hepatocellular carcinoma, with special reference to the des-gamma-carboxy prothrombin. Liver Transpl Surg 1995;1:249–55.

25. Tsai SL, Huang GT, Yang PM, et al. Plasma des-gamma-carboxyprothrombin in the early stage of hepatocellular carcinoma. Hepatology 1990;11:481–8.

26. Suehiro T, Sugimachi K, Matsumata T, et al. Protein induced by vitamin K absence or antagonist II as a prognostic marker in hepatocellular carcinoma. Comparison with alpha-fetoprotein. Cancer 1994;73:2464–71.

27. Marrero JA, Su GL, Wei W, et al. Des-gamma carboxyprothrombin can differentiate hepatocellular carcinoma from nonmalignant chronic liver disease in American patients. Hepatology 2003;37:1114–21.

28. Singal A, Volk ML, Waljee A, et al. Meta-analysis: surveillance with ultrasound for early-stage hepatocellular carcinoma in patients with cirrhosis. Aliment Pharmacol Ther 2009;30(1):37–47.

29. Bolondi L, Sofia S, Siringo S, et al. Surveillance programme of cirrhotic patients for early diagnosis and treatment of hepatocellular carcinoma: a cost-effectiveness analysis. Gut 2001;48:251–9.

30. Chen TH, Chen CJ, Yen MF, et al. Ultrasound screening and risk factors for death from hepatocellular carcinoma in a high risk group in Taiwan. Int J Cancer 2002; 98:257–61.

31. Larcos G, Sorokopud H, Berry G, et al. Sonographic screening for hepatocellular carcinoma in patients with chronic hepatitis or cirrhosis: an evaluation. AJR Am J Roentgenol 1998;171:433–5.

32. Snowberger N, Chinnakotla S, Lepe RM, et al. Alpha fetoprotein, ultrasound, computerized tomography and magnetic resonance imaging for detection of hepatocellular carcinoma in patients with advanced cirrhosis. Aliment Pharmacol Ther 2007;26:1187–94.

33. Zhang B, Yang B. Combined alpha fetoprotein testing and ultrasonography as a screening test for primary liver cancer. J Med Screen 1999;6:108–10.

34. Kim DY, Han KH, Ahn SH, et al. Semiannual surveillance for hepatocellular carcinoma improved patient survival compared to annual surveillance (Korean experience). Hepatology 2007;46(Suppl 1):403A.

35. Stravitz RT, Heuman DM, Chand N, et al. Surveillance for hepatocellular carcinoma in patients with cirrhosis improves outcome. Am J Med 2008;121(2):119–26.

36. Welch HG, Black WC. Overdiagnosis in cancer. J Natl Cancer Inst 2010;102(9): 605–13.

37. Okuda K, Kubo Y. Clinical types of hepatocellular carcinoma and correlation between liver pathology and clinical manifestations. Kurume Med J 1979;26(3): 247–60.

38. Leung TW, Tang AM, Zee B, et al. Construction of the Chinese University Prognostic Index for hepatocellular carcinoma and comparison with the TNM staging system, the Okuda staging system, and the Cancer of the Liver Italian Program staging system: a study based on 926 patients. Cancer 2002;94(6):1760–9.

39. Minagawa M, Ikai I, Matsuyama Y, et al. Staging of hepatocellular carcinoma: assessment of the Japanese TNM and AJCC/UICC TNM systems in a cohort of 13,772 patients in Japan. Ann Surg 2007;245(6):909–22.

40. The Cancer of the Liver Italian Program (CLIP) Investigators. Prospective validation of the CLIP score: a new prognostic system for patients with cirrhosis and hepatocellular carcinoma. Hepatology 2000;31(4):840–5.

41. Chevret S, Trinchet JC, Mathieu D, et al. A new prognostic classification for predicting survival in patients with hepatocellular carcinoma. J Hepatol 1999;31(1): 133–41.

42. Sala M, Forner A, Varela M, et al. Prognostic prediction in patients with hepatocellular carcinoma. Semin Liver Dis 2005;25(2):171–80.

43. Vauthey JN, Lauwers GY, Esnaola NF, et al. Simplified staging for hepatocellular carcinoma. J Clin Oncol 2002;20(6):1527–36.

44. Kudo M, Chung H, Haji S, et al. Validation of a new prognostic staging system for hepatocellular carcinoma: the JIS score compared with the CLIP score. Hepatology 2004;40(6):1396–405.

45. Llovet JM, Ricci S, Mazzaferro V, et al. Sorafenib in advanced hepatocellular carcinoma. N Engl J Med 2008;359(4):378–90.
46. Cheng AL, Kang YK, Chen Z, et al. Efficacy and safety of sorafenib in patients in the Asia-Pacific region with advanced hepatocellular carcinoma: a phase III randomised, double-blind, placebo-controlled trial. Lancet Oncol 2009;10(1):25–34.
47. Llovet JM, Bustamante J, Castells A, et al. Natural history of untreated nonsurgical hepatocellular carcinoma: rationale for the design and evaluation of therapeutic trials. Hepatology 1999;29(1):62–7.

Imaging of Hepatocellular Carcinoma: Practical Guide to Differential Diagnosis

Munazza Anis, MD*, Abid Irshad, MD

KEYWORDS

- Hepatocellular cancer • Imaging of HCC
- Focal HCC • Diffuse HCC

An estimated 80% to 90% of patients with hepatocellular carcinoma (HCC) in the United States have cirrhosis,[1] with a handful of cases presenting in the noncirrhotic liver. Cirrhosis is characterized by bridging fibrosis and a spectrum of hepatocellular nodules, most of which are benign and regenerative. However, degeneration into dysplastic nodules or HCC can occur through the sequential steps of hepatocarcinogenesis.[2]

IMAGING OF HCC

The main goals of imaging in HCC are: (1) to make the diagnosis and exclude competing causes; (2) to assess the number and size(s) of tumor(s), which have important implications for medical or surgical therapy, such as liver transplantation; and (3) to locate the masses anatomically and describe the vascular relationships for surgical or interventional treatment planning. The practice guidelines of the American Association for the Study of Liver Diseases (AASLD) include recommendations for periodic surveillance by imaging in patients with cirrhosis.[3]

Several imaging modalities are available for the evaluation of hepatocellular carcinoma. The role of each is discussed in this article.

Ultrasonography

Despite its inherent limitations in evaluating chronic liver disease, routine gray-scale ultrasound (US) is still widely used for the initial evaluation of patients suspected of having liver disease, as well as for HCC screening in patients with known cirrhosis

The authors have nothing to disclose.
Department of Radiologic Sciences, Medical University of South Carolina, 96 Jonathan Lucas Street, MSC 323, Charleston, SC 29425, USA
* Corresponding author.
E-mail address: anis@musc.edu

Clin Liver Dis 15 (2011) 335–352
doi:10.1016/j.cld.2011.03.014
1089-3261/11/$ – see front matter © 2011 Elsevier Inc. All rights reserved.

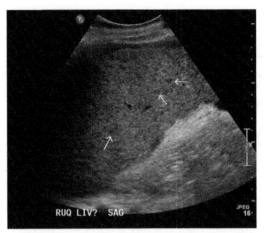

Fig. 1. Sagittal gray-scale ultrasound (US) image through the right lobe of liver shows coarsened liver texture and surface irregularity. The parenchyma shows numerous small hypoechoic nodules scattered throughout the liver (*arrows*), likely representing regenerative nodules.

(**Figs. 1** and **2**). There have been recent advances in digital technology and US imaging software that have significantly improved image quality and resolution. This progress has enabled sonographers to identify subtle changes in the liver texture and delineate small masses in the liver with greater success than before.[4]

New techniques such as tissue harmonic imaging (THI), a relatively new ultrasound technique that uses higher secondary US frequencies (harmonic frequencies) to improve the resolution of the ultrasound image and decrease artifacts, spatial compounding, and 3-dimensional US have been recently introduced. On gray-scale imaging, THI has improved image quality and has decreased the number of image artifacts.[5] The sensitivity and specificity for the detection of HCC with US varies widely in the literature, which is likely related to variation in sonographer skill, patient's body habitus, the size of the nodule, and the background coarseness of the cirrhotic liver,[6] as shown in **Fig. 3**.

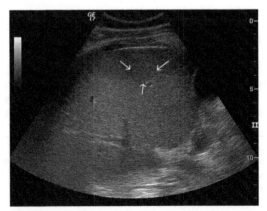

Fig. 2. Gray-scale US image through the left lobe of liver shows an HCC (*arrows*) seen as a subtle change in the texture that is apparent, due to a relatively normal background parenchyma.

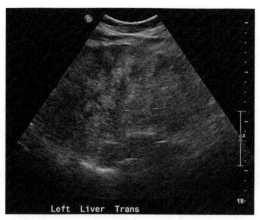

Fig. 3. Gray-scale US transverse image through the left lobe of liver shows diffuse large nodular architectural changes throughout the liver. Finding a small HCC in this case may be extremely difficult.

Imaging features

HCC may present as a solitary mass (see **Fig. 2**), as several nodules, or with a diffuse infiltrative pattern (**Fig. 4**). Although HCC can be hypoechoic, isoechoic, or hyperechoic (**Fig. 5**), most of the smaller (<5 cm) HCCs are hypoechoic compared with the liver parenchyma.[7] A thin hypoechoic halo may be seen around a small HCC (**Fig. 6**).[7] Occasionally a small tumor may become hyperechoic because of internal fatty metamorphosis, resulting in an appearance similar to that of a hemangioma. Larger tumors tend to be more heterogeneous (see **Fig. 5**), which is secondary to hemorrhage, fibrosis, or focal fat infiltration. Calcifications are uncommon in HCC but are sometimes seen in the fibrolamellar type, which typically shows a central scar. HCC has a propensity to invade the portal or hepatic veins.[7] Neovascularity within the thrombus in the portal or hepatic veins on Doppler US is considered diagnostic of hepatocellular carcinoma. Recently, the US elastography technique has shown promising results for differentiating HCC from non-HCC nodules.[8]

The diagnosis of HCC in cirrhotic patients typically involves identifying hypervascularity in the focal nodules that may be confirmed on contrast-enhanced US, computed

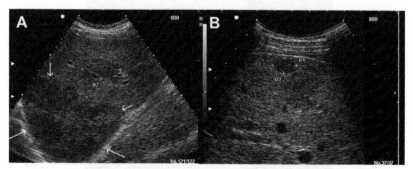

Fig. 4. (*A, B*) Multicentric HCC. (*A*) Gray-scale US transverse image through the right lobe of liver showing a large irregular hypoechoic infiltrative mass posteriorly (*arrows*). There is an additional mass more anteriorly (*calipers*). (*B*) Image through the left lobe of liver shows another small hypoechoic mass in the anterior part of the left lobe.

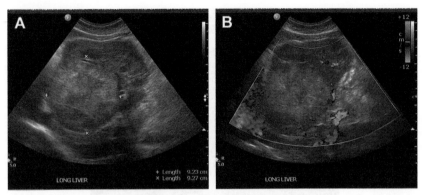

Fig. 5. (*A*) Gray-scale US longitudinal view through the right lobe of liver showing a large exophytic mass (*calipers*). The mass is slightly hyperechoic compared with the liver parenchyma, and shows slight internal heterogeneity. (*B*) Color Doppler image through the same mass shows no significant color flow within the mass.

tomography (CT) scan, magnetic resonance imaging (MRI), or angiography. Increased vascularity and blood flow within the mass may be detected by using various US techniques such as color Doppler or power Doppler examination. Color Doppler is an ultrasound technique by which the blood flow, direction of flow, and velocity within the vessels can be detected. More vascular tumors show more color flow on Doppler US. Power Doppler is similar but is more sensitive to detect slower flow or vascularity, but does not detect the direction of flow (**Fig. 7**). However, the sensitivity of Doppler in detecting flow is not as great as that of contrast-enhanced US, CT, or MRI. A color signal may be absent in some nodules with slow flow or small vessels, especially if the lesions are deep within the liver. Contrast-enhanced US has shown promise in demonstrating increased vascularity in these nodules. This technique is now frequently being used in many countries around the world to identify HCC and to differentiate it from other benign lesions.[9] In the United States, where these contrast agents are not approved by the Food and Drug Administration for routine clinical use in liver imaging, further diagnosis of HCC relies on subsequent contrast-enhanced CT or MRI after a suspicious solid mass is identified by US.

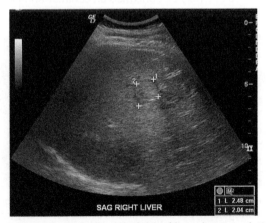

Fig. 6. Gray-scale US image through the right lobe of liver shows a relatively isoechoic HCC (*calipers*), which only becomes more visible because of a surrounding hypoechoic halo.

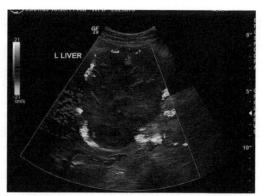

Fig. 7. Color Doppler image through a large HCC in the left lobe of liver shows increased vascular flow in the periphery as well as within the central areas of the mass.

Focal masses such as hemangiomas, lipomas, or angiomyolipomas may have a characteristic appearance ultrasonographically, and can be categorized as benign with a high degree of certainty in normal livers. On liver US, lesions that are less than 3 cm in size, hyperechoic, homogeneous in appearance, and show well-defined margins are considered benign if these patients do not have cirrhosis or other known malignancy. Approximately 67% to 79% of all hemangiomas are hyperechoic while 58% to 73% are homogeneous in appearance.[7] Incidentally found typical benign-appearing hemangiomas on US examination in noncirrhotic patients with no other malignancy have a less than 1% chance of being malignant.[10] In general, no further follow-up is necessary for these patients. However, in patients with known cirrhosis, only 50% of hyperechoic lesions are hemangiomas.[11] Consequently, in patients who have an increased risk of HCC, abnormal liver tests, atypical US appearance of the lesion, or a known malignancy, further evaluation with contrast-enhanced CT, MRI, red cell scintigraphy or contrast-enhanced US is recommended.

Cystic masses may also be confidently identified on US. Other solid masses such as focal nodular hyperplasia (FNH), adenoma, dysplastic nodules, or HCC have overlapping imaging features on gray-scale and Doppler US. US has not been shown to accurately differentiate between dysplastic nodules and HCC.

Computed Tomography

With the current multidetector CT scanners the entire liver can be imaged in a few seconds, thereby allowing the capture of distinct phases of imaging, such as nonenhanced arterial, portal, and delayed venous phases (**Fig. 8**). However, this technique raises concerns about radiation-induced cancer, which is particularly relevant in young individuals. In addition, significant debate is present in the radiology literature regarding whether there is improved detection of small HCC with multiphasic CT versus biphasic or triple-phase CT scanning.[12–14]

Imaging features

HCC nodules are usually seen as hyperenhancing masses on a background of a minimally enhanced liver parenchyma during the hepatic arterial phase, which is the key phase for making the diagnosis (see **Fig. 8**; **Fig. 9**). A precontrast CT may reveal a focal hypodense area or, on rare occasions, minimal fat within the HCC lesion. Cases in which chemoembolization with ethiodized oil has been performed previously require a baseline precontrast sequence to look for areas of enhancement that would indicate

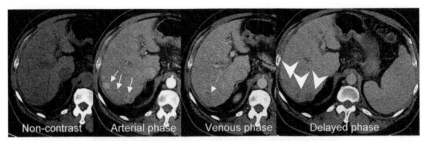

Fig. 8. Four-phase liver CT scan reveals a multifocal HCC on the background of cirrhosis. These masses are isodense on noncontrast phase, demonstrate arterial enhancement (*arrows*), slight washout on the venous phase (*dashed arrow*), and significant washout masses on the delayed phase (*arrowheads*).

recurrence. The arterial phase may be further split into an early phase, which is useful for mapping out arterial anatomy, and a late arterial phase, which is essential for detecting HCC. However, there are limitations regarding the visualization of very small tumors,[15–17] due to several variables that may affect the optimal timing of the hepatic arterial dominant phase, including patient size and cardiovascular status.[15] When the portovenous phase shows typical washout within the tumor and a surrounding capsule, these are features diagnostic of HCC (see **Fig. 8**). However, some cases of hypoenhancing HCC are better seen on this phase than on the arterial phase. In addition, the portovenous phase is also useful for demonstrating portal venous thrombosis (**Fig. 10**) and differentiating neoplasms from vessels, and in the identification of varices and shunts. There are limited data related to the usefulness of the delayed phase in HCC diagnosis, even though some investigators report that HCCs are often more conspicuous on delayed-phase than on portovenous-phase images (see **Fig. 8**).

Positron Emission Tomography

Positron emission tomography (PET) imaging detects lesions that have increased glucose metabolism, as detected by the uptake of 2-fluorodeoxy-D-glucose-6-phosphate (FDG) uptake. FDG normally is dephosphorylated and exits the cell, but this is impaired in cancer cells, leading to the accumulation of the FDG tracer.

PET scanning is very sensitive in detecting metastases, but the sensitivity for HCC is only about 50%. The sensitivity for extrahepatic metastases related to HCC and

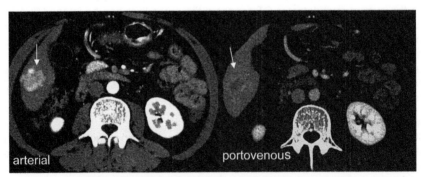

Fig. 9. Arterial-phase and portovenous-phase CT images demonstrate arterial-phase enhancing mass (*arrow*) in a cirrhotic liver, which demonstrates washout and a subtle surrounding capsule (*arrow*) on the portovenous phase.

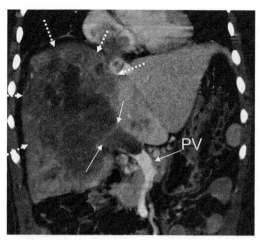

Fig. 10. Coronal CT image in portovenous phase depicting a large diffuse mass (*dashed arrows*) replacing the right lobe of the liver, with enhancing tumor thrombus in the intra-hepatic portal vein (PV) (*arrows*).

especially poorly differentiated HCC is somewhat better. In addition, there is some role for PET in monitoring response to therapy in PET-positive HCC-related metastases.

Magnetic Resonance Imaging

MRI has better lesion-to-liver contrast in comparison with CT scanning, and is useful for assessing tissue properties such as intracellular lipid and hemorrhage. In addition, a wider variety of contrast agents are available for MRI than for CT. Therefore, MRI has emerged as an important modality for the assessment of cirrhosis-associated hepatic nodules.[16–18]

A typical liver protocol includes T1-weighted sequences such as gradient-recalled echo (GRE) with out-of-phase and in-phase image acquisition, which are helpful in delineating the intracellular lipid content within the liver or in focal mass a cirrhotic liver, which is suggestive of HCC. T2 sequences include those with and without fat saturation in axial and coronal planes, which aids in the detection of nodules with hyperintense or hypointense signals. T2* sequences are T2 sequences altered in such a way that information is acquired that measures the iron content within the hepatic parenchyma, and this increases the conspicuity of non–iron-containing hepatic masses such as HCC. Diffusion-weighted imaging appearances are variable. Depending on histology, well-differentiated tumors are often isointense, whereas moderately to poorly differentiated tumors are more often hyperintense.[19,20] These sequences are critical in diagnosing HCC in patients who cannot receive intravenous gadolinium.

T1-weighted images are acquired before and dynamically after the administration of the gadolinium chelate, using volumetric 3-dimensional fat-saturated spoiled GRE sequences. Critical dynamic imaging phases include the hepatic arterial phase to detect these hypervascular nodules followed by images from the portovenous phase, delayed venous phase, and then equilibrium phase to better assess venous washout.[21] Precise timing and breath holding during image acquisition are crucial, because of the transient nature of gadolinium-related enhancement. It must be noted that some well-differentiated HCCs and some dysplastic nodules may be portally perfused, thus avoiding detection on the arterial phase.

Three different types of MR contrast agents are available for assessing cirrhosis-associated hepatocellular nodules: extracellular agents such as the gadolinium chelates, hepatocyte-specific agents that are excreted by hepatocytes into bile, and superparamagnetic iron oxide (SPIO) particles.[22] Gadolinium chelates are extracellular contrast agents that provide information about tumor vascularity. Hepatocyte-specific agents are useful in assessing hepatocellular masses on images acquired after an appropriate delay. Two such agents have been manufactured commercially: gadobenate dimeglumine (Gd-BOPTA) and gadoxetic acid disodium (Gd-EOB-DTPA). Gadobenate dimeglumine, 5% of which is excreted into the bile, is the only mixed extracellular and hepatocellular agent currently approved for use in the United States. Delayed imaging at 60 to 120 minutes is needed for characterization of hepatocellular masses. By contrast, 50% of the gadoxetic acid disodium is excreted by the liver and 50% by the kidneys. This distribution provides robust hepatocyte-phase imaging at approximately 90 minutes, which has been shown to increase the sensitivity for the detection of HCC nodules.[23]

SPIO particles have been falling out of favor recently, due to the introduction of hepatocyte-specific agents. SPIO particles cause shortening of T2* (darkening) and, to a lesser degree, T2, which results in loss of signal within the regenerative nodules, some dysplastic nodules, and regions of surrounding liver parenchyma. As most HCCs lack Kupffer cells, they do not accumulate SPIO particles, and therefore appear hyperintense relative to the liver parenchyma.

HCC is a malignant neoplasm composed of dedifferentiated hepatocytes. The pathologic classification of HCC includes "massive" (ie, single large mass with or without satellite nodules), "nodular" (ie, solitary or discrete nodules), or "diffuse" (ie, multiple indistinct masses throughout the liver).[24]

Radiologically, however, HCC presents as focal or diffuse. Focal tumors can be solitary or multiple.

1. Focal
   a. Solitary
      i. Small HCC
      ii. Large HCC
   b. Multifocal HCC
2. Diffuse HCC, also known as infiltrative HCC.

The imaging diagnosis of HCC is related to the gradual reduction of the normal hepatic arterial and portal venous supply to the nodule and an increase in the abnormal arterial supply via neoangiogenesis.[2,25] This process of neoangiogenesis or arterial recruitment dictates the main imaging feature of HCC, which is arterial enhancement.[2,26] Arterial enhancement (hypervascularity) is considered an essential characteristic of HCC, and is used as the only radiologic feature on contrast-enhanced CT or MR images approved by the United Network for Organ Sharing (UNOS) for the noninvasive diagnosis of HCC prior to listing.[27]

In addition to arterial-phase enhancement, the size and number of the tumors is of utmost importance because it affects further management, that is, transplantation or radiofrequency ablation versus systemic therapy. Solitary tumors less than 5 cm in size, or 2 to 3 hepatocellular tumors each smaller than 3 cm, are amenable to transplantation. Other salient information needed for treatment decisions and provided by imaging includes the degree of lymphadenopathy and portal vein involvement.

IMAGING FEATURES OF HCC
Focal HCC

Small HCC is defined as a tumor measuring 2 cm or smaller. The signal typically is isointense (**Fig. 11**) on T1-weighted MR imaging for lesions smaller than 1.5 cm,

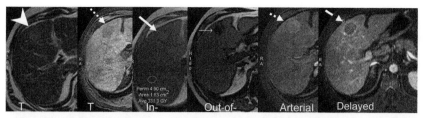

Fig. 11. Typical features of HCC on MRI examination revealing hyperintense signal on T2 (*arrowhead*), hypointense signal on T1 (*dotted arrow*), slightly hyperintense on in-phase (*thick arrow*), marked signal dropout on out-of-phase image (*arrow*), arterial-phase enhancement (*dashed arrow*), and washout with a capsule (*dot-dash arrow*) on delayed-phase images on the background of cirrhosis.

whereas larger lesions may be hyperintense because of lipid, copper, or glycogen content (**Fig. 12**).[28,29] Fatty change in a cirrhotic nodule is suspicious for HCC. T2-weighted imaging shows most HCC lesions as hyperintense masses, although some well-differentiated tumors may be isointense. Post-gadolinium sequences reveal an arterially enhancing mass that demonstrates washout of the lesion relative to the surrounding parenchyma on delayed phases, and formation of a surrounding tumor capsule. These features are highly specific for HCC,[28,29] with a reported overall sensitivity of 89% and specificity of 96% for delayed hypointensity.[30] Rarely, HCCs may remain hyperintense relative to adjacent liver parenchyma on venous and delayed-phase images. Occasionally early-stage HCC, especially tumors smaller than 2 cm, can be isointense or hypointense in the arterial phase. Breathing artifacts, particularly in patients with ascites, can also create difficulty in detection.

Diffuse HCC

Diffuse HCC generally presents with nonspecific heterogeneous areas on noncontrast T1-weighted and T2-weighted MR images; typically mildly hypointense on T1-weighted and hyperintense on T2-weighted images. Diffuse areas of enhancement on the early-phase and heterogeneous areas of washout on the late-phase images are diagnostic for malignant tumor (**Figs. 13–15**).[31]

Diffuse-type HCC constitutes a fraction of cases and appears as a heterogeneous, infiltrative hepatic mass with portal venous tumor thrombosis (see **Fig. 14** and **Fig. 15**), often associated with an elevated serum α-fetoprotein level. Portal vein invasion is an important feature of HCC and is thought to be related to its portal venous drainage.[32]

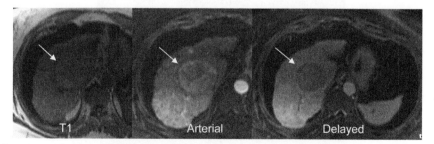

Fig. 12. Axial MR images demonstrate a rounded slightly T1 hyperintense hepatic mass (*arrow*) in the background of cirrhosis, which demonstrates slightly heterogeneous enhancement (*arrow*) on the arterial phase, with complete washout and a capsule on the delayed postcontrast phase (*arrow*).

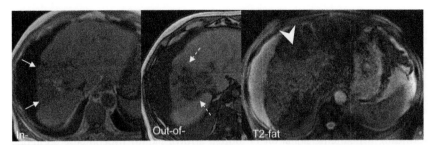

Fig. 13. MR examination demonstrates a large geographic area in the right lobe of the liver with scattered hyperintense area (*arrow*) compatible with diffuse HCC, which reveals marked signal dropout on out-of-phase images (*dashed arrows*) in a cirrhotic liver. This area demonstrates T2 hyperintense signal (*arrowhead*).

Benign portal vein thrombosis (**Fig. 16**) in cirrhotic patients occurs secondary to portal hypertension, venous stasis, and often a hypercoagulable state, whereas malignant portal vein thrombosis is attributable to direct invasion of the vein. Increased T2-weighted signal intensity is highly suggestive of malignant thrombosis. In addition, dramatic expansion of the vein diameter, compared with near-normal caliber of veins in bland thrombosis and the presence of neovascularity, is also highly specific for malignant thrombosis.[32]

DIFFERENTIAL DIAGNOSIS
Cirrhosis-Related Nodules

Regenerative nodules are present in all cirrhotic livers, are surrounded by fibrous septa, and are classified into micronodular (<3 mm), macronodular (>3 mm), and mixed types (**Fig. 17**).[17,33] The blood supply of a regenerative nodule continues to largely originate from the portal vein, with minimal contribution from the hepatic artery.[26] This vascular distribution explains why there is no enhancement during the hepatic arterial phase on MR images. Large regenerative nodules can measure 5 cm or more and may mimic a mass.[34] Because they consist of proliferating normal liver cells surrounded by a fibrous stroma, these nodules are indistinct on T1-weighted and T2-weighted images. Less commonly, they can be hyperintense to the surrounding liver on T1-weighted images,

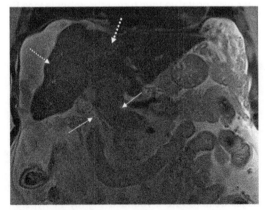

Fig. 14. Coronal T2 image demonstrates cirrhotic liver with ascites demonstrating central T2 hyperintense area (*dashed arrows*) compatible with HCC and extending into the portal, which is markedly distended (*arrows*).

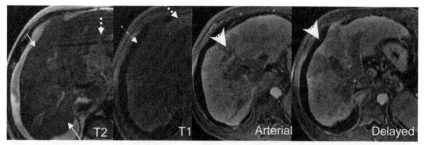

Fig. 15. MR examination demonstrating diffuse T2 hyperintense signal in the cirrhotic liver parenchyma (*arrows*) with a more central T2 hyperintense signal (*dashed arrow*) at the portal vein bifurcation. This area demonstrates T1 hypointense signal compared with the liver parenchyma (*dashed arrows*). Post-gadolinium images demonstrate heterogeneous areas compatible with HCC extending into the portal vein (*arrowheads*).

probably because of the presence of lipid, protein, or possibly copper.[29] Regenerative nodules that contain iron (siderotic nodules) may have decreased signal intensity on both T1-weighted and T2-weighted images, owing to susceptibility effects (see **Fig. 17**), that is, the spoiling of the signal by heavy metals.

Dysplastic nodules are usually isointense to surrounding liver on T1-weighted and T2-weighted images (see **Fig. 17**; **Fig. 18**). Some dysplastic nodules retain copper, so they have high signal intensity on T1-weighted images. Siderotic nodules are hypointense to surrounding liver on T1-weighted and T2-weighted images. Low-grade dysplastic nodules are normally supplied by the portal vein and therefore are isointense to liver during the arterial phase. The signal-intensity characteristics of some high-grade dysplastic nodules, which receive increasing supply from the hepatic artery, may overlap with those of HCC nodules. Occasionally both regenerative and dysplastic nodules can infarct, leading to high signal intensity on T2-weighted images.[34] Such nodules are often mistaken for HCC. A dysplastic nodule with a central focus of HCC was first described on T2-weighted images as "a nodule within a nodule."[35] The classic MR appearance is a focus of high signal intensity within a low-signal-intensity nodule on T2-weighted images. This focus of HCC may also enhance in the arterial phase.[35]

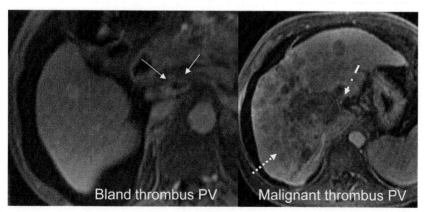

Fig. 16. Two MR images. (*Left*) Bland thrombus in the portal vein confluence (*arrows*) in a cirrhotic liver with ascites. (*Right*) diffuse HCC (*dotted arrow*) causing malignant thrombus extension into the portal vein (*dot-dash arrow*).

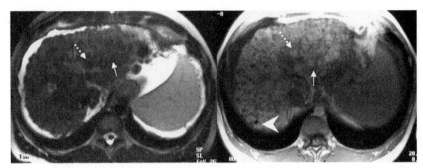

Fig. 17. Axial T2 and T1 MR images demonstrate cirrhotic liver with innumerable T2 isointense nodules (*arrows*), which are isointense on T1 (*arrow*), compatible with regenerative nodules. Several T2 hypointense, T1 hyperintense nodules (*dashed arrows*) are compatible with dysplastic nodules. A T2 and T1 hypointense nodule compatible with siderotic nodule (*arrowhead*) are also evident.

Small (≤2 cm) Hepatic Arterial Phase–Enhancing Lesions

Transient focal arterial enhancement due to arterioportal shunts or focal obstruction of a distal portal vein branch is commonly seen in the cirrhotic liver. Usually these shunts are isointense to surrounding parenchyma on T1-weighted and T2-weighted images (**Fig. 19**).[36] Recent studies with intravenous gadoxetic acid have shown slightly increased detection and improved sensitivity for distinguishing hepatic arterial phase–enhancing (HAPE) lesions from small HCC on MRI examination.[23] Shunts are commonly peripheral and wedge shaped, but can be nodular or irregular. Small arteriovenous shunts and pseudoaneurysms can occur following liver biopsy and can demonstrate enhancement that is similar to the blood pool on contrast-enhanced images. Aberrant venous drainage and early drainage by a subcapsular vein has also been found to appear as hypervascular lesions mimicking small HCCs. Detection of lesions smaller than 1 cm that may be tiny HCCs is important, as curative treatments at this stage can potentially improve outcome.[29,36] General recommendations for HAPE lesions include short-term follow-up or biopsy. UNOS requires documentation of tumors every 3 months, as increase in size has been shown to be highly predictive for HCC. Biopsy becomes important if the imaging diagnosis of HCC is doubtful, especially in patients for whom its presence expedites transplantation. The AASLD recommendations for hypervascular nodules smaller than 1 cm detected on contrast-enhanced images are less clear. In general, 6-month follow-up should be

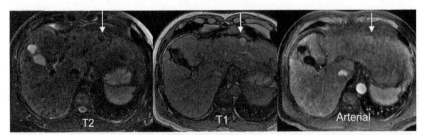

Fig. 18. Axial MR images demonstrate a cirrhotic liver with several nodules; the dominant nodule in the left lobe of the liver demonstrates T2 hypointense signal (*arrow*), T1 hyperintense signal (*arrow*), and no enhancement after gadolinium compatible with a dysplastic nodule.

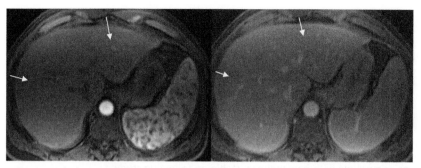

Fig. 19. Arterial-phase and venous-phase MR images in a cirrhotic liver reveal 2 tiny foci of arterial enhancement (*arrows*), which are not apparent on venous-phase or on T2 images.

obtained for nodules with subcapsular foci smaller than 5 mm.[37] Round or oval enhancing foci in the central parenchyma, or in the presence of a dominant mass, should be followed up at 3-monthly intervals.

Confluent Hepatic Fibrosis

Focal confluent hepatic fibrosis (CHF) seen in end-stage liver disease can be mass-like and mistaken for HCC.[38] CHF presents as areas of inflammatory fibrosis that are wedge shaped, with the wide base toward the liver capsule located in the hepatic dome (**Fig. 20**), usually associated with atrophy of the affected segment, and capsular retraction. Confluent fibrosis is usually of low signal intensity relative to the liver on T1-weighted images and hyperintense on T2-weighted images. Delayed contrast enhancement of fibrosis is characteristic, but occasionally confluent fibrosis can demonstrate early contrast, simulating a neoplasm. Such cases require biopsy for confirmation.

Hemangiomas

Hemangiomas are commonly found in normal livers but are rare in end-stage cirrhosis, probably because cirrhosis obliterates existing hemangiomas. If present in cirrhosis, hemangiomas, also known as sclerosed or sclerosing hemangiomas, are often atypical in appearance and contain large regions of fibrosis that alter the typical features of peripheral nodular enhancement with centripetal filling (**Fig. 21**). Prior studies and stability in size on follow-up studies are also helpful in making the diagnosis.

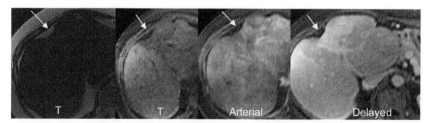

Fig. 20. MR examination of a cirrhotic patient reveals a subtle wedge-shaped area of T2 hyperintense signal in the liver with capsular retraction, which demonstrates T1 hypointense signal (*arrow*), no arterial enhancement (*arrow*), and mild delayed enhancement compatible with confluent hepatic fibrosis (*arrow*).

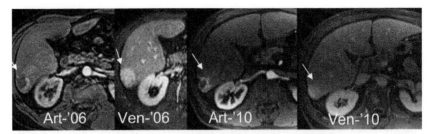

Fig. 21. Serial MR images of a cirrhotic patient from 2006 and 2010 in arterial and venous phases demonstrate a focal peripherally enhancing mass with centripetal filling on delayed images, compatible with hemangioma, stable on follow-up study.

Cysts

Small cysts are often seen in cirrhosis, and do not pose a diagnostic challenge. Simple cysts exhibit low signal intensity on T1-weighted images, high signal intensity on T2-weighted images, and no enhancement.

Intrahepatic Cholangiocarcinoma

Intrahepatic cholangiocarcinoma usually shows thin or thick rim enhancement in the arterial and venous phases, with progressive and concentric filling of contrast material in the later phases. This pattern of enhancement is atypical for HCC. Intrahepatic biliary duct dilation proximal to the tumor and associated capsular retraction are features more commonly associated with intrahepatic cholangiocarcinoma and are rarely seen in HCC. Narrowing or obstruction of the portal vein associated with intrahepatic cholangiocarcinoma is usually attributable to external compression.

Multifocal Hepatic Masses

Metastases (**Fig. 22**) are the most common malignant hepatic tumor, occurring much more frequently than primary neoplasms. These tumors most commonly manifest as multifocal, discrete lesions, but sometimes present as a solitary mass or confluent masses. The imaging appearance depends on the degree of underlying hepatic arterial supply. Hypovascular metastases show decreased enhancement relative to normal liver, and are most conspicuous on portal venous-phase images. Hypervascular metastases demonstrate arterial-phase enhancement, and show washout on delayed images that can be a diagnostic challenge for the radiologist to differentiate from multifocal HCC. These metastases typically arise from primary neuroendocrine tumors (eg, pancreatic islet cell tumors and carcinoid tumors), renal cell carcinoma,

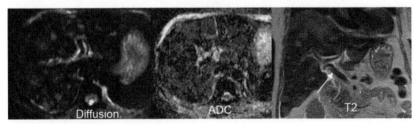

Fig. 22. Diffusion-weighted images and T2-weighted coronal image demonstrate multiple hepatic masses of target appearance, showing restricted diffusion compatible with metastases. Note the patency of the portal vein (*arrow*).

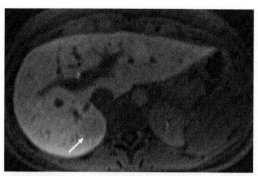

Fig. 23. MR image obtained during hepatocyte phase (120 minutes delay image) after gadoxetic acid administration reveals a hypointense mass in the posterior liver (*arrow*) compatible with an adenoma.

thyroid carcinoma, and melanoma. On post-gadolinium sequences, metastases demonstrate a "target" appearance on delayed images, in addition to the fact that the origin of the primary is generally known. A multifocal pattern of metastatic disease can be discerned from the diffuse infiltrating pattern of HCC, except with infiltrating metastases that can be seen with breast cancer; again, in such cases the primary tumor may be known. Also, portal venous thrombosis is rare in patients with metastatic disease, whereas it is commonly seen with diffuse HCC.

Others

Benign lesions such as FNH or FNH-like nodules and hepatic adenomas are rare in the cirrhotic liver but can be difficult to distinguish from HCC.

It may be difficult or impossible to distinguish HCC from adenoma (**Fig. 23**) on the basis of imaging findings alone that are identical on arterial-phase enhancement and delayed washout with a surrounding capsule. Adenomas almost always occur in the setting of oral contraceptive or anabolic steroid use, or abnormal carbohydrate metabolism (eg, glycogen storage diseases or diabetes).

FNH is characterized by a T2 hyperintense central scar in an otherwise "stealth" lesion that is isointense on T1 or T2. The central scar retains contrast on delayed post-contrast images (**Fig. 24**). This scar can be readily differentiated from HCC, in which

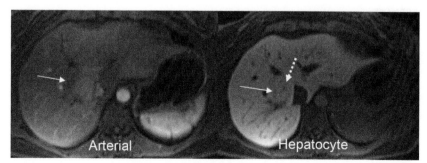

Fig. 24. Immediate post–gadoxetic acid arterial phase demonstrates homogeneous enhancement of a focal mass, which on the delayed hepatocyte phase demonstrates persistent enhancement (*arrow*) and a central scar (*dashed arrow*) compatible with a focal nodular hyperplasia.

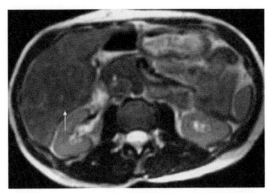

Fig. 25. Axial T2 image in a patient with Budd-Chiari syndrome depicting regenerative nodules (*arrow*) that appear mass like. In some cases these nodules may demonstrate arterial-phase enhancement, although washout or capsule is not seen on delayed sequences.

there is washout of the lesion on delayed imaging and formation of a capsule. It is also important to distinguish HCC from large benign regenerative nodules, which occur secondary to liver damage without cirrhosis, for example in Budd-Chiari syndrome (**Fig. 25**), or severe disease of the portal veins or hepatic sinusoids. These nodules often appear as many, well-defined, arterially enhancing nodules with high signal intensity on T2-weighted images and sometimes delayed hypointensity. The nodules sometimes contain a central scar. Unlike regenerative nodules of cirrhosis, regenerative nodules in Budd-Chiari syndrome do not have fibrosis around the nodules.

SUMMARY

Hepatocellular cancer is most commonly seen in patients with cirrhosis. Criteria for diagnosis include arterial-phase enhancement, venous-phase washout, and a capsule on delayed sequences. Tiny HCC are best detected with MRI using the new hepatocyte-specific gadolinium agents; otherwise, short-term follow-up versus biopsy is considered. Diffuse HCC can be difficult to diagnose because of the inherent heterogeneous hepatic parenchyma in cirrhosis; however, portal vein expansion due to thrombosis is a helpful sign.

REFERENCES

1. Llovet JM, Burroughs A, Bruix J. Hepatocellular carcinoma. Lancet 2003;362: 1907–17.
2. Efremidis SC, Hytiroglou P. The multistep process of hepatocarcinogenesis in cirrhosis with imaging correlation. Eur Radiol 2002;12:753–64.
3. Bruix J, Sherman M. Practice Guidelines Committee, American Association for the Study of Liver Diseases. Management of hepatocellular carcinoma. Available at: http://www.aasld.org/practiceguidelines/Documents/Bookmarked%20Practice%20Guidelines/HCCUpdate2010.pdf. Accessed February 7, 2011.
4. Harvey CJ, Albrecht T. Ultrasound of focal liver lesions. Eur Radiol 2001;11: 1578–93.
5. Shapiro RS, Wagreich J, Parsons RB, et al. Tissue harmonic imaging sonography: evaluation of image quality compared with conventional sonography. AJR Am J Roentgenol 1998;171:1203–6.

6. Teefey SA, Hildeboldt CC, Dehdashti F, et al. Detection of primary hepatic malignancy in liver transplant candidates: prospective comparison of CT, MR imaging, US, and PET. Radiology 2003;226:533–42.

7. Wilson SR, Withers CE. The liver. In: Rumack CM, Wilson SR, Charboneau JW, editors. Diagnostic ultrasound. 3rd edition. St Louis (MO): CV Mosby Co; 2005. p. 77–146.

8. Gheorghe L, Iacob S, Iacob R, et al. Real time elastography—a non-invasive diagnostic method of small hepatocellular carcinoma in cirrhosis. J Gastrointestin Liver Dis 2009;18(4):439–46.

9. Lencioni R, Piscaglia F, Bolondi L. Contrast-enhanced ultrasound in the diagnosis of hepatocellular carcinoma. J Hepatol 2008;48:848–57.

10. Leifer DM, Middleton WD, Teefey SA, et al. Follow-up of patients at low risk for hepatic malignancy with a characteristic hemangioma at US. Radiology 2000; 214(1):167–72.

11. Caturelli E, Pompili M, Bartolucci F, et al. Hemangioma-like lesions in cirrhotic liver disease: diagnostic evaluation in patients. Radiology 2001;220(2):337–42.

12. Miller FH, Butler RS, Hoff FL, et al. Using triphasic helical CT to detect focal hepatic lesions in patients with neoplasms. AJR Am J Roentgenol 1998;171: 643–9.

13. Laghi A, Iannaccone R, Rossi P, et al. Hepatocellular carcinoma: detection with triple-phase multi-detector row helical CT in patients with chronic hepatitis. Radiology 2003;226:543–9.

14. Baron RL, Oliver JH III, Dodd GD III, et al. Hepatocellular carcinoma: evaluation with biphasic, contrast enhanced, helical CT. Radiology 1996;199:505–11.

15. Mitsuzaki K, Yamashita Y, Ogata I, et al. Multiple-phase helical CT of the liver for detecting small hepatomas in patients with liver cirrhosis: contrast-injection protocol and optimal timing. AJR Am J Roentgenol 1996;167:753–7.

16. Semelka RC, Martin DR, Balci C, et al. Focal liver lesions: comparison of dual-phase CT and multisequence multiplanar MR imaging including dynamic gadolinium enhancement. J Magn Reson Imaging 2001;13(3):397–401.

17. Baron RL, Peterson MS. From the RSNA refresher courses: screening the cirrhotic liver for hepatocellular carcinoma with CT and MR imaging: opportunities and pitfalls. Radiographics 2001;21:S117–32.

18. Larson RE, Semelka RC, Bagley AS, et al. Hypervascular malignant liver lesions: comparison of various MR imaging pulse sequences and dynamic CT. Radiology 1994;192(2):393–9.

19. Parikh T, Drew SJ, Lee VS, et al. Focal liver lesion detection and characterization with diffusion-weighted MR imaging: comparison with standard breath-hold T2-weighted imaging. Radiology 2008;246(3):812–22.

20. Nasu K, Kuroki Y, Tsukamoto T, et al. Diffusion-weighted imaging of surgically resected hepatocellular carcinoma: imaging characteristics and relationship among signal intensity, apparent diffusion coefficient, and histopathologic grade. AJR Am J Roentgenol 2009;193:438–44.

21. Willatt MJ, Hussain KH, Adusumilli S, et al. MR imaging of hepatocellular carcinoma in the cirrhotic liver: challenges and controversies. Radiology 2008;247: 311–30.

22. Gandhi S, Brown MA, Wong JG, et al. MR contrast agents for liver imaging: what, when, how. Radiographics 2006;26:1621–36.

23. Motosugi U, Ichikawa T, Sou H, et al. Distinguishing hypervascular pseudolesions of the liver from hypervascular hepatocellular carcinomas with gadoxetic acid-enhanced MR imaging. Radiology 2010;256(1):151–8.

24. Edmondson HA, Steiner PE. Primary carcinoma of the liver: a study of 100 cases among 48,900 necropsies. Cancer 1954;7:462–503.

25. Park YN, Yang CP, Fernandez GJ, et al. Neoangiogenesis and sinusoidal "capillarization" in dysplastic nodules of the liver. Am J Surg Pathol 1998;22:656–62.

26. Kitao A, Zen Y, Matsui O, et al. Hepatocarcinogenesis: multistep changes of drainage vessels at CT during arterial portography and hepatic arteriography—radiologic-pathologic correlation. Radiology 2009;252:605–14.

27. United Network for Organ Sharing. Policy 3.6, organ distribution: allocation of livers. Organ procurement and transplantation network web site. Available at: http://optn.transplant.hrsa.gov/. Accessed September 18, 2007.

28. Grazioli L, Morana G, Caudana R, et al. Hepatocellular carcinoma: correlation between gadobenate dimeglumine-enhanced MRI and pathologic findings. Invest Radiol 2000;35:25–34.

29. Ebara M, Fukuda H, Kojima Y, et al. Small hepatocellular carcinoma: relationship of signal intensity to histopathologic findings and metal content of the tumor and surrounding hepatic parenchyma. Radiology 1999;210:81–8.

30. Marrero JA, Hussain HK, Nghiem HV, et al. Improving the prediction of hepatocellular carcinoma in cirrhotic patients with an arterially-enhancing liver mass. Liver Transpl 2005;11(3):281–9.

31. Kanematsu M, Semelka RC, Leonardou P, et al. Hepatocellular carcinoma of diffuse type: MR imaging findings and clinical manifestations. J Magn Reson Imaging 2003;18:189–95.

32. Tublin ME, Dodd GD 3rd, Baron RL. Benign and malignant portal vein thrombosis: differentiation by CT characteristics. AJR Am J Roentgenol 1997;168: 719–23.

33. Terminology of nodular hepatocellular lesions. International Working Party. Hepatology 1995;22:983–93.

34. Kim T, Baron RL, Nalesnik MA. Infarcted regenerative nodules in cirrhosis: CT and MR imaging findings with pathologic correlation. AJR Am J Roentgenol 2000;175: 1121–5.

35. Earls JP, Theise ND, Weinreb JC, et al. Dysplastic nodules and hepatocellular carcinoma: thin-section MR imaging of explanted cirrhotic livers with pathologic correlation. Radiology 1996;201:207–14.

36. Holland A, Hecht EM, Hahn WY, et al. Importance of small (≤20-mm) enhancing lesions seen only during the hepatic arterial phase at MR imaging of the cirrhotic liver: evaluation and comparison with whole explanted liver. Radiology 2005;237: 938–44.

37. Itai Y, Moss AA, Goldberg HI. Transient hepatic attenuation difference of lobar or segmental distribution detected by dynamic computed tomography. Radiology 1982;144:835–9.

38. Ohtomo K, Baron RL, Dodd GD, et al. Confluent hepatic fibrosis in advanced cirrhosis: appearance at CT. Radiology 1993;188:31–5.

Conventional Surgical Treatment of Hepatocellular Carcinoma

T. Mark Earl, MD, William C. Chapman, MD*

KEYWORDS

- Hepatocellular carcinoma • Surgical resection
- Cirrhosis • Liver cancer

Numerous treatment modalities for hepatocellular carcinoma (HCC) exist, but resection remains the standard therapy. Few patients, however, are candidates due to advanced stage or, more commonly, advanced chronic liver disease.[1] Liver transplantation offers excellent outcomes with 5-year disease-free survival rates of approximately 70% because it eliminates the tumor and associated diseased liver.[2–4] Transplantation, however, is restricted to those with small, early-stage lesions, and donor organ availability further limits its broader applicability. Although improvements in HCC screening among cirrhotics and use of Model for End-Stage Liver Disease (MELD) exemptions have improved transplantation rates and survival among patients with HCC, the majority of patients continue to present outside of the Milan criteria (namely, a single tumor up to 5 cm in diameter or up to 3 tumors, the largest being 3 cm in diameter).[1,5–11] Due to limitations in donor organ availability and high costs as well as improvements in patient selection, operative and anesthetic techniques, and postoperative care, there has been renewed interested in resection for HCC.[12–16] The results of liver resection for HCC depend in large part on the functional capacity of the remnant liver, comorbid illness of the patient, tumor size/stage, and intraoperative factors, such as blood loss.

DIAGNOSIS

HCC commonly remains asymptomatic until there is right upper quadrant pain, fullness or constitutional symptoms (such as fatigue) are noted, or there is evidence of hepatic decompensation. In the absence of chronic liver disease, patients often

WCC Is a founder of Pathfinder Therapeutics, Inc. Otherwise, the authors have no financial conflicts of interest to disclose.

Section of Transplantation, Department of Surgery, Washington University School of Medicine, Washington University, 660 South Euclid Avenue, Campus Box 8109, St Louis, MO 63130, USA
* Corresponding author.
E-mail address: chapmanw@wustl.edu

present with large, advanced-stage tumors.[17] Presentation with ascites, jaundice, or other signs of hepatic decompensation usually heralds an unresectable tumor. The majority of patients with HCC have histologic or radiographic evidence of chronic liver disease and these patients often present with pain or decompensated liver function.[18] Due to better surveillance and improved adherence to surveillance recommendations, patients with chronic liver disease and HCC are presenting at an earlier, asymptomatic phase when curative therapy may be used.[19,20]

Detection of HCC often begins with ultrasound either as part of a screening program or due to new-onset right upper quadrant symptoms. α-Fetoprotein (AFP) is a useful adjunct and is a recommended part of routine screening; however, it lacks sufficient sensitivity and specificity for stand-alone use.[21–23] Once a liver lesion has been demonstrated by ultrasound or an AFP level greater than 200 ng/mL is detected in a patient with chronic liver disease, the next step is high-resolution cross-sectional imaging usually in the form of triple-phase contrasted CT or contrast-enhanced MRI. This allows for more precise detection of multifocal disease, macrovascular invasion, portal hypertension, and evidence of extrahepatic malignancy. Screening for HCC is discussed in the article by Sherman elsewhere in this issue and imaging is discussed in the article by Anis and Irshad elsewhere in this issue; these topics are not discussed further in this article. The role of biopsy for confirmation has diminished greatly as imaging techniques and understanding of the natural history of the disease have improved. Arguments now include histologic analysis in HCC evaluation, as discussed in the article by Roskams elsewhere in this issue.

RESECTION VERSUS TRANSPLANTATION

Liver transplantation remains the best theoretic option for HCC because it removes the tumor and underlying diseased liver. In patients with advanced liver disease who are not candidates for resection, transplantation represents the only option with a significant chance of cure. Deceased donor organ shortages and poor outcomes in advanced cases, however, have limited transplant applicability only to early-stage disease,[2] with less than 30% of patients eligible for transplantation at presentation.[24,25] Although transplantation in patients with stage III tumors (outside of Milan criteria) is offered at some institutions either through expanded criteria, such as the University of California, San Francisco (UCSF) citeria,[26,27] or using downstaging strategies,[28,29] these strategies have not been uniformly adopted. These approaches are discussed in the article by Masuoka and Rosen elsewhere in this issue.

HCC in the absence of chronic liver disease accounts for approximately 10% to 20% of cases.[17,30] The fibrolamellar variant most commonly occurs in young white women often with lymph node metastasis and without elevations of AFP.[31] Patients with fibrolamellar and sporadic HCC commonly present when tumors have grown large and symptomatic. When feasible, resection is the mainstay of therapy and is often well tolerated due to the ability of the healthy remnant liver to regenerate.[32] As expected, 5-year survival rates for patients without chronic liver disease are as high as 50% despite the often advanced stage at presentation, highlighting the significant role that the presence or absence of underlying liver disease plays in both management and outcome.[15,33]

Every patient with early-stage HCC cannot be offered transplantation and another form of extirpative therapy must be considered for select patients (**Fig. 1**). Liver resection is immediately available, requires no waiting time, allows complete pathologic evaluation of the tumor, and does not, in theory, preclude future transplantation. Patients without chronic liver disease should undergo resection when technically

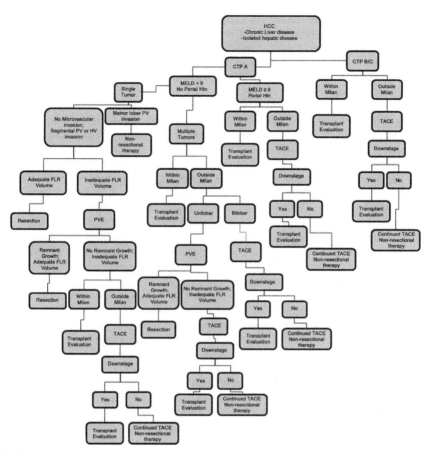

Fig. 1. Decision tree for the surgical management of HCC in patients with chronic liver disease and hepatic-confined disease.

feasible. Patients with end-stage liver disease, Child-Turcotte-Pugh (CTP) class B or C, should undergo transplantation if available, as should patients with relatively preserved hepatic function but multifocal disease that is within Milan criteria. The difficulty lies in deciding which patients with chronic liver disease and small (<5 cm) solitary tumors are best served by resection and which should proceed with transplant evaluation; this topic is the focus of this article.

DETERMINATION OF CANDIDACY
Tumor Characteristics

The major definitive contraindication to resection of HCC is the presence of extrahepatic disease. HCC commonly spreads to lymph nodes, lungs, and bone[34] although the likelihood of extrahepatic spread is dependent on the size of the tumor and evidence of vascular invasion.[35,36] In addition to cross-sectional abdominal imaging, chest CT to evaluate for pulmonary metastases is generally recommended before consideration of resection and is required by the United Network for Organ Sharing (UNOS) before listing for transplantation.[37] The role of bone scanning is somewhat controversial and is no longer required by UNOS for transplant listing. In an evaluation of the utility of chest CT and bone scan before listing for liver transplantation for stages I and II, Koneru and colleagues[35] found no positive scans among 117 patients evaluated. Twenty-nine patients had indeterminate scans, but none was denied listing based on chest CT or bone scan findings. The indeterminate scans led to 6 invasive procedures from which 1 patient died as a direct result of percutaneous biopsy of a mediastinal mass that proved nonmalignant. In general, fluorodeoxyglucose-6-phosphate–position emission tomography (FDG-PET) has been thought to have a low sensitivity of 55% in patients with HCC,[38] which is likely due to variability in tumoral FDG-6-phosphatase expression. In tumors with higher stage or grade where extrahepatic spread is more likely and thus evaluation is more critical, FDG avidity rates are likely higher. Several reports have shown increased FDG avidity rates of up to 100% of patients with primary hepatic tumors greater than 5 cm.[36,39] Thus, FDG-PET is a useful adjunct to chest CT and bone scan for evaluation of extrahepatic disease when resection of large tumors is under consideration. This topic is discussed elsewhere in this issue in the article by Anis and Irshad.

In the absence of extrahepatic disease, the resectability of HCC depends primarily on the extent of hepatic disease and the function of the proposed liver remnant (discussed later). Large tumor size, major vascular or biliary invasion, and bilobar tumors are often considered relative contraindications; however, each case must be considered individually. Several groups have documented excellent outcomes after resection of large (>10 cm) tumors albeit less so than those for smaller tumors.[32] One recent report by Young and colleagues[40] demonstrated 5-year disease-free and overall survival rates of 43% and 45%, respectively, in patients with tumors greater than 10 cm. Mortality for resection of these large tumors varies widely but is reported to be 5% in an international cooperative study of more than 300 patients, more than half of whom had moderate to severe fibrosis of the remnant liver.[41] Multinodular tumors, alternatively, carry a significantly worse prognosis,[42] likely due to a field defect within the liver and subsequent oncogenesis. Despite the worse prognosis, resection and possibly staged resection may be considered when transplantation is not an option. Recurrence rates are as high as 80% to 100%. Five-year overall survival rates, however, of up to 30% have been reported.[43]

Resection for patients with invasion of the vena cava, portal vein, and/or hepatic vein is controversial due to poor outcomes, with a 5-year survival rate of only 10% and a reported median survival of 11 months in resected patients.[44,45] Although overall results of resection for patients with venous invasion and tumor thrombus are poor, rare patients with small tumors, thrombosis of secondary portal branches, or hepatic venous tributaries and preserved liver function may benefit from resection.[44] In the report by Pawlik and colleagues,[45] 23% of patients with no to minimal fibrosis survived 5 years compared with 5% of those with moderate to severe fibrosis. As with macrovascular invasion, major bile duct involvement generally carries a poor prognosis and invasion of the biliary confluence almost always precludes resection. When biliary tumor thrombi are present, 5-year survival is approximately 5% with a median survival of 11.4 months (reported by Ikenaga and colleagues).[46,47] As such, patients with major vascular or bile duct involvement are rarely candidates for resection.

Liver Characteristics

As discussed previously, in the absence of chronic liver disease, resection is the mainstay of therapy. When chronic liver disease is present, however, the degree of portal hypertension, remnant volume, and regenerative capacity of the remnant liver must be considered before embarking on resection. To better quantify the degree of hepatic impairment and risk of postresection mortality and/or hepatic decompensation, several scoring systems have been devised. The first and most widely used scoring system to estimate hepatic functional impairment is the CTP system.[48] Historically, patients with CTP class A, B, or C have operative mortality rates of 10%, 30%, and 80%, respectively, although more recent reports indicate a fairly significant improvement.[49–51] In general, CTP class A patients may be considered for major hepatectomy. More detailed stratification, however, is necessary to determine tolerance of this large operation. CTP classes B and C are generally considered to pose a contraindication to hepatectomy; transplantation or other hepatic directed therapy should be considered when feasible for these more decompensated patients.

Because of the subjective nature of several components of the CTP score and its categorical nature, a continuous and objective system for stratifying liver disease was sought. The MELD scoring system was introduced to evaluate survival after transjugular intrahepatic portosystemic shunt placement. In 2002, UNOS adopted MELD scoring as the basis for organ allocation in the United States because of its ability to predict survival and inclusion of solely objective data; the continuous nature of MELD scores compared well with the prior waiting time/status-based liver allocation protocol. In an effort to improve on the trichotomized CTP system, MELD has also been used to predict outcomes after nonshunt abdominal operations, including hepatectomy. Like CTP, MELD scores correlate with postoperative outcomes and in some cases are superior to CTP.[52–54] When applied specifically to partial hepatectomy for HCC, several reports have demonstrated the ability of MELD to aid in the differentiation of which CTP class A patients can withstand hepatectomy.[55–58] The exact value of MELD at which resection leads to excess risk varies among reported series, but it generally lies between 8 and 11. For example, in a series of 155 cirrhotic patients (93% CTP class A) undergoing resection, Cucchetti and colleagues[57] found a MELD score of 11 to be 82% sensitive and 89% specific for postoperative liver failure. Patients with MELD scores less than 9 had no episodes of liver failure and a reportedly low morbidity rate of 8.1%. Hsu and colleagues[56] reported on 1017 patients who underwent resection and found that those with a MELD score greater than 8 had significantly higher mortality (4% vs 0.6%) and higher rates of postoperative liver failure (16.1 vs 4.3%) than those with a MELD score less than 6. In an American series from Mayo Clinic, Teh and colleagues[58] found a MELD score cutoff of 9 was associated with a significant mortality difference of 16% versus 29% for MELD score greater than 9 versus less than or equal to 9. Although most of the resections in these series were minor (<3 segments), it seems that MELD scores greater than or equal to 9 represent the point at which morbidity and mortality of any hepatectomy increases significantly and other therapeutic modalities should be considered. Moreover, MELD aids in further defining which CTP class A patients are at risk for postoperative death and liver-related complications.

The volume of liver remaining postresection is standardized to patient size. The functional liver remnant (FLR) required for safe resection varies for individual patients, depending on comorbid illness, age, and, most important, severity of liver disease. In patients without chronic liver disease (ie, normal background liver), an FLR of greater than or equal to 20% is sufficient to minimize the risk of postoperative hepatic decompensation.[59–61] Patients with chronic liver disease but not cirrhosis require a larger FLR of at least 30% to allow for safe resection and those with cirrhosis without portal hypertension generally require an FLR of at least 40%.[62] When the FLR as predicted on preoperative imaging is of inadequate size, portal vein embolization (PVE) can be used to increase volume of the FLR (discussed later). Moreover, response to PVE can be used to determine the ability of the liver remnant to hypertrophy after resection and, in turn, predict risk of hepatic decompensation. Patients with a normal background liver and FLR less than or equal to 20% whose remnant grows to greater than 20% after PVE have a low likelihood of hepatic failure after resection.[61] Those who have growth of the FLR greater than 5% likewise have low risk of postresection hepatic failure.[60]

Although measurement of liver remnant volume is widely used in Western centers, indocyanine green (ICG) clearance at 15 minutes is used by many Eastern centers to augment CTP and/or MELD in determining hepatic functional reserve. The dye is given at a dose of 0.5 mg/kg and is excreted into the bile. Elimination is measured either by venipuncture or, more recently, by transcutaneous spectrophotometry.[63] Impaired clearance is most often defined as retention of 15% or more of the dye 15 minutes after administration.[64] Although ICG retention does correlate with CTP score and results of several series demonstrate its discriminatory ability, its utility as a predictor of liver failure postresection varies widely.[64,65] When applied to minor resections, ICG clearance fares well because the functional liver to be removed is small. When major resections are performed or when large amounts of functional liver are removed, ICG clearance is less reliable as a predictor of hepatic decompensation because it does not account for the volume of the remnant liver.

In cirrhotics with relatively preserved synthetic function, other methods, such as hepatic venous pressure gradient (HVPG) measurement, have been used to better discern the presence of portal hypertension and predict postresection hepatic failure. In a study of 29 patients with CTP class A cirrhosis, Bruix and colleagues[66] found that the mean HVPG was significantly higher in those patients who had persistent decompensation 3 months after resection compared with those whose symptoms resolved (13.9 ± 2.4 vs 7.4 ± 3.5; P<.001). In multivariate analysis, HVPG was the only factor to predict persistent decompensation with an odds ratio of 1.90 (95% CI, 1.12–3.22; P = .0001). Although measuring HVPG is likely a useful adjunct in stratifying which CTP class A patients are resection candidates, it is an invasive procedure that predicts the presence of portal hypertension, which can generally be determined by noninvasive means (splenomegaly, thrombocytopenia, presence of varices, and so forth), although these clinical assessments have measurable false negativity. Moreover, the contribution of portal pressure determination, either invasive or noninvasive, to the resolution that MELD provides in predicting postresection liver failure is unknown. Cucchetti and colleagues[67] found that MELD and extent of liver resection were the only significant predictors of postoperative hepatic decompensation in 241 patients who underwent resection for HCC. Portal hypertension, defined as varices on endoscopy or splenomegaly with thrombocytopenia, was associated with worse outcomes. The patients in this report, however, also had significantly elevated MELD scores. In a matched series using propensity score analysis of 78 patients each, with and without portal hypertension (taken from the same cohort), there was no significant difference in the intraoperative course or postoperative outcome, including liver failure, morbidity, length of stay, or survival.

In addition to MELD and CTP, other factors have been identified for risk stratification/prediction in cirrhotic patients undergoing major operations. These include elevated creatinine, chronic obstructive pulmonary disease, male gender, and American Society of Anesthesiologists (ASA) class IV or V.[68] Teh and colleagues[69] further demonstrated ASA class as a useful marker to further stratify the comorbid illness in cirrhotic patients preoperatively. This case-controlled study of cirrhotic patients who underwent major nontransplant operations identified MELD, ASA, and age as predictors of perioperative mortality. An ASA class IV was equivalent to the addition of 5.5 MELD points in added risk, and age greater than 70 years was equivalent to 3 additional MELD points. A single-point increase in MELD score was associated with a 15% increase in perioperative mortality. ASA class V was the strongest predictor of 7-day mortality and MELD score is the most robust predictor beyond 7 days. The median survival of patients in this series was 4.8 years for MELD scores 0 to 7, 3.4 years for MELD scores 8 to 11, 1.6 years for MELD scores 12 to 15, 64 days for MELD scores 16 to 20, 23 days for MELD scores 21 to 25, and 14 days for MELD scores greater than or equal to 26, respectively.

PREOPERATIVE THERAPY
PVE

PVE was initially used to prevent portal vein tumor extension in patients with HCC[70] but is now widely used to increase the volume of the FLR in all patients who undergo trisegmentectomy or, in those with chronic liver disease, right hemihepatectomy or when the FLR is less than 40%.[71,72] Meta-analysis of 37 studies has established the safety of PVE and its ability to increase FLR volume.[73] A prospective trial by Farges and colleagues[74] confirmed the benefit of PVE in cirrhotics undergoing right hepatectomy. Those patients who underwent PVE had a significantly reduced ICU stay, incidence of liver failure, and ascites and pulmonary complications. The investigators also confirmed that a good growth response in the FLR portends a low risk of hepatic failure.

In a recent small series, Palavecino and coworkers[75] demonstrated a reduced rate of major complications (35% vs 10%; $P = .028$) and death (18% vs 0%; $P = .038$) in patients who underwent PVE before major hepatectomy compared with patients who did not undergo this intervention preoperatively. Five patients in the non-PVE group died as a result of hepatic failure and subsequent multiorgan failure. Based on these data, it seems that PVE has a beneficial effect when FLR volumes are insufficient, depending on the severity of liver disease, and can convert patients at high risk of postresection hepatic failure to relatively low risk. Relative contraindications to PVE include portal invasion/occlusion in the segment to be embolized, hyperbilirubinemia, biliary obstruction of the FLR (due to the reduced ability of the obstructed liver to hypertrophy), the risk of infectious complications in the obstructed portion of the liver, uncorrectable coagulopathy, and renal failure.[76]

Transarterial Chemoembolization

The use of transarterial chemoembolization (TACE) as neoadjuvant therapy before resection has been extensively reported. The data are conflicting, although the majority of studies found no improvement in disease-free or overall survival. A recent trial randomized 108 patients with resectable HCC greater than or equal to 5 cm to preoperative TACE versus no TACE, and no improvement was found in disease-free or overall survival at 1, 3, and 5 years (disease-free with TACE 48.9%, 25.5%, and 12.8%, respectively, versus non-TACE 39.2%, 21.4%, and 8.9%, respectively; overall survival with TACE 73.1%, 40.4%, and 30.7%, respectively, versus non-TACE 69.6%, 32.1%, and 21.1%, respectively).[77] Additionally, 5 patients (9.6%) in the preoperative TACE group did not proceed to resection because of subsequent discovery of extrahepatic metastases or liver failure. The inability of neoadjuvant TACE to improve outcomes after resection of HCC has been further validated in a meta-analysis by Chua and colleagues.[78] Eighteen studies were included, with 3 being randomized trials. Despite a higher rate of tumor necrosis in patients undergoing TACE, no consistent improvement in disease-free survival could be ascertained.

Operative Details

Morbidity and mortality of hepatic resection have greatly improved in recent decades due in large part to better patient selection. Significant improvements in operative technique, primarily via reduction of intraoperative hemorrhage, have contributed as well.[79,80] The use of low central venous pressure anesthetic strategies has contributed to minimization of blood loss.[81] Several studies have attempted to ascertain the best method of parenchymal transection and no consistently superior method has been identified despite much technical innovation.[82] A Cochrane Review published in 2009[83] analyzed data from 7 trials that included 556 patients, focusing on comparisons of crush-clamp, Cavitron Ultrasonic Surgical Aspirator (CUSA), radiofrequency dissecting sealer (RFDS), and hydrojet. Blood loss was greater with RFDS than with crush-clamp, and blood transfusion was greater with CUSA and hydrojet than with crush-clamp. No difference in resultant ICU and hospital stay was noted for the different techniques. Operating times were shorter with crush-clamp than with CUSA, RFDS, and hydrojet and crush-clamp was 2 to 6 times cheaper, leading the investigators to recommend the crush-clamp method for parenchymal transection, given its speed, reduction in blood loss or transfusion requirement, and decreased cost. Several other methods of parenchymal dissection have been described, including radiofrequency energy, microwave coagulation, and linear staplers, and data can be found touting the superiority of all of them. The ultimate decision seems to reside with availability, preference, and experience of the individual hepatic surgeon.

Historically, portal triad clamping (Pringle maneuver) has not been advocated in patients with chronic liver disease undergoing resection due to concern over liver remnant ischemia contributing to postresection liver dysfunction. Blood loss, however, has been shown to correlate with overall and oncologic outcome[79,84] although this result is not consistent.[85] In a randomized trial of 100 patients, 60% of whom had chronic liver disease, Man and colleagues[86] demonstrated that intermittent clamping of the hepatoduodenal ligament was well tolerated. There was no significant difference in postoperative liver function, morbidity, or mortality and patients who underwent Pringle clamping had less blood loss, fewer transfusions, and decreased time for parenchymal transection than with other methods.

Anatomic resections have been advocated by some surgeons based on the belief that this resulted in superior oncologic outcomes. Other series have not supported this, however.[33,87,88] Larger resections have been favored due to the belief that hepatic recurrence is largely due to micrometastases or tumor emboli from the portal vein feeding the tumor. This potential benefit must be balanced by the need to minimize operative magnitude and preserve hepatic mass. In 2000, Poon and colleagues[89] published a series of 288 patients who underwent resection for HCC and compared outcomes based on resection margins less than 1 cm or greater. No difference in survival or recurrence was demonstrated in those with smaller margins. This contrasts with results in a trial by Shi and colleagues,[90] who randomized 169 patients to either 1-cm or 2-cm margins. Patients with a 2-cm intended margin had increased recurrence-free survival and significantly improved overall survival ($P<.008$). These findings have led to the general recommendation that wide margins should used whenever feasible without significantly altering the risk of postresection hepatic decompensation.[91] This is most feasible with small, peripheral tumors. With large or deep-seated tumors, formal anatomic resection that sacrifices substantial liver parenchyma may be necessary to obtain negative margins. When possible, consideration should be given to performance of more complex resections such as formal segmentectomy, central hepatectomy (segments IV, V, and VIII), or sectionectomy (eg, VI and VII or V and VIII) (**Fig. 2**).[92] It is in these cases that intraoperative ultrasound and selective pedicular control can prove most useful to minimize blood loss and define resection planes. It is also important in these settings to perform preoperative planning with accurate prediction of remnant liver volumes and consideration of preoperative PVE, if indicated (**Fig. 3**).

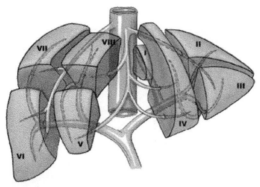

Fig. 2. Segmental liver anatomy.

Anterior Approach

Patients with large tumors confined to the right hemiliver can prove challenging, due to difficulty in exposure when dissecting the bare area and retrohepatic vena cava. Moreover, excessive traction and manipulation of the right liver can lead to hemorrhage from avulsion of hepatic veins and the risk of tumor rupture or dissemination. The difficulty of resection of these large, right-sided lesions led Lai and colleagues[93] to develop the anterior approach, in which the hepatic parenchyma is divided under inflow control before dissection of the right triangular ligament. A subsequent randomized trial from the same group in Hong Kong evaluated the effect of anterior approach hepatectomy on perioperative and survival outcomes.[94] There was no significant difference in blood loss between the anterior approach compared with conventional right hepatectomy. There was a high incidence of excessive hemorrhage (>2 L) in the conventional group, leading to higher rates of blood transfusion in this treatment arm. There was no difference in morbidity, and in-hospital mortality occurred in 1.7% versus 10% ($P = .114$) in anterior versus conventional resection, respectively. Median disease-free survival was also not significantly different (13.9 months conventional versus 15.5 months anterior; $P = .882$). Overall survival was significantly better with the anterior approach (>68.1 months vs 22.6 months; $P = .006$) due to a higher likelihood of treatable (ie, solitary or nondisseminated) recurrence. On multivariate analysis, anterior approach hepatectomy was associated with improved overall survival.

The anterior approach, however, is technically demanding due to the risk of injury to the middle hepatic vein and vena cava during deep parenchymal transection. To aid in the dissection and reduce the risk of caval injury, Belghiti and colleagues[95] described the liver hanging maneuver in 2001. In this technique, the right hilar structures are controlled and a space between the middle and right hepatic veins is developed. The anterior surface of the infrahepatic vena cava is exposed and a clamp is passed bluntly along the midplane of the vena cava that exits between the middle and right hepatic veins. A tape is then passed through the space and subsequently used to elevate the liver from the vena cava during parenchymal transection. This technique allows better protection of the inferior vena cava, easier hemostasis during deeper parenchymal transection, and a more linear transection plane.[96] Wu and colleagues[97] retrospectively analyzed 71 patients who underwent resection of less than or equal to 5 cm HCC, using either conventional right hepatectomy or anterior approach with the liver hanging maneuver. The patient groups were similar except that those undergoing anterior approach hepatectomy had significantly larger tumors (12 cm vs 9.7 cm; $P = .019$) although stage distribution was similar between the groups. The anterior approach

A

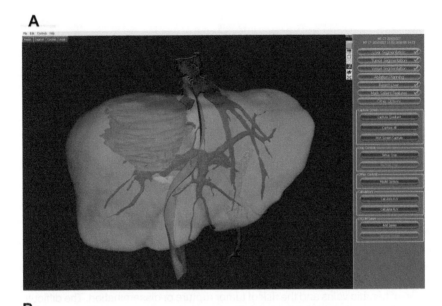

B

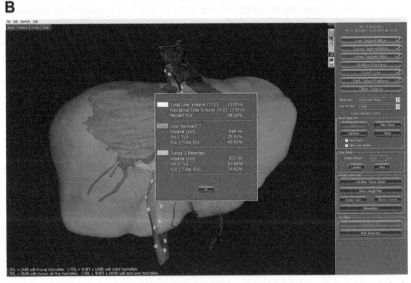

Fig. 3. (*A*) 3-D liver anatomy and proposed resection of a large HCC arising in the right hemiliver. (*B*) Volumetric analysis of proposed resection. (*Courtesy of* Pathfinder Therapeutics, Inc., Nashville, TN.)

group had a lower incidence of blood transfusion and lower recurrence rate (36.4% vs 71.1%; $P = .003$). Disease-free survival was better with the anterior approach (median 40.3 vs 7.1 months) but there was no difference in overall survival.

Outcomes

Although rates of disease recurrence remain high, overall survival has improved over the past several decades, with 5-year patient survival rates ranging from 25% to 55%, in large part likely due to improved therapy of intrahepatic recurrence (**Table 1**).[13–15,88,98–105]

Table 1
Representative series of resected HCC from Western and Eastern series

Author	Year	Study Period	N	% Cirrhosis	Misc	Recurrence Free Survival (years)			Overall Survival (years)		
						1	3	5	1	3	5
Nagasue[102]	1993	1980–1990	229	77.3%		60% death due to recurrence			79%	51%	28%
Vauthey[104]	1995	1970–1992	106	33%	68% vascular invasion						41%
Chen[101]	1997	1983–1994	382	45%	60% >5 cm				71%	52%	46%
Llovet[13]	1999	1989–1997	77	100%	3.3 cm mean tumor size				85%	62%	51%
Poon[14]	2001	1989–1994	136	50%	72% major resection	73%	39%	25%	68%	47%	36%
		1994–1999	241	43%	63% major resection	42%	23%	16%	82%	62%	49%
Belghiti[15]	2002	1990–1999	328	50%	42% major resection	60%	38%	25%	61%	57%	37%
Ercolani[105]	2003	1983–1999	224	100%	17% CTP B/C	70%	43%	27%	83%	63%	43%
Cha[100]	2003	1990–2001	164	40%	85% hemihepatectomy			25%	79%	51%	40%
Ikai[99]	2007	1992–2003	27,062	43%	26.6% multinodular				88%	69%	53%
Dahiya[88]	2010	1983–2002	373	100% (all tumors <5 cm)	Major Resection	70%	43%	32%	82%	63%	44%
					Minor Resection	67%	43%	32%	86%	65%	51%
Huang[98]	2010	2003–2005	115	65.2%	Within Milan	98%	92%	75%	85%	61%	51%

The largest series published to date is the 17th report of the Liver Cancer Study Group of Japan, which includes 27,062 patients treated with hepatic resection for HCC between 1992 and 2003.[99] In this series, 1-year, 3-year, 5-year, and 10-year overall survival rates were 87.8%, 69.2%, 53.4%, and 27.7%, respectively. Comparable results have been reported worldwide without marked differences between Western and Asian centers.[106] In well-selected patients (ie, well-compensated liver disease and small [<2 cm] solitary tumors without vascular invasion), resection can offer 5-year survival rates as high as 68%.[99] This is a small proportion of the patients who present with HCC; however, these results are similar to those of liver transplantation for early-stage HCC.[2]

Tumor recurrence after resection remains common despite great advances in patient selection and operative and anesthetic techniques, with 5-year recurrence rates ranging from 60% to 100% in larger series.[13,85,105] Recurrence most commonly occurs within the remnant liver, and clonality analysis of the recurrent tumor indicates that approximately one-third result from multicentric occurrence rather than intrahepatic metastasis.[107,108] Many factors influence the likelihood of intrahepatic recurrence, including the state of the native liver, tumor size, multicentricity, macrovascular or microvascular invasion, and, in some series, the need for blood transfusion.[105,109,110] There is no standard therapy for intrahepatic recurrence after resection. When feasible, repeat resection should be considered although this approach is often not possible due to multicentric recurrence and/or progression of chronic liver disease.[111] Several reports document the use of salvage transplantation for intrahepatic recurrence after resection.[109,112,113] The implications of this approach, especially for patients within the Milan criteria, are far-reaching and affected by many factors, including waiting time and regional deceased donor organ availability. Although this approach is attractive for patients with small tumors, groups in Paris and Bologna have shown that a substantial proportion of patients with recurrence do not proceed to liver transplantation (approximately 75% in the Bologna series).[112,113] Despite this, an intention-to-treat analysis in the Bologna series demonstrated similar 5-year survivals in the resection with salvage transplant group compared with patients listed for primary transplant. For patients with intrahepatic recurrence who are neither re-resection nor transplant candidates, several percutaneous options exist, including TACE, radiofrequency ablation, cryoablation, and percutaneous ethanol injection. These interventions are discussed in detail in the article by Guimaraes and Uflacker elsewhere in this issue. The modality of choice depends on tumor anatomy and center experience.

SUMMARY

Liver resection remains the standard therapy for solitary HCC in patients with preserved hepatic function. In well-selected patients, 5-year survival rates are good and can approach that of liver transplantation for early-stage disease. The role of resection in more advanced stages of disease (such as multicentric tumors, major vascular or biliary invasion, or with more advanced hepatic dysfunction) is controversial. Patient selection is critical to optimizing therapeutic benefit, and the health of the native liver must be considered in addition to tumor characteristics. Several modalities exist to aid in determining resection candidacy, including measurement of ICG clearance, FLR, CTP, MELD, and HVPG. Prior to resection, PVE can be used to predict the likelihood of hepatic failure and to reduce the likelihood of postresection morbidity and mortality in patients with and without chronic liver disease. Hepatic recurrence after resection is common. Several modalities can be used, however, to treat recurrent disease, including ablative therapy, TACE, re-resection and transplantation.

REFERENCES

1. Llovet JM, Beaugrand M. Hepatocellular carcinoma: present status and future prospects. J Hepatol 2003;38(Suppl 1):S136–49.
2. Mazzaferro V, Regalia E, Doci R, et al. Liver transplantation for the treatment of small hepatocellular carcinomas in patients with cirrhosis. N Engl J Med 1996; 334(11):693–9.
3. Tsoulfas G, Kawai T, Elias N, et al. Long-term experience with liver transplantation for hepatocellular carcinoma. J Gastroenterol 2011;46(2):249–56.
4. Island ER, Pomposelli J, Pomfret EA, et al. Twenty-year experience with liver transplantation for hepatocellular carcinoma. Arch Surg 2005;140(4):353–8.
5. Trevisani F, Cantarini MC, Labate AM, et al. Surveillance for hepatocellular carcinoma in elderly Italian patients with cirrhosis: effects on cancer staging and patient survival. Am J Gastroenterol 2004;99(8):1470–6.
6. Tong MJ, Blatt LM, Kao VW. Surveillance for hepatocellular carcinoma in patients with chronic viral hepatitis in the United States of America. J Gastroenterol Hepatol 2001;16(5):553–9.
7. Zhang BH, Yang BH, Tang ZY. Randomized controlled trial of screening for hepatocellular carcinoma. J Cancer Res Clin Oncol 2004;130(7):417–22.
8. Yuen MF, Cheng CC, Lauder IJ, et al. Early detection of hepatocellular carcinoma increases the chance of treatment: Hong Kong experience. Hepatology 2000;31(2):330–5.
9. Sharma P, Balan V, Hernandez JL, et al. Liver transplantation for hepatocellular carcinoma: the MELD impact. Liver Transpl 2004;10(1):36–41.
10. Washburn K. Model for end stage liver disease and hepatocellular carcinoma: a moving target. Transplant Rev (Orlando) 2010;24(1):11–7.
11. Bruix J, Llovet JM. Prognostic prediction and treatment strategy in hepatocellular carcinoma. Hepatology 2002;35(3):519–24.
12. Bismuth H, Chiche L, Adam R, et al. Liver resection versus transplantation for hepatocellular carcinoma in cirrhotic patients. Ann Surg 1993;218(2):145–51.
13. Llovet JM, Fuster J, Bruix J. Intention-to-treat analysis of surgical treatment for early hepatocellular carcinoma: resection versus transplantation. Hepatology 1999;30(6):1434–40.
14. Poon RT, Fan ST, Lo CM, et al. Improving survival results after resection of hepatocellular carcinoma: a prospective study of 377 patients over 10 years. Ann Surg 2001;234(1):63–70.
15. Belghiti J, Regimbeau JM, Durand F, et al. Resection of hepatocellular carcinoma: a European experience on 328 cases. Hepatogastroenterology 2002; 49(43):41–6.
16. Cha CH, Ruo L, Fong Y, et al. Resection of hepatocellular carcinoma in patients otherwise eligible for transplantation. Ann Surg 2003;238(3):315–21 [discussion: 321–3].
17. Bralet MP, Regimbeau JM, Pineau P, et al. Hepatocellular carcinoma occurring in nonfibrotic liver: epidemiologic and histopathologic analysis of 80 French cases. Hepatology 2000;32(2):200–4.
18. Trevisani F, D'Intino PE, Caraceni P, et al. Etiologic factors and clinical presentation of hepatocellular carcinoma. Differences between cirrhotic and noncirrhotic Italian patients. Cancer 1995;75(9):2220–32.
19. Trevisani F, De NS, Rapaccini G, et al. Semiannual and annual surveillance of cirrhotic patients for hepatocellular carcinoma: effects on cancer stage and patient survival (Italian experience). Am J Gastroenterol 2002;97(3):734–44.

20. Wong LL, Limm WM, Severino R, et al. Improved survival with screening for hepatocellular carcinoma. Liver Transpl 2000;6(3):320–5.
21. Pateron D, Ganne N, Trinchet JC, et al. Prospective study of screening for hepatocellular carcinoma in Caucasian patients with cirrhosis. J Hepatol 1994;20(1): 65–71.
22. Sherman M. Alphafetoprotein: an obituary. J Hepatol 2001;34(4):603–5.
23. Lencioni R. Surveillance and early diagnosis of hepatocellular carcinoma. Dig Liver Dis 2010;42(Suppl 3):S223–7.
24. Bilimoria MM, Lauwers GY, Doherty DA, et al. Underlying liver disease, not tumor factors, predicts long-term survival after resection of hepatocellular carcinoma. Arch Surg 2001;136(5):528–35.
25. Llovet JM, Fuster J, Bruix J. The Barcelona approach: diagnosis, staging, and treatment of hepatocellular carcinoma. Liver Transpl 2004;10(2 Suppl 1):S115–20.
26. Yao FY, Bass NM, Nikolai B, et al. Liver transplantation for hepatocellular carcinoma: analysis of survival according to the intention-to-treat principle and dropout from the waiting list. Liver Transpl 2002;8(10):873–83.
27. Yao FY, Ferrell L, Bass NM, et al. Liver transplantation for hepatocellular carcinoma: expansion of the tumor size limits does not adversely impact survival. Hepatology 2001;33(6):1394–403.
28. Bharat A, Brown DB, Crippin JS, et al. Pre-liver transplantation locoregional adjuvant therapy for hepatocellular carcinoma as a strategy to improve longterm survival. J Am Coll Surg 2006;203(4):411–20.
29. Chapman WC, Majella Doyle MB, Stuart JE, et al. Outcomes of neoadjuvant transarterial chemoembolization to downstage hepatocellular carcinoma before liver transplantation. Ann Surg 2008;248(4):617–25.
30. Grando-Lemaire V, Guettier C, Chevret S, et al. Hepatocellular carcinoma without cirrhosis in the West: epidemiological factors and histopathology of the non-tumorous liver. Groupe d'Etude et de Traitement du Carcinome Hepatocellulaire. J Hepatol 1999;31(3):508–13.
31. El-Serag HB, Davila JA. Is fibrolamellar carcinoma different from hepatocellular carcinoma? A US population-based study. Hepatology 2004;39(3):798–803.
32. Poon RT, Fan ST, Wong J. Selection criteria for hepatic resection in patients with large hepatocellular carcinoma larger than 10 cm in diameter. J Am Coll Surg 2002;194(5):592–602.
33. Belghiti J, Kianmanesh R. Surgical treatment of hepatocellular carcinoma. HPB (Oxford) 2005;7(1):42–9.
34. Yuki K, Hirohashi S, Sakamoto M, et al. Growth and spread of hepatocellular carcinoma. A review of 240 consecutive autopsy cases. Cancer 1990;66(10): 2174–9.
35. Koneru B, Teperman LW, Manzarbeitia C, et al. A multicenter evaluation of utility of chest computed tomography and bone scans in liver transplant candidates with stages I and II hepatoma. Ann Surg 2005;241(4):622–8.
36. Yoon KT, Kim JK, Kim do Y, et al. Role of 18F-fluorodeoxyglucose positron emission tomography in detecting extrahepatic metastasis in pretreatment staging of hepatocellular carcinoma. Oncology 2007;72(Suppl 1):104–10.
37. UNOS Liver Allocation Policy 3.6.4.4(i). In: UNOS, editor. UNOS; 2010.
38. Khan MA, Combs CS, Brunt EM, et al. Positron emission tomography scanning in the evaluation of hepatocellular carcinoma. J Hepatol 2000;32(5):792–7.
39. Wolfort RM, Papillion PW, Turnage RH, et al. Role of FDG-PET in the evaluation and staging of hepatocellular carcinoma with comparison of tumor size, AFP level, and histologic grade. Int Surg 2010;95(1):67–75.

40. Young AL, Malik HZ, Abu-Hilal M, et al. Large hepatocellular carcinoma: time to stop preoperative biopsy. J Am Coll Surg 2007;205(3):453–62.
41. Pawlik TM, Poon RT, Abdalla EK, et al. Critical appraisal of the clinical and pathologic predictors of survival after resection of large hepatocellular carcinoma. Arch Surg 2005;140(5):450–7 [discussion: 457–8].
42. Ng KK, Vauthey JN, Pawlik TM, et al. Is hepatic resection for large or multinodular hepatocellular carcinoma justified? Results from a multi-institutional database. Ann Surg Oncol 2005;12(5):364–73.
43. Wang BW, Mok KT, Liu SI, et al. Is hepatectomy beneficial in the treatment of multinodular hepatocellular carcinoma? J Formos Med Assoc 2008;107(8):616–26.
44. Ikai I, Yamamoto Y, Yamamoto N, et al. Results of hepatic resection for hepatocellular carcinoma invading major portal and/or hepatic veins. Surg Oncol Clin N Am 2003;12(1):65–75, ix.
45. Pawlik TM, Poon RT, Abdalla EK, et al. Hepatectomy for hepatocellular carcinoma with major portal or hepatic vein invasion: results of a multicenter study. Surgery 2005;137(4):403–10.
46. Yeh CN, Jan YY, Lee WC, et al. Hepatic resection for hepatocellular carcinoma with obstructive jaundice due to biliary tumor thrombi. World J Surg 2004;28(5):471–5.
47. Ikenaga N, Chijiiwa K, Otani K, et al. Clinicopathologic characteristics of hepatocellular carcinoma with bile duct invasion. J Gastrointest Surg 2009;13(3):492–7.
48. Franco D, Capussotti L, Smadja C, et al. Resection of hepatocellular carcinomas. Results in 72 European patients with cirrhosis. Gastroenterology 1990; 98(3):733–8.
49. Garrison RN, Cryer HM, Howard DA, et al. Clarification of risk factors for abdominal operations in patients with hepatic cirrhosis. Ann Surg 1984;199(6):648–55.
50. Mansour A, Watson W, Shayani V, et al. Abdominal operations in patients with cirrhosis: still a major surgical challenge. Surgery 1997;122(4):730–5 [discussion: 735–6].
51. Telem DA, Schiano T, Goldstone R, et al. Factors that predict outcome of abdominal operations in patients with advanced cirrhosis. Clin Gastroenterol Hepatol 2010;8(5):451–7 [quiz: e458].
52. Befeler AS, Palmer DE, Hoffman M, et al. The safety of intra-abdominal surgery in patients with cirrhosis: model for end-stage liver disease score is superior to Child-Turcotte-Pugh classification in predicting outcome. Arch Surg 2005; 140(7):650–4 [discussion: 655].
53. Farnsworth N, Fagan SP, Berger DH, et al. Child-Turcotte-Pugh versus MELD score as a predictor of outcome after elective and emergent surgery in cirrhotic patients. Am J Surg 2004;188(5):580–3.
54. Perkins L, Jeffries M, Patel T. Utility of preoperative scores for predicting morbidity after cholecystectomy in patients with cirrhosis. Clin Gastroenterol Hepatol 2004;2(12):1123–8.
55. Delis SG, Bakoyiannis A, Biliatis I, et al. Model for end-stage liver disease (MELD) score, as a prognostic factor for post-operative morbidity and mortality in cirrhotic patients, undergoing hepatectomy for hepatocellular carcinoma. HPB (Oxford) 2009;11(4):351–7.
56. Hsu KY, Chau GY, Lui WY, et al. Predicting morbidity and mortality after hepatic resection in patients with hepatocellular carcinoma: the role of Model for End-Stage Liver Disease score. World J Surg 2009;33(11):2412–9.
57. Cucchetti A, Ercolani G, Vivarelli M, et al. Impact of model for end-stage liver disease (MELD) score on prognosis after hepatectomy for hepatocellular carcinoma on cirrhosis. Liver Transpl 2006;12(6):966–71.

58. Teh SH, Christein J, Donohue J, et al. Hepatic resection of hepatocellular carcinoma in patients with cirrhosis: model of end-stage liver disease (MELD) score predicts perioperative mortality. J Gastrointest Surg 2005;9(9):1207–15 [discussion: 1215].

59. Vauthey JN, Pawlik TM, Abdalla EK, et al. Is extended hepatectomy for hepato-biliary malignancy justified? Ann Surg 2004;239(5):722–30 [discussion: 730–2].

60. Ribero D, Abdalla EK, Madoff DC, et al. Portal vein embolization before major hepatectomy and its effects on regeneration, resectability and outcome. Br J Surg 2007;94(11):1386–94.

61. Kishi Y, Abdalla EK, Chun YS, et al. Three hundred and one consecutive extended right hepatectomies: evaluation of outcome based on systematic liver volumetry. Ann Surg 2009;250(4):540–8.

62. Dixon E, Abdalla E, Schwarz RE, et al. AHPBA/SSO/SSAT Sponsored Consensus Conference on Multidisciplinary Treatment of Hepatocellular Carcinoma. HPB (Oxford) 2010;12(5):287–8.

63. Okochi O, Kaneko T, Sugimoto H, et al. ICG pulse spectrophotometry for peri-operative liver function in hepatectomy. J Surg Res 2002;103(1):109–13.

64. Lau H, Man K, Fan ST, et al. Evaluation of preoperative hepatic function in patients with hepatocellular carcinoma undergoing hepatectomy. Br J Surg 1997;84(9):1255–9.

65. Lam CM, Fan ST, Lo CM, et al. Major hepatectomy for hepatocellular carcinoma in patients with an unsatisfactory indocyanine green clearance test. Br J Surg 1999;86(8):1012–7.

66. Bruix J, Castells A, Bosch J, et al. Surgical resection of hepatocellular carcinoma in cirrhotic patients: prognostic value of preoperative portal pressure. Gastroenterology 1996;111(4):1018–22.

67. Cucchetti A, Ercolani G, Vivarelli M, et al. Is portal hypertension a contraindication to hepatic resection? Ann Surg 2009;250(6):922–8.

68. Ziser A, Plevak DJ, Wiesner RH, et al. Morbidity and mortality in cirrhotic patients undergoing anesthesia and surgery. Anesthesiology 1999;90(1):42–53.

69. Teh SH, Nagorney DM, Stevens SR, et al. Risk factors for mortality after surgery in patients with cirrhosis. Gastroenterology 2007;132(4):1261–9.

70. Kinoshita H, Sakai K, Hirohashi K, et al. Preoperative portal vein embolization for hepatocellular carcinoma. World J Surg 1986;10(5):803–8.

71. Kubota K, Makuuchi M, Kusaka K, et al. Measurement of liver volume and hepatic functional reserve as a guide to decision-making in resectional surgery for hepatic tumors. Hepatology 1997;26(5):1176–81.

72. Shirabe K, Shimada M, Gion T, et al. Postoperative liver failure after major hepatic resection for hepatocellular carcinoma in the modern era with special reference to remnant liver volume. J Am Coll Surg 1999;188(3):304–9.

73. Abulkhir A, Limongelli P, Healey AJ, et al. Preoperative portal vein embolization for major liver resection: a meta-analysis. Ann Surg 2008;247(1):49–57.

74. Farges O, Belghiti J, Kianmanesh R, et al. Portal vein embolization before right hepatectomy: prospective clinical trial. Ann Surg 2003;237(2):208–17.

75. Palavecino M, Chun YS, Madoff DC, et al. Major hepatic resection for hepatocellular carcinoma with or without portal vein embolization: perioperative outcome and survival. Surgery 2009;145(4):399–405.

76. Vauthey JN, Dixon E, Abdalla EK, et al. Pretreatment assessment of hepatocellular carcinoma: expert consensus statement. HPB (Oxford) 2010;12(5):289–99.

77. Zhou WP, Lai EC, Li AJ, et al. A prospective, randomized, controlled trial of preoperative transarterial chemoembolization for resectable large hepatocellular carcinoma. Ann Surg 2009;249(2):195–202.

78. Chua TC, Liauw W, Saxena A, et al. Systematic review of neoadjuvant transarterial chemoembolization for resectable hepatocellular carcinoma. Liver Int 2010; 30(2):166–74.
79. Fan ST, Lo CM, Liu CL, et al. Hepatectomy for hepatocellular carcinoma: toward zero hospital deaths. Ann Surg 1999;229(3):322–30.
80. Bryant R, Laurent A, Tayar C, et al. Liver resection for hepatocellular carcinoma. Surg Oncol Clin N Am 2008;17(3):607–33, ix.
81. Chen H, Merchant NB, Didolkar MS. Hepatic resection using intermittent vascular inflow occlusion and low central venous pressure anesthesia improves morbidity and mortality. J Gastrointest Surg 2000;4(2):162–7.
82. Pamecha V, Gurusamy KS, Sharma D, et al. Techniques for liver parenchymal transection: a meta-analysis of randomized controlled trials. HPB (Oxford) 2009;11(4):275–81.
83. Gurusamy KS, Pamecha V, Sharma D, et al. Techniques for liver parenchymal transection in liver resection. Cochrane Database Syst Rev 2009;1:CD006880.
84. Katz SC, Shia J, Liau KH, et al. Operative blood loss independently predicts recurrence and survival after resection of hepatocellular carcinoma. Ann Surg 2009;249(4):617–23.
85. Poon RT, Fan ST, Lo CM, et al. Intrahepatic recurrence after curative resection of hepatocellular carcinoma: long-term results of treatment and prognostic factors. Ann Surg 1999;229(2):216–22.
86. Man K, Fan ST, Ng IO, et al. Prospective evaluation of Pringle maneuver in hepatectomy for liver tumors by a randomized study. Ann Surg 1997;226(6):704–11 [discussion: 711–3].
87. Chen J, Huang K, Wu J, et al. Survival after anatomic resection versus nonanatomic resection for hepatocellular carcinoma: a meta-analysis. Dig Dis Sci 2010. [Epub ahead of print].
88. Dahiya D, Wu TJ, Lee CF, et al. Minor versus major hepatic resection for small hepatocellular carcinoma (HCC) in cirrhotic patients: a 20-year experience. Surgery 2010;147(5):676–85.
89. Poon RT, Fan ST, Ng IO, et al. Significance of resection margin in hepatectomy for hepatocellular carcinoma: a critical reappraisal. Ann Surg 2000;231(4):544–51.
90. Shi M, Guo RP, Lin XJ, et al. Partial hepatectomy with wide versus narrow resection margin for solitary hepatocellular carcinoma: a prospective randomized trial. Ann Surg 2007;245(1):36–43.
91. Jarnagin W, Chapman WC, Curley S, et al. Surgical treatment of hepatocellular carcinoma: expert consensus statement. HPB (Oxford) 2010;12(5):302–10.
92. Chouillard E, Cherqui D, Tayar C, et al. Anatomical bi- and trisegmentectomies as alternatives to extensive liver resections. Ann Surg 2003;238(1):29–34.
93. Lai EC, Fan ST, Lo CM, et al. Anterior approach for difficult major right hepatectomy. World J Surg 1996;20(3):314–7 [discussion: 318].
94. Liu CL, Fan ST, Cheung ST, et al. Anterior approach versus conventional approach right hepatic resection for large hepatocellular carcinoma: a prospective randomized controlled study. Ann Surg 2006;244(2):194–203.
95. Belghiti J, Guevara OA, Noun R, et al. Liver hanging maneuver: a safe approach to right hepatectomy without liver mobilization. J Am Coll Surg 2001;193(1):109–11.
96. Meng WC, Shao CX, Mak KL, et al. Anatomical justification of Belghiti's 'liver hanging manoeuvre' in right hepatectomy with anterior approach. ANZ J Surg 2003;73(6):407–9.

97. Wu TJ, Wang F, Lin YS, et al. Right hepatectomy by the anterior method with liver hanging versus conventional approach for large hepatocellular carcinomas. Br J Surg 2010;97(7):1070–8.

98. Huang J, Yan L, Cheng Z, et al. A randomized trial comparing radiofrequency ablation and surgical resection for HCC conforming to the Milan criteria. Ann Surg 2010;252(6):903–12.

99. Ikai I, Arii S, Okazaki M, et al. Report of the 17th nationwide follow-up survey of primary liver cancer in Japan. Hepatol Res 2007;37(9):676–91.

100. Cha C, Fong Y, Jarnagin WR, et al. Predictors and patterns of recurrence after resection of hepatocellular carcinoma. J Am Coll Surg 2003;197(5):753–8.

101. Chen MF, Jeng LB. Partial hepatic resection for hepatocellular carcinoma. J Gastroenterol Hepatol 1997;12(9–10):S329–34.

102. Nagasue N, Kohno H, Chang YC, et al. Liver resection for hepatocellular carcinoma. Results of 229 consecutive patients during 11 years. Ann Surg 1993; 217(4):375–84.

103. Shimozawa N, Hanazaki K. Longterm prognosis after hepatic resection for small hepatocellular carcinoma. J Am Coll Surg 2004;198(3):356–65.

104. Vauthey JN, Klimstra D, Franceschi D, et al. Factors affecting long-term outcome after hepatic resection for hepatocellular carcinoma. Am J Surg 1995;169(1):28–34 [discussion: 34–5].

105. Ercolani G, Grazi GL, Ravaioli M, et al. Liver resection for hepatocellular carcinoma on cirrhosis: univariate and multivariate analysis of risk factors for intrahepatic recurrence. Ann Surg 2003;237(4):536–43.

106. Esnaola NF, Mirza N, Lauwers GY, et al. Comparison of clinicopathologic characteristics and outcomes after resection in patients with hepatocellular carcinoma treated in the United States, France, and Japan. Ann Surg 2003;238(5): 711–9.

107. Li Q, Wang J, Juzi JT, et al. Clonality analysis for multicentric origin and intrahepatic metastasis in recurrent and primary hepatocellular carcinoma. J Gastrointest Surg 2008;12(9):1540–7.

108. Ng IO, Guan XY, Poon RT, et al. Determination of the molecular relationship between multiple tumour nodules in hepatocellular carcinoma differentiates multicentric origin from intrahepatic metastasis. J Pathol 2003;199(3):345–53.

109. Poon RT, Fan ST, Lo CM, et al. Long-term survival and pattern of recurrence after resection of small hepatocellular carcinoma in patients with preserved liver function: implications for a strategy of salvage transplantation. Ann Surg 2002; 235(3):373–82.

110. Imamura H, Matsuyama Y, Tanaka E, et al. Risk factors contributing to early and late phase intrahepatic recurrence of hepatocellular carcinoma after hepatectomy. J Hepatol 2003;38(2):200–7.

111. Poon RT, Fan ST, O'Suilleabhain CB, et al. Aggressive management of patients with extrahepatic and intrahepatic recurrences of hepatocellular carcinoma by combined resection and locoregional therapy. J Am Coll Surg 2002;195(3): 311–8.

112. Del Gaudio M, Ercolani G, Ravaioli M, et al. Liver transplantation for recurrent hepatocellular carcinoma on cirrhosis after liver resection: university of bologna experience. Am J Transplant 2008;8(6):1177–85.

113. Adam R, Azoulay D. Is primary resection and salvage transplantation for hepatocellular carcinoma a reasonable strategy? Ann Surg 2005;241(4):671–2.

Laparoscopic Liver Resection in the Treatment of Hepatocellular Carcinoma

Jens Mittler, MD[1], John W. McGillicuddy, MD[1,*],
Kenneth D. Chavin, MD, PhD

KEYWORDS

- Laparoscopic hepatic resection • Hepatocellular carcinoma
- Cirrhosis • Noncirrhotic HCC

Laparoscopic liver resection is an emerging technique in liver surgery. Although laparoscopy is well established for several abdominal procedures and is for some even considered the preferred approach, laparoscopic hepatic resection has been introduced into clinical practice more widely since 2000. Although the feasibility and efficacy of laparoscopic resections has been reported often, these procedures are performed only in experienced centers and only in a select group of patients. While initially performed only for benign hepatic lesions, the indications for laparoscopic resection have gradually broadened to encompass all kinds of malignant hepatic lesions, including hepatocellular carcinoma (HCC) in patients with cirrhosis. It is in cirrhotic patients that the advantages of the minimally invasive approach may be most evident.

The roles of transplantation, local ablation, chemoembolization, and chemotherapy in the treatment of HCC are addressed elsewhere in this issue. Surgical resection is the oldest therapeutic approach to hepatic malignancy. The treatment algorithm has grown increasingly complex over the years, and reflects both the complexity of the disease and the myriad of therapeutic options. For HCC, more than for any other abdominal malignancy, the role of each treatment option remains controversial, and for many patients there is no one correct answer. The decision has to take into account not only the extent of disease and patient-specific factors but the availability of other treatments and donor organ availability as well as the criteria for liver transplantation.

The purpose of this article is to report the worldwide experience with laparoscopic resection for HCC and to delineate its role compared with the "open" or laparotomy

Division of Transplant Surgery, Department of Surgery, Medical University of South Carolina (MUSC), 96 Jonathan Lucas Street Charleston, SC 29425, USA
[1] J.M. and J.W.McG. contributed equally to this article.
* Corresponding author.
E-mail address: mcgillij@musc.edu

Clin Liver Dis 15 (2011) 371–384
doi:10.1016/j.cld.2011.03.009
1089-3261/11/$ – see front matter © 2011 Elsevier Inc. All rights reserved.

approach. The anatomic and surgical terminology in this article follows the International Hepato-Pancreato-Biliary Association (IHPBA) consensus *Brisbane 2000 Terminology of Liver Anatomy and Resections* as reviewed by Strasberg.[1] The terminology regarding technical aspects and types of laparoscopic resections is in concordance with the 2008 International Position on Laparoscopic Liver Surgery, namely The Louisville Statement 2008.[2]

HISTORY OF LAPAROSCOPIC LIVER RESECTION

The initial development of laparoscopic liver surgery was mostly driven by groups in France, Italy, and Great Britain. The first laparoscopic liver resection was reported by Gagner and colleagues[3] in 1992, who performed a wedge resection of a focal nodular hyperplasia. A few reports on laparoscopic wedge resections of rather peripheral and mostly benign lesions then ensued. The first reported resection of an HCC was published in 1995 by Hashizume and colleagues,[4] and the first anatomic laparoscopic resection, a left-lateral sectionectomy in 1996, by Azagra and colleagues.[5]

From a technical standpoint, these first efforts were all resections limited to the anterior, or "laparoscopic", liver segments 2, 3, 4b, 5, and 6, which are comparatively easier to access laparoscopically than the more posterior segments 1, 4a, 7, and 8. The first laparoscopic hemihepatectomy was performed by Huscher and colleagues in 1998.[6] It was not until 2000 that Cherqui and colleagues[7] published a prospective cohort of 30 laparoscopic resections, which was the first in a series of larger studies demonstrating the feasibility and safety of the laparoscopic approach. Since then, highly specialized centers have published their experience with laparoscopic wedge and minor resections, laparoscopic hemihepatectomies, extended resections, trisectionectomies, and resections in the laparoscopically difficult posterior segments (**Table 1**). In 2000, Fong and colleagues[8] described the hand-assisted laparoscopic approach to manually examine the liver for additional tumors and to rule out extrahepatic metastases, and Inagaki and colleagues[9] performed the first hand-assisted left-lateral sectionectomy in a cirrhotic patient. The first laparoscopic procurement of a living donor graft was reported in France in 2002.[10] The Glissonian approach, a selective intraparenchymal dissection to gain control of the vasculobiliary pedicle, was safely demonstrated by Topal and colleagues,[11] and a single-incision laparoscopic technique was first introduced in 2010.[12,13]

The development of laparoscopic liver resection and its clinical application has been closely linked to technical innovations especially regarding parenchymal transection. The first use of a disposable stapler to laparoscopically transect the hepatic parenchyma was published in 1993.[14] Mechanical fragmentation and argon beam coagulation were reported in 1994,[15] use of a hydrojet dissector and a Cavitron Ultrasonic Surgical Aspirator (CUSA; Tyco, Mansfield, MA) both in 1995,[16,17] the ultrasonic scalpel in 1998,[18] and the LigaSure device (Covidien, Boulder, CO) in 2005.[16,19] As in open liver surgery, the choice of one or other transection technique is mostly center-specific or surgeon-specific, and no single method has been show to be superior.

TERMINOLOGY AND TYPES OF LAPAROSCOPIC LIVER RESECTIONS

According to the 2008 International Louisville Consensus, there are 3 types of laparoscopic liver resections[2]:

1. Pure laparoscopic procedures
2. Hand-assisted laparoscopic liver resections
3. The hybrid technique.

In the pure laparoscopic approach, the entire operation is performed through laparoscopic ports, and only a small incision is made to extract the specimen. If the unplanned placement of a hand-port is required for management of intraoperative complications or because of failure to making progress, the procedure is labeled "pure laparoscopy with hand-port conversion."

The hand-assisted approach includes the elective placement of a hand-port to facilitate the operation and for the purpose of a manual examination of the liver.

The hybrid technique describes a procedure that is begun as either pure or hand-assisted laparoscopy, but in which the actual parenchymal transection is accomplished through a mini-laparotomy.

As far as the extent of the resection is concerned, the literature distinguishes between minor and major laparoscopic procedures. Wedge resections and segmentectomies in the more easily approached segments 2, 3, 4b, 5, and 6 are usually referred to as minor resections. A left-lateral sectionectomy (bisegmentectomy 2 and 3) is also considered a minor resection.

By contrast, hemihepatectomies, extended hemihepatectomies, and trisectionectomies are classified as major laparoscopic procedures. Resections in the difficult to access posterior liver segments 1, 4a, 7, and 8 demand a high degree of laparoscopic skill and are therefore also considered major procedures.

MINOR LAPAROSCOPIC LIVER RESECTIONS

The vast majority of laparoscopic liver resections for HCC reported thus far are minor hepatic procedures (see **Table 1**), which are mostly performed as wedge resections, segmentectomies in segments 2 to 6, or left-lateral sectionectomies for peripherally located solitary tumors not larger than 5 cm. At the 2009 International Consensus Meeting in Louisville, left-lateral sectionectomy was found to be the most straightforward moderately sized laparoscopic procedure, and all participants agreed that the laparoscopic approach should be considered the standard of care for this procedure.[2]

Anatomic resection has been shown to provide superior oncological outcomes compared with wedge resection. Removal of the tumor along with its portal territory (ie, the surrounding liver segment) should be attempted whenever possible.[20] A recent large meta-analysis comparing results of anatomic with nonanatomic liver resection for HCC in more than 1500 patients showed better disease-free survival, but no difference in overall survival in the anatomic resection group.[21]

MAJOR LAPAROSCOPIC LIVER RESECTIONS

As previously mentioned, major laparoscopic resections are defined as hemihepatectomies (**Fig. 1**, for example), extended hemihepatectomies, trisectionectomies, and resections in the laparoscopically difficult liver segments 1, 4a, 7, or 8. Almost all have been performed at a small number of highly experienced centers. Although Huscher reported the first laparoscopic right hemihepatectomy as early as 1998,[6] the experience with major laparoscopic resections is still limited. These procedures are being performed only in a small number of centers, and therefore cannot yet be considered the standard of care. An international review of laparoscopic liver resections from 2009 found that in only 16% of 2804 patients were major resections performed (9% right hemihepatectomies, 7% left hemihepatectomies).[22]

An analysis of 210 hemihepatectomies (136 right hemihepatectomies and 74 left hemihepatectomies) that were performed in 6 centers worldwide (3 European, 2 United States, and 1 Australian) demonstrated the feasibility, safety, and efficacy of major laparoscopic liver resections.[23] HCC was the indication in 36 cases and 16 patients

Table 1
Reports with greater than 10 laparoscopic liver resections for HCC

Reference	Year	No. of HCC Cases/Total Cases	Major LLR (%)	Cirrhosis Present (%)	Tumor Size (cm)	Surgical Margin (cm)	Perioperative Morbidity (%)	Perioperative Mortality (%)	OS 1 y/5 y (%)	RFS 1 y/5 y (%)	OS Mean (mo)	RFS mean (mo)
Dagher et al[61]	2010	163	10	73.6	3.6	1.2	22	1.2	92.6/64.9	77.5/32.2	—	—
Aldrighetti et al[60]	2010	16	—	56.2	4 + 2.2	1.1	25	0	—	—	40.2	23.3
Nitta et al[69]	2010	15/43	100	80	4.5	—	11.6	0	—	—	—	—
Yoon et al[62]	2010	69	30	55	3.1	1.5	21.7	0	90.4 (3 y)	60.4 (3 year)	—	—
Zhen et al[70]	2010	29	0	55.2	4.7	>1.0	27.6	—	—	—	—	—
Zhang et al[71]	2009	33/78	9	26.4	6.2	1.2	0	0	—	—	—	—
Vigano et al[72]	2010	69/174	33	26.4	3.5	1.1	21.2	0	—	—	—	—
Tranchart et al[73]	2010	42	12	73	3.6	1.1	9.5	—	93.1/59.5	81.6/45.6	—	—
Endo et al[74]	2009	10/21	0	100	3.0	1.7	30	0	100/57	72 /31	—	—
Cherqui et al[29]	2009	37/274	6	74	—	1.1	34	0	—/72	—/44	—	—
Belli et al[75]	2009	54/125	6	100	3.8	—	19	2	94/67 (3 y)	78/52 (3 y)	63	38
Lai et al[76]	2009	30	1	93	2.8	—	20	0	95/50	90/36	33.6	33.6
Ito et al[77]	2009	10/65	0	7.7	—	—	13.8	0	72.3 (3 y)	57 (1 y)	—	22
Itano et al[78]	2009	13/17	0	8	3	1.1	24	0	—	100	—	18
Bryant et al[79]	2009	64/166	19	28	3.5	1.15	15.1	0	70 (3 y)/65 (5 y)	46 (3 y)/34 (5 y)	26	26

Study	Year											
Sarpel et al[80]	2009	20/56	—	45	4.3	—	5	—	100/95 (4 y)	90/50 (4 y)	24	24
Lai et al[76]	2009	25/33	—	92	2.5	1.3	16	0	100/38	100/52	—	29
Cho et al[81]	2009	27/40	30	89	3.4	—	28	0	—	—	—	—
Inagaki et al[82]	2009	36/68	0.05	42	2.9	—	26	0	100/79.3	—	—	—
Sasaki et al[58]	2009	37/82	0	73	02.5	0.7	5	—	97/52.7	50 (2.5 y)	36	30
Buell et al[59]	2008	36/253	5	56	4.6	0.7	16	1.6	90/80	23 (2 y)	28	28
Chen et al[57]	2008	116/116	3	100	2.1	>1	6	0	90/61	—	—	—
Cho et al[83]	2008	57/128	32	80.7	3.5	1.6	18	0	—	—	—	—
Dagher et al[84]	2008	32	9	69	3.8	1.4	15.6	3.1	95/72 (3 y)	80/55 (3 y)	26	26
Cai et al[85]	2008	24/31	9.7	16	3.99	>1	0	0	95.4/56.2	—	29.8	—
Belli et al[86]	2007	23	0	100	3.1	1.0	22	4.3	93/85 (2 y)	—	46.3	46.3
Santambrogio et al[87]	2009	19/22	0	100	2.8	1	10.5	0	85/50 (4 y)	60/24 (4 y)	11.5	11.5
Vibert et al[54]	2006	16/89	—	50	6.5	—	21	1	85/66 (3 y)	76/68 (3 y)	40	40
Tang et al[88]	2006	17/40	0	94	—	>1	20	0	86/59 (2 y)	53 (2 y)	—	26
Kaneko et al[89]	2005	30/40	0	100	3.0	—	10	0	97/61	87/31	—	—
Teramoto et al[90]	2005	11/11	0	67	2.0	—	26	0	100/80 (3 y)	75/40 (3 y)	—	—
Shimada et al[66]	2001	17/38	0	76.5	2.6	0.8	5.9	—	85/48	80/40 (4 y)	—	—

Abbreviations: LLR, laparoscopic liver resection; OS, overall survival; RFS, recurrence-free survival.

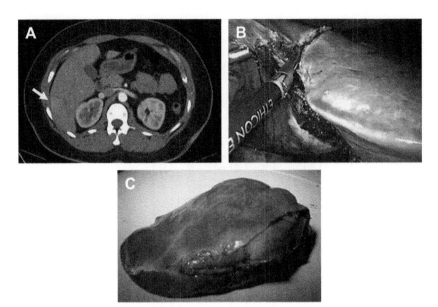

Fig. 1. (*A*) Abdominal computed tomography (arterial phase) demonstrating right-lobe HCC in a noncirrhotic liver (*arrow*). (*B*) Parenchymal transection using a Harmonic Scalpel. (*C*) Hemihepatectomy specimen (surgical margin 9 mm).

had cirrhosis. United States centers tended to use the hand-assist technique whereas European centers favored the pure laparoscopic approach. The conversion rate to open surgery was 12%. The investigators emphasized the importance of careful patient selection (ie, tumors well clear of the line of resection and not too close to major vessels, small tumors, and otherwise healthy livers without parenchymal changes). Comparing the first 15 patients in each center with the following 20, surgical outcomes regarding operative time, blood loss, conversion rate, use of a Pringle maneuver, and length of stay improved significantly with growing experience. Similarly, a report on 43 patients (15 with HCC, 12 with cirrhosis) from a single Japanese center emphasized the importance of patient selection and demonstrated a clear learning curve as center experience grew. Of note in this study, a laparoscopic hanging maneuver, in analogy to the hanging maneuver as described by Belghiti and colleagues[24] for open procedures, was used to facilitate parenchymal transection.

TECHNICAL CONSIDERATIONS IN MAJOR RESECTIONS
Assessment of the Future Liver Remnant

Postoperative morbidity and mortality associated with liver resection, especially after major hepatectomies, are largely attributable to hemorrhage and postoperative liver failure. Bleeding complications have become considerably less frequent with improved operative techniques and instrumentation, and advances in perioperative anesthesia management.[25] The degree of postoperative liver dysfunction and failure is determined by the functional capacity of the liver remnant.

When planning a major resection, it is critical to attempt to preoperatively predict the size and function of the future liver remnant. Advanced radiologic imaging can be used to study the hepatic anatomy, to define the relation of the tumor to the intrahepatic structures, and to measure volumes of resected and remnant liver tissue just as it is for open hepatic resection.[26] In the setting of chronic underlying liver disease and cirrhosis, analysis of reports in the literature suggests that a liver remnant of at least 40% provides an adequate margin of safety.[27]

Portal Vein Embolization

The technique of inducing parenchymal hypertrophy through embolization of the contralateral portal vein branch appears to be of value even in the setting of cirrhosis.[27] Although cirrhotic livers have limited regenerative capacity, cirrhotic patients developed volume hypertrophy of their future liver remnant, averaging 9% compared with 16% in the noncirrhotic group, after preoperative embolization of the contralateral portal vein branch.[28] Failure to demonstrate adequate hypertrophy following portal vein embolization was seen in approximately 10% to 20% of cirrhotics, and was considered a contraindication to a major hepatectomy. Similarly, a French group reported good results with routine portal vein embolization prior to right hemihepatectomy in chronically diseased (cirrhotic and noncirrhotic) livers.[29]

INDICATIONS

In 70% to 90% of cases HCC develops on a background of hepatic cirrhosis or chronic inflammation,[30] and is particularly prevalent in patients with chronic hepatitis B virus (52% of all HCC cases worldwide) or hepatitis C virus infection (20% of all cases).[31] This high association with underlying chronic liver disease differentiates HCC from other hepatic lesions and has considerable impact on surgical decision making.

HCC in the Absence of Chronic Liver Disease or Cirrhosis

HCC without cirrhosis is uncommon but not rare, as 5% to 15% of all HCCs are found in patients with an otherwise normal liver.[32] In contrast to cirrhotic patients, these noncirrhotic HCC (NC-HCC) are often found in young, otherwise healthy women. Diagnosis is often made late, most often not until after the development of symptoms.

Because these livers are otherwise healthy and not considered to be precancerous, even extended resection can be performed safely in most patients, and is the treatment of choice. Of interest, results of several studies have suggested that outcome after resection for NC-HCC is much less dependent on tumor size than for cirrhotic patients.[33,34] Reported overall 5-year survival rates after resection of NC-HCC range between 45% and 70%, with recurrence-free survival rates between 25% and 50%.[35–38] In selected patients and at specialized centers, resections of NC-HCC have been successfully performed laparoscopically.[39] For unresectable NC-HCC liver transplantation can be considered in selected patients, as 5-year survival rates are between 50% and 70%.[40]

HCC in Well-Compensated Cirrhosis (Child-Turcotte-Pugh Class A)

HCC within the Milan criteria (transplantable HCC)

For solitary tumors of less than 5 cm diameter, there is ongoing debate about whether a patient should first be offered resection or transplantation. For HCC in well-compensated cirrhosis (Child-Turcotte-Pugh [CTP] Class A), liver resection offers a 5-year overall survival of up to 50% with an operative mortality as low as 0% to 6.4% at major hepatobiliary centers worldwide.[41–44] This outcome compares with a reported disease-free survival of 70% after liver transplantation if the cancer meets the so-called Milan criteria, namely, a single lesion smaller than 5 cm or up to 3 lesions all smaller than 3 cm.[45] Liver transplantation removes not only the malignant lesion but also the background precancerous state. Its use is limited, however, by the availability of donor organs.

With advanced surgical technique and perioperative care, outcome after liver resection for HCC has improved.[46] Resection allows histologic assessment of the tumor, but still carries a high risk of recurrence due to the precancerous nature of the liver remnant.[47] Patients need to be followed closely to detect recurrence early for possible rescue liver transplantation, re-resection, or other treatment modality. Cherqui and colleagues[29] demonstrated overall and disease-free 5-year survival rates of 72% and 44%, respectively, in transplantable patients (ie, those with tumors within Milan criteria and age less than 65 years). The rates of recurrence, transplantable recurrence, and intention-to-treat salvage liver transplantation were 59%, 80%, and 61%. Five-year survival after salvage liver transplantation was 70% when calculated from the time of transplant and 87% when calculated from the time of resection. Salvage transplantation was technically easier when the previous resection was done laparoscopically, due to fewer adhesions.[29]

For patients with multifocal HCC within the Milan criteria, North American and European centers tend to transplant rather than resect.[48] South-Eastern Asian centers, however, have reported their experience with resections of 2 to 3 tumors all smaller than 3 cm, and have reported overall 5-year survival rates that range from 50% to 60%.[49–52]

HCC outside the Milan criteria
In many Western countries, patients with HCC that fall outside the Milan criteria are not eligible for deceased donor liver transplantation because of higher recurrence rates and poorer survival. Transarterial chemoembolization (TACE) offers 5-year survival rates of less than 10%, and living-donor liver transplantation is only exceptionally considered in these patients.

Several studies of laparoscopic liver resection have reported that average tumor diameters of greater than 5 cm, and even tumors larger than 10 cm, have been successfully resected laparoscopically. Hwang and colleagues[53] reviewed the worldwide experience in hepatic resection for HCC greater than 10 cm and reported 5-year survival rates of 16.7% to 38.5%. In this group's experience overall and disease-free survivals were 31% and 20%.[47] A French group reported successful laparoscopic resection of HCC lesions up to 18 cm in size.[54]

Despite its limitations, resection, if feasible, is the best treatment option for large HCC lesions. However, laparoscopic resection of these large lesions is possible only in the minority of cases, and the total reported experience is limited. Some groups have recommended against the laparoscopic approach for lesions larger than 5 cm, due to concern for the difficulty of tumor mobilization, the risk of tumor rupture, and the adequacy of margins.[39]

HCC in Advanced Cirrhosis
All types of surgery carry a substantially higher risk of morbidity and mortality in cirrhotic patients; the risk increases with the severity of the liver disease.[55] Nonetheless, laparoscopic liver resections have been successfully performed in patients with advanced cirrhosis (CTP Class B/C). A first article by a French group in 1999 reported good outcomes after laparoscopic resection in 3 patients with HCC and advanced cirrhosis, who were felt to have contraindications to open surgery.[56] Chen and colleagues[57] reported their experience with laparoscopic resections in 116 patients

with HCC, 16 of whom also had advanced cirrhosis. A study by Sasaki and colleagues[58] reported on 39 patients with HCC, 27 of whom had cirrhosis and 4 of whom had advanced disease, who underwent laparoscopic resection. Neither report, however, specified the outcomes for the patients with advanced cirrhosis.

Overall, the experience with laparoscopic resections in patients with advanced cirrhosis is limited, and these patients are usually better served with liver transplantation unless it is contraindicated.

LAPAROSCOPIC VERSUS OPEN LIVER RESECTION
Oncological Outcome

The real measure of any potentially curative operation for cancer is its oncological outcome as measured by tumor-free margins, disease-free survival, and patient survival. There have been no prospective randomized trials addressing the relative merits of the laparoscopic approach, so all of the relevant data have come from case series.

In a systematic review of the literature, Vigano and colleagues[39] reported in 2009 that in most studies on the topic, there were equivalent oncological outcomes. Taken as a whole, disease-free 3-year and 5-year survival rates were 65% to 75% and 50% to 70%, respectively, in the laparoscopic groups, and 50% to 70% and 35% to 50%, respectively, in the open surgery groups. Resection margin widths were adequate (>10 mm) in most studies, and port site metastasis, with the exception of one reported case, was not a problem.[59] More recently, there has been equivalent or slightly improved survival with the laparoscopic approach.[60,61] The analysis by Cherqui and colleagues[29] in 2009 (see earlier discussion) showed overall and disease-free 5-year survival rates of 70% and 42% in transplantable (within Milan criteria and younger than 65 years) HCC patients. Yoon and colleagues[62] reported overall and disease-free 3-year survival rates of 90.4% and 60.4%, respectively.

Comparing these data with outcomes after open surgery for HCC raises two concerns. First, none of these studies were prospective trials and second, as for every new technique, there is the possibility of a significant selection bias as patients picked to undergo laparoscopic resection have been very carefully selected.

One possible advantage of the laparoscopic approach is that it may be feasible for patients in whom an open surgery for HCC has been deemed too morbid. Such diminished morbidity was reported as early as 1999 by Abdel-Atty, who found that the development or exacerbation of ascites and the development of liver failure were less common after laparoscopy than after laparotomy.[56] These findings have been subsequently confirmed.[63,64] Laparoscopic resection of HCC also facilitates salvage transplantation in cases of transplantable recurrence, because adhesions are less severe.[65] Comparing 12 laparoscopically resected patients undergoing salvage transplantation to 12 patients undergoing transplantation after open resection, Laurent and colleagues[65] saw shorter operating times, less blood loss, and lower transfusion rates in the laparoscopy group (**Box 1**).

Secondary Outcome Benefits to Laparoscopy

Other potential benefits of the laparoscopic approach include less postoperative pain, a shorter length of stay in hospital, and an earlier return of functional status.[63,64,66,67] It has also been suggested that there are financial savings with laparoscopic resection, as the cost of the relatively expensive laparoscopic instruments is outweighed by shorter operating times.[67] Comparing laparoscopic with open left-lateral sectionectomies, a Canadian group showed greater cost efficiency with laparoscopy.[68]

Box 1
Advantages and disadvantages of the laparoscopic compared with the open approach for liver resections

- Advantages
  - ○ Less postoperative ascites production
  - ○ Reduced postoperative pain
  - ○ Feasible in selected cirrhotics who have contraindications to open surgery
  - ○ Less intra-abdominal adhesions (easier salvage transplantation)
  - ○ Shorter recovery time
  - ○ Shorter length of stay
  - ○ Reduced financial cost
- Disadvantages
  - ○ No manual palpation or exploration of the liver parenchyma possible (with the pure laparoscopic approach)
  - ○ High demand in surgical skill (especially major resections)

SUMMARY

Hepatic resections are highly complex procedures that demand a high level of surgical competency, and this is especially true for laparoscopic liver resections because they require, in addition, expert laparoscopic skills. While laparoscopic left-lateral sectionectomy is the most straightforward of the laparoscopic procedures and is now considered the standard of care for some indications, major laparoscopic resections are still performed only at highly specialized centers in carefully selected patients. The ability to provide equivalent oncologic outcomes with diminished liver-specific morbidity makes the laparoscopic approach to HCC particularly attractive in patients with concomitant cirrhosis. In the absence of randomized control trial data, results to date must be interpreted in the light of selection bias. Prospective trials are needed to clarify the utility and safety of laparoscopic HCC resection.

REFERENCES

1. Strasberg SM. Nomenclature of hepatic anatomy and resections: a review of the Brisbane 2000 system. J Hepatobiliary Pancreat Surg 2005;12(5):351–5.
2. Buell JF, Cherqui D, Geller DA, et al. The international position on laparoscopic liver surgery: the Louisville Statement, 2008. Ann Surg 2009;250(5):825–30.
3. Gagner M, Lacroix A, Bolte E. Laparoscopic adrenalectomy in Cushing's syndrome and pheochromocytoma. N Engl J Med 1992;327(14):1033.
4. Hashizume M, Takenaka K, Yanaga K, et al. Laparoscopic hepatic resection for hepatocellular carcinoma. Surg Endosc 1995;9(12):1289–91.
5. Azagra JS, Goergen M, Gilbart E, et al. Laparoscopic anatomical (hepatic) left lateral segmentectomy-technical aspects. Surg Endosc 1996;10(7):758–61.
6. Huscher CG, Lirici MM, Chiodini S. Laparoscopic liver resections. Semin Laparosc Surg 1998;5(3):204–10.
7. Cherqui D, Husson E, Hammoud R, et al. Laparoscopic liver resections: a feasibility study in 30 patients. Ann Surg 2000;232(6):753–62.
8. Fong Y, Jarnagin W, Conlon KC, et al. Hand-assisted laparoscopic liver resection: lessons from an initial experience. Arch Surg 2000;135(7):854–9.

9. Inagaki H, Kurokawa T, Nonami T, et al. Hand-assisted laparoscopic left lateral segmentectomy of the liver for hepatocellular carcinoma with cirrhosis. J Hepatobiliary Pancreat Surg 2003;10(4):295–8.

10. Cherqui D, Soubrane O, Husson E, et al. Laparoscopic living donor hepatectomy for liver transplantation in children. Lancet 2002;359(9304):392–6.

11. Topal B, Aerts R, Penninckx F. Laparoscopic intrahepatic Glissonian approach for right hepatectomy is safe, simple, and reproducible. Surg Endosc 2007;21(11):2111.

12. Gaujoux S, Kingham TP, Jarnagin WR, et al. Single-incision laparoscopic liver resection. Surg Endosc 2011;25(5):1489–94.

13. Aldrighetti L, Guzzetti E, Ferla G. Laparoscopic hepatic left lateral sectionectomy using the LaparoEndoscopic Single Site approach: evolution of minimally invasive liver surgery. J Hepatobiliary Pancreat Sci 2011;18(1):103–5.

14. Trede M. [Use of a laparoscopic disposable surgical stapler in liver resection]. Chirurg 1993;64(5):406–7 [in German].

15. Croce E, Azzola M, Russo R, et al. Laparoscopic liver tumour resection with the argon beam. Endosc Surg Allied Technol 1994;2(3–4):186–8.

16. Kato K, Matsuda M, Onodera K, et al. An ultrasonically powered instrument for laparoscopic surgery: a brief technical report of preliminary success. J Laparoendosc Surg 1995;5(1):31–6.

17. Rau HG, Meyer G, Cohnert TU, et al. Laparoscopic liver resection with the water-jet dissector. Surg Endosc 1995;9(9):1009–12.

18. Trupka A, Hallfeldt K, Kalteis T, et al. [Open and laparoscopic liver resection with a new ultrasound scalpel]. Chirurg 1998;69(12):1352–6 [in German].

19. Constant DL, Slakey DP, Campeau RJ, et al. Laparoscopic nonanatomic hepatic resection employing the LigaSure device. JSLS 2005;9(1):35–8.

20. Regimbeau JM, Kianmanesh R, Farges O, et al. Extent of liver resection influences the outcome in patients with cirrhosis and small hepatocellular carcinoma. Surgery 2002;131(3):311–7.

21. Chen J, Huang K, Wu J, et al. Survival after anatomic resection versus nonanatomic resection for hepatocellular carcinoma: a meta-analysis. Dig Dis Sci 2011;56(6):1626–33.

22. Nguyen KT, Gamblin TC, Geller DA. World review of laparoscopic liver resection-2,804 patients. Ann Surg 2009;250(5):831–41.

23. Dagher I, O'Rourke N, Geller DA, et al. Laparoscopic major hepatectomy: an evolution in standard of care. Ann Surg 2009;250(5):856–60.

24. Belghiti J, Guevara OA, Noun R, et al. Liver hanging maneuver: a safe approach to right hepatectomy without liver mobilization. J Am Coll Surg 2001;193(1):109–11.

25. Cunningham JD, Fong Y, Shriver C, et al. One hundred consecutive hepatic resections. Blood loss, transfusion, and operative technique. Arch Surg 1994;129(10):1050–6.

26. Lang H, Radtke A, Hindennach M, et al. Impact of virtual tumor resection and computer-assisted risk analysis on operation planning and intraoperative strategy in major hepatic resection. Arch Surg 2005;140(7):629–38 [discussion: 638].

27. Truty MJ, Vauthey JN. Uses and limitations of portal vein embolization for improving perioperative outcomes in hepatocellular carcinoma. Semin Oncol 2010;37(2):102–9.

28. Farges O, Belghiti J, Kianmanesh R, et al. Portal vein embolization before right hepatectomy: prospective clinical trial. Ann Surg 2003;237(2):208–17.

29. Cherqui D, Laurent A, Mocellin N, et al. Liver resection for transplantable hepatocellular carcinoma: long-term survival and role of secondary liver transplantation. Ann Surg 2009;250(5):738–46.

30. Schutte K, Bornschein J, Malfertheiner P. Hepatocellular carcinoma—epidemiological trends and risk factors. Dig Dis 2009;27(2):80–92.
31. Bosch FX, Ribes J, Díaz M, et al. Primary liver cancer: worldwide incidence and trends. Gastroenterology 2004;127(5 Suppl 1):S5–16.
32. Llovet JM, Burroughs A, Bruix J. Hepatocellular carcinoma. Lancet 2003; 362(9399):1907–17.
33. Laurent C, Blanc JF, Nobili S, et al. Prognostic factors and longterm survival after hepatic resection for hepatocellular carcinoma originating from noncirrhotic liver. J Am Coll Surg 2005;201(5):656–62.
34. Dupont-Bierre E, Compagnon P, Raoul JL, et al. Resection of hepatocellular carcinoma in noncirrhotic liver: analysis of risk factors for survival. J Am Coll Surg 2005;201(5):663–70.
35. Lang H, Sotiropoulos GC, Brokalaki EI, et al. Survival and recurrence rates after resection for hepatocellular carcinoma in noncirrhotic livers. J Am Coll Surg 2007; 205(1):27–36.
36. Bismuth H, Chiche L, Castaing D. Surgical treatment of hepatocellular carcinomas in noncirrhotic liver: experience with 68 liver resections. World J Surg 1995;19(1):35–41.
37. Eguchi S, Ijtsma AJ, Slooff MJ, et al. Outcome and pattern of recurrence after curative resection for hepatocellular carcinoma in patients with a normal liver compared to patients with a diseased liver. Hepatogastroenterology 2006;53(70):592–6.
38. Fong Y, Sun RL, Jarnagin W, et al. An analysis of 412 cases of hepatocellular carcinoma at a Western center. Ann Surg 1999;229(6):790–9 [discussion: 799–800].
39. Vigano L, Tayar C, Laurent A, et al. Laparoscopic liver resection: a systematic review. J Hepatobiliary Pancreat Surg 2009;16(4):410–21.
40. Mergental H, Porte RJ. Liver transplantation for unresectable hepatocellular carcinoma in patients without liver cirrhosis. Transpl Int 2010;23(7):662–7.
41. Esnaola NF, Mirza N, Lauwers GY, et al. Comparison of clinicopathologic characteristics and outcomes after resection in patients with hepatocellular carcinoma treated in the United States, France, and Japan. Ann Surg 2003;238(5):711–9.
42. Fan ST, Lo CM, Liu CL, et al. Hepatectomy for hepatocellular carcinoma: toward zero hospital deaths. Ann Surg 1999;229(3):322–30.
43. Fuster J, García-Valdecasas JC, Grande L, et al. Hepatocellular carcinoma and cirrhosis. Results of surgical treatment in a European series. Ann Surg 1996; 223(3):297–302.
44. Wu CC, Cheng SB, Ho WM, et al. Liver resection for hepatocellular carcinoma in patients with cirrhosis. Br J Surg 2005;92(3):348–55.
45. Mazzaferro V, Regalia E, Doci R, et al. Liver transplantation for the treatment of small hepatocellular carcinomas in patients with cirrhosis. N Engl J Med 1996;334(11):693–9.
46. Taketomi A, Kitagawa D, Itoh S, et al. Trends in morbidity and mortality after hepatic resection for hepatocellular carcinoma: an institute's experience with 625 patients. J Am Coll Surg 2007;204(4):580–7.
47. Tung-Ping Poon R, Fan ST, Wong J. Risk factors, prevention, and management of postoperative recurrence after resection of hepatocellular carcinoma. Ann Surg 2000;232(1):10–24.
48. Bruix J, Sherman M. Management of hepatocellular carcinoma. Hepatology 2005; 42(5):1208–36.
49. Ishizawa T, Hasegawa K, Aoki T, et al. Neither multiple tumors nor portal hypertension are surgical contraindications for hepatocellular carcinoma. Gastroenterology 2008;134(7):1908–16.

50. Poon RT, Fan ST, Lo CM, et al. Long-term survival and pattern of recurrence after resection of small hepatocellular carcinoma in patients with preserved liver function: implications for a strategy of salvage transplantation. Ann Surg 2002; 235(3):373–82.
51. Makuuchi M, Kokudo N, Arii S, et al. Development of evidence-based clinical guidelines for the diagnosis and treatment of hepatocellular carcinoma in Japan. Hepatol Res 2008;38(1):37–51.
52. Ho MC, Huang GT, Tsang YM, et al. Liver resection improves the survival of patients with multiple hepatocellular carcinomas. Ann Surg Oncol 2009;16(4): 848–55.
53. Hwang S, Moon DB, Lee SG. Liver transplantation and conventional surgery for advanced hepatocellular carcinoma. Transpl Int 2010;23(7):723–7.
54. Vibert E, Perniceni T, Levard H, et al. Laparoscopic liver resection. Br J Surg 2006;93(1):67–72.
55. Teh SH, Nagorney DM, Stevens SR, et al. Risk factors for mortality after surgery in patients with cirrhosis. Gastroenterology 2007;132(4):1261–9.
56. Abdel-Atty MY, Farges O, Jagot P, et al. Laparoscopy extends the indications for liver resection in patients with cirrhosis. Br J Surg 1999;86(11):1397–400.
57. Chen HY, Juan CC, Ker CG. Laparoscopic liver surgery for patients with hepatocellular carcinoma. Ann Surg Oncol 2008;15(3):800–6.
58. Sasaki A, Nitta H, Otsuka K, et al. Ten-year experience of totally laparoscopic liver resection in a single institution. Br J Surg 2009;96(3):274–9.
59. Buell JF, Thomas MT, Rudich S, et al. Experience with more than 500 minimally invasive hepatic procedures. Ann Surg 2008;248(3):475–86.
60. Aldrighetti L, Guzzetti E, Pulitanò C, et al. Case-matched analysis of totally laparoscopic versus open liver resection for HCC: short and middle term results. J Surg Oncol 2010;102(1):82–6.
61. Dagher I, Belli G, Fantini C, et al. Laparoscopic hepatectomy for hepatocellular carcinoma: a European experience. J Am Coll Surg 2010;211(1):16–23.
62. Yoon YS, Han HS, Cho JY, et al. Total laparoscopic liver resection for hepatocellular carcinoma located in all segments of the liver. Surg Endosc 2010;24(7):1630–7.
63. Laurent A, Cherqui D, Lesurtel M, et al. Laparoscopic liver resection for subcapsular hepatocellular carcinoma complicating chronic liver disease. Arch Surg 2003;138(7):763–9 [discussion: 769].
64. Belli G, Fantini C, D'Agostino A, et al. Laparoscopic versus open liver resection for hepatocellular carcinoma in patients with histologically proven cirrhosis: short- and middle-term results. Surg Endosc 2007;21(11):2004–11.
65. Laurent A, Tayar C, Andréoletti M, et al. Laparoscopic liver resection facilitates salvage liver transplantation for hepatocellular carcinoma. J Hepatobiliary Pancreat Surg 2009;16(3):310–4.
66. Shimada M, Hashizume M, Maehara S, et al. Laparoscopic hepatectomy for hepatocellular carcinoma. Surg Endosc 2001;15(6):541–4.
67. Koffron AJ, Auffenberg G, Kung R, et al. Evaluation of 300 minimally invasive liver resections at a single institution: less is more. Ann Surg 2007;246(3):385–92 [discussion: 392–4].
68. Vanounou T, Steel JL, Nguyen KT, et al. Comparing the clinical and economic impact of laparoscopic versus open liver resection. Ann Surg Oncol 2010; 17(4):998–1009.
69. Nitta H, Sasaki A, Fujita T, et al. Laparoscopy-assisted major liver resections employing a hanging technique: the original procedure. Ann Surg 2010;251(3): 450–3.

70. Zhen ZJ, Lau WY, Wang FJ, et al. Laparoscopic liver resection for hepatocellular carcinoma in the left liver: Pringle maneuver versus tourniquet method. World J Surg 2010;34(2):314–9.

71. Zhang L, Chen YJ, Shang CZ, et al. Total laparoscopic liver resection in 78 patients. World J Gastroenterol 2009;15(45):5727–31.

72. Vigano L, Laurent A, Tayar C, et al. The learning curve in laparoscopic liver resection: improved feasibility and reproducibility. Ann Surg 2009;250(5):772–82.

73. Tranchart H, Di Giuro G, Lainas P, et al. Laparoscopic resection for hepatocellular carcinoma: a matched-pair comparative study. Surg Endosc 2010;24(5):1170–6.

74. Endo Y, Ohta M, Sasaki A, et al. A comparative study of the long-term outcomes after laparoscopy-assisted and open left lateral hepatectomy for hepatocellular carcinoma. Surg Laparosc Endosc Percutan Tech 2009;19(5):e171–4.

75. Belli G, Limongelli P, Fantini C, et al. Laparoscopic and open treatment of hepatocellular carcinoma in patients with cirrhosis. Br J Surg 2009;96(9):1041–8.

76. Lai EC, Tang CN, Ha JP, et al. Laparoscopic liver resection for hepatocellular carcinoma: ten-year experience in a single center. Arch Surg 2009;144(2):143–7 [discussion: 148].

77. Ito K, Ito H, Are C, et al. Laparoscopic versus open liver resection: a matched-pair case control study. J Gastrointest Surg 2009;13(12):2276–83.

78. Itano O, Chiba N, Maeda S, et al. Laparoscopic-assisted limited liver resection: technique, indications and results. J Hepatobiliary Pancreat Surg 2009;16(6):711–9.

79. Bryant R, Laurent A, Tayar C, et al. Laparoscopic liver resection-understanding its role in current practice: the Henri Mondor Hospital experience. Ann Surg 2009;250(1):103–11.

80. Sarpel U, Hefti MM, Wisnievsky JP, et al. Outcome for patients treated with laparoscopic versus open resection of hepatocellular carcinoma: case-matched analysis. Ann Surg Oncol 2009;16(6):1572–7.

81. Cho JY, Han HS, Yoon YS, et al. Outcomes of laparoscopic liver resection for lesions located in the right side of the liver. Arch Surg 2009;144(1):25–9.

82. Inagaki H, et al. Results of laparoscopic liver resection: retrospective study of 68 patients. J Hepatobiliary Pancreat Surg 2009;16(1):64–8.

83. Cho JY, Han HS, Yoon YS, et al. Experiences of laparoscopic liver resection including lesions in the posterosuperior segments of the liver. Surg Endosc 2008;22(11):2344–9.

84. Dagher I, Lainas P, Carloni A, et al. Laparoscopic liver resection for hepatocellular carcinoma. Surg Endosc 2008;22(2):372–8.

85. Cai XJ, Yang J, Yu H, et al. Clinical study of laparoscopic versus open hepatectomy for malignant liver tumors. Surg Endosc 2008;22(11):2350–6.

86. Belli G, Fantini C, D'Agostino A, et al. Laparoscopic liver resections for hepatocellular carcinoma (HCC) in cirrhotic patients. HPB (Oxford) 2004;6(4):236–46.

87. Santambrogio R, Aldrighetti L, Barabino M, et al. Laparoscopic liver resections for hepatocellular carcinoma. Is it a feasible option for patients with liver cirrhosis? Langenbecks Arch Surg 2009;394(2):255–64.

88. Tang CN, Tsui KK, Ha JP, et al. A single-centre experience of 40 laparoscopic liver resections. Hong Kong Med J 2006;12(6):419–25.

89. Kaneko H, Takagi S, Otsuka Y, et al. Laparoscopic liver resection of hepatocellular carcinoma. Am J Surg 2005;189(2):190–4.

90. Teramoto K, Kawamura T, Takamatsu S, et al. Laparoscopic and thoracoscopic approaches for the treatment of hepatocellular carcinoma. Am J Surg 2005;189(4):474–8.

Liver Transplantation for Hepatocellular Carcinoma: Expanding Frontiers and Building Bridges

Howard C. Masuoka, MD, PhD[a], Charles B. Rosen, MD[b],*

KEYWORDS

- Hepatocellular carcinoma • Liver transplantation
- Organ allocation • Cirrhosis

Despite the significant advances there have been made in nonsurgical treatments of hepatocellular carcinoma (HCC) over recent decades, these approaches rarely result in resolution of this tumor. Surgical treatment remains the mainstay of curative therapy for HCC, and liver transplantation, in particular, has become one of the most important therapeutic modalities. There are several questions, however, regarding HCC surveillance, the choice of simple surgical resection versus transplantation, the role of chemotherapy, the optimal selection criteria for transplantation, and pretransplant ablative therapies to downsize tumors.

HCC SURVEILLANCE, LIVER TRANSPLANTATION, AND ORGAN ALLOCATION

Because curative interventions are currently only possible in early-stage disease, early detection of HCC is a critical component of successful treatment. The current screening protocol in patients with cirrhosis involves abdominal ultrasound every 6 months combined with serum α-fetoprotein (AFP) level (see article elsewhere in this issue by Morris Sherman). The majority of patients with cirrhosis, however, do not undergo regular surveillance for HCC. One series from the United States found that fewer than 20% of patients over 65 years of age with previously documented cirrhosis undergo screening with ultrasound and AFP at the recommended interval, with approximately 45% of these patients having no screening before the diagnosis

[a] Division of Gastroenterology and Hepatology, William J. von Liebig Transplant Center, Mayo Clinic and Mayo Clinic College of Medicine, Rochester, MN 55905, USA
[b] Division of Transplantation Surgery, William J. von Liebig Transplant Center, Mayo Clinic and Mayo Clinic College of Medicine, Rochester, MN 55905, USA
* Corresponding author.
E-mail address: rosen.charles@mayo.edu

Clin Liver Dis 15 (2011) 385–393
doi:10.1016/j.cld.2011.03.005
1089-3261/11/$ – see front matter © 2011 Elsevier Inc. All rights reserved.

liver.theclinics.com

of HCC.[1] Thus, patients with HCC typically present at an advanced stage of disease, and if the tumor burden is moderate it may not be clearly amenable to transplantation.

Initial outcomes of transplantation for HCC were disappointing due to high recurrence rates, resulting in poor patient survival.[2] It was recognized, however, that patients with early HCC could undergo liver transplantation with acceptable outcomes that were similar to other indications for transplantation and superior to outcomes from resection. Thus, HCC is one of the few malignancies for which solid organ transplantation has been used as treatment. Liver transplantation for early HCC has several advantages over surgical resection in patients with cirrhosis. It removes both the entire tumor and the surrounding cirrhotic parenchyma, which is at risk for harboring additional lesions. Transplantation also obviates development of new HCC and avoids the risk of hepatic decompensation associated with resection.

Transplantation is unique as a surgical therapy in that there are other issues to consider in addition to the benefit, morbidity, and mortality of the procedure. Organ availability and disease progression must be considered while patients await transplantation. Furthermore, recurrent HCC often follows a more aggressive course likely secondary to immunosuppression as well as the underlying tumor biology. Patients with hepatitis C as the underlying cause for cirrhosis are at risk for recurrent hepatitis disease after transplantation, even if their cirrhosis was well compensated before transplantation, because hepatitis C viremia persists almost universally after transplantation and can readily infect the graft.

Selection of patients who do not have recurrence of HCC is important from several perspectives. From a societal viewpoint, transplant physicians are stewards of a scarce resource, namely donor livers. Even though an individual patient may have a survival benefit with transplantation, this benefit might be much lower than that for other patients awaiting transplantation. Transplantation followed by HCC recurrence with patient death is a lost opportunity for another patient to have had a higher benefit of transplantation. Even from an individual patient's standpoint, transplantation with subsequent recurrence is associated with the procedural risks, pain and discomfort, psychological strain, and impaired quality of life with no improvement in life expectancy. It is best to avoid transplantation for patients destined to develop recurrent disease. Conversely, it is important to have transplantation criteria that are not too stringent to avoid excluding patients with tumor characteristics that do not adversely affect survival.

THE MILAN AND RECENTLY EXPANDED LIVER TRANSPLANTATION CRITERIA

Liver transplantation was initially performed for patients with large, unresectable, and advanced-staged HCC, and results were disappointing. Five-year survival rates were only approximately 25% for patients who underwent transplantation during the period from 1987 to 1991.[3]

In their landmark study, Mazzaferro and colleagues[4] reported much better survival for patients with early compared with late-stage HCC. They defined criteria now known as the Milan criteria: a single lesion less than 5 cm or up to 3 lesions all less than 3 cm, no macrovascular invasion, and no extrahepatic spread. Transplantation of HCC within these criteria yielded a 5-year patient survival of 70% with a recurrence rate of 8%.[5] This outcome is similar to results achieved with other benign indications for liver transplantation.

In the United States, current United Network for Organ Sharing policy permits a Model for End-stage Liver Disease (MELD) score exception for patients with HCC within the Milan criteria. Irrespective of the MELD score based on laboratory values, patients are initially assigned a score of 22, which is equivalent to an estimated 3-month mortality rate of 15%. Patients awaiting transplantation receive additional MELD points equivalent to an increased mortality of 10% every 3 months provided that the HCC remains within the Milan criteria.

The Milan criteria are viewed by many in transplantation as too conservative because there are some patients with HCC exceeding the criteria who would still do well after transplantation. Thus, there has been a great deal of interest in expanding HCC transplant criteria to enable more patients to undergo transplantation without incurring a significant risk of disease recurrence.

The best-characterized of these expanded criteria are those proposed by the University of California, San Francisco (UCSF criteria), which allow transplantation for a solitary HCC up to 6.5 cm in diameter or up to 3 nodules, none larger than 4.5 cm, with a cumulative diameter up to 8 cm and no gross vascular invasion.[6] Post-transplantation survival is similar between patients satisfying either the Milan or UCSF criteria when assessed by pathologic examination of the explanted liver (which was how the UCSF criteria were derived). Tumor size and number of nodules are underestimated, however, by pretransplant imaging in up to 45% of patients with HCC.[7] When pretransplant imaging is used, the 5-year survival of patients beyond Milan criteria but within UCSF criteria was found in one series to be significantly lower than that for patients within the Milan criteria (46% vs 60%).[8] Another series found no significant difference in 5-year survival between patients who were within Milan criteria and those who exceeded Milan but were still within UCSF criteria, although this series used locoregional therapy to downsize tumors.[9]

The up-to-seven limit has been recently been proposed, which permits transplantation for patients with a sum of the largest tumor diameter in centimeters added to the number of tumors that is less than 7.[10] These criteria were derived from data in a retrospective study. These findings suggest that size is more important than the number of lesions, but the model has yet to be extensively evaluated prospectively.

BRIDGING/ABLATIVE THERAPIES

The risk of dropout (ie, removal from the transplant waiting list because of disease progression beyond transplant criteria) is approximately 20% during the first 6 months after listing. Dropout of patients due to progression of tumor beyond criteria has become a significant clinical problem, especially for patients at transplant centers with long waiting times. Within 1 year of diagnosis, at least 70% of patients with untreated HCC have tumor growth, 20% develop vascular invasion, and 9% develop metastases.[11] Hence, there is strong interest in used therapies that can reduce tumor burden and the risk of dropout.

There are several ablative therapies that have been used in the treatment of HCC either as a bridge to transplantation or as destination therapy in patients who are not transplant candidates. These treatments have been used with increasing frequency to downsize tumors and prevent lesions from exceeding transplantable criteria while patients await transplantation. Even in the initial publication by Mazzaferro and colleagues[4] that proposed the Milan criteria, 67% of patients underwent treatment for the tumor, mainly chemoembolization, before transplantation. The results of several studies have differed with respect to whether locoregional therapy improves survival after transplantation or has no significant effect.[12–15] The differing results may be due to selection bias because pretransplant ablative therapy is typically used in patients with relatively well-compensated disease and limited tumor burden. Ultimately, locoregional therapy does not seem to increase the risk of recurrent disease after transplantation compared with individuals who have not undergone an ablative procedure. Intention-to-treat analyses suggest that such bridge therapy is effective for patients with anticipated waiting times longer than 6 months.[16] Thus, for patients within Milan criteria, ablative therapies are typically only used if the expected waiting time until transplantation is greater than 6 months.

Ablative procedures have also been used to downsize tumors, which exceed Milan criteria such that patients may eventually undergo transplantation. Such an approach represents an attractive alternative to expanding the Milan criteria.[13,17] Most studies have demonstrated that patients with HCC initially beyond Milan criteria that have a response to locoregional therapy with downsizing to within Milan criteria and who do not show subsequent tumor progression, have excellent survival rates that are comparable to those initially within Milan criteria.[12,13,18] Results of other studies, however, have failed to demonstrate a survival benefit from successful downsizing of tumors from within the UCSF criteria to within the Milan criteria.[19] It remains to be determined which patients with downsized tumors are at increased risk of recurrent HCC disease relative to those who do not exceed criteria. One advantage of using locoregional therapy is the ability to assess the tumor biology (ie, lack of progression after locoregional therapy indicating that the tumor is not aggressive). It seems prudent to observe such patients for a period up to 6 months after ablation, to assess the biology of individual tumors, and to potentially exclude patients whose tumors show more aggressive tumor growth.

Several procedures have been used as bridge therapy to transplantation: transarterial chemoembolization (TACE) or bland transarterial embolization that does not incorporate chemotherapy with the embolization material, percutaneous ethanol injection or radiofrequency ablation (RFA), and surgical resection. The efficacies of these therapies remain controversial and are discussed in detail in the article elsewhere in this issue by Guimares and Uflacker. The choice of which ablative procedure to pursue has typically been dependent on tumor location and local expertise.

CHEMOTHERAPY

Several chemotherapeutic regimens have been used in the treatment of HCC and are described in detail in the article elsewhere in this issue by Wrzesinski and coworkers. Despite some significant advances in recent years, the development of truly effective chemotherapy for this cancer remains elusive. One of the most promising agents is the multikinase inhibitor, sorafenib, which has antiangiogenic and antiproliferative properties. It is the first agent to demonstrate a modest but statistically significant improvement in overall survival of patients with advanced HCC.[20] One question that has not been addressed is whether sorafenib or another chemotherapeutic agent might be of use in a select subset of patients to decrease the risk of drop out before transplantation or to reduce the risk of recurrence after transplantation.

SURGICAL RESECTION AND SALVAGE TRANSPLANTATION

Surgical resection has been the gold standard treatment of patients with HCC. Resection requires that a tumor is in a location amenable to resection and that patients have adequate hepatic function immediately afterward. The best resection candidates are those with a single lesion in a noncirrhotic background or in well-compensated cirrhosis with a normal bilirubin and no portal hypertension.

Unfortunately, surgical resection is associated with a high rate of both early recurrence (likely due to failure to completely resect the primary tumor or synchronous tumors) and late recurrence (likely due to the residual hepatic tissue being predisposed to neoplasia [ie, a field effect]). There have been no large randomized trials comparing transplantation to resection for early HCC. Observational studies suggest a survival advantage for cirrhotic patients treated with transplantation.[21–23]

Salvage liver transplantation (transplantation for recurrent HCC and/or liver failure after resection) remains highly controversial. Liver resection as a bridge to transplantation has the advantages of potentially decreasing the need for donor livers for patients with HCC, avoiding disease progression while awaiting transplantation, and permitting histopathologic examination of the resected tumor that could affect a transplant decision. Subsequent transplantation can then be avoided for patients with pathologic findings, such as microvascular invasion, that pose a high risk for recurrence, and patients with good prognostic factors and higher risk for metachronous lesions could undergo transplantation. Although transplantation is clearly technically feasible after resection, intention-to-treat analyses have demonstrated significantly worse outcomes with salvage compared with primary liver transplantation.[24,25] Additional experience and study is necessary to identify what group of patients will benefit from resection and salvage transplantation.

TUMOR PATHOLOGY AND MOLECULAR PROFILING

Commonly used selection criteria do not consider tumor histology or molecular characteristics. Tumor characteristics, such as size and number, are actually surrogates for molecular characteristics and the presence of microvascular invasion. Poor differentiation has been shown to be a predictor of microvascular invasion and is an independent risk factor for tumor recurrence.[26,27] There is a poor correlation between the tumor grade on pretransplant percutaneous fine-needle biopsy, however, and the grade determined by pathologic examination of the explanted liver.[28] This phenomenon is discussed elsewhere in this issue by Roskams. In addition, the risk of tumor seeding with biopsy has been reported as approximately 2%.[29] The development of surrogate markers for microvascular invasion would be valuable if shown to be accurate and obtainable without risk of tumor seeding. An example is serum des-gamma-carboxy prothrombin; high levels have been shown be associated with an increased risk of microvascular invasion and recurrence after transplantation.[30,31]

In the future, it is possible that molecular profiling though gene expression analysis or proteomics could provide prognostic information, such as the risk for an individual patient to be removed from the waiting list because of tumor progression, the potential for the tumor to respond to downsizing therapies, or the risk of recurrence after transplantation. Such information could allow adjustments to be made in prioritization for transplantation or exclusion of patients at high risk for recurrence. For patients with HCC treated with resection, a gene-expression signature present in liver tissue adjacent to the tumor, but not the tumor itself, correlated with late recurrence and survival.[32] The profile of the tissue surrounding the HCC might identify patients with a field effect, who should undergo pre-emptive transplantation before the development of recurrent or metachronous lesions. Even if useful molecular tumor profiles were established, there would remain several significant challenges to their application, including the need for tumor biopsy with the risks of morbidity and tumor seeding, and sampling effects due to tumor heterogeneity. Noninvasive techniques, such as levels of novel serum markers or magnetic resonance spectroscopy, would have the advantages of examining the entire tumor (obviating sampling error) and avoiding the risk of tumor seeding.

IMMUNOSUPPRESSION AFTER TRANSPLANTATION

Immunosuppression after transplantation may be a factor in disease progression for patients with recurrent disease. The addition or substitution of an agent with antiproliferative effects may slow the rate of tumor growth. Mammalian target of rapamycin inhibitors, such as sirolimus and everolimus, have been used at some centers due to their potential antiproliferative effect. Controlled trials, however, are necessary to demonstrate actual efficacy for routine use of mammalian target of rapamycin inhibitors in this setting.

ASSESSING THE RISK OF PROGRESSION OR RECURRENCE AND MONITORING FOR RECURRENT DISEASE

Transplant criteria, such as the Milan criteria, have been designed to select individuals least likely to develop recurrent disease after transplantation. Unknown is whether other characteristics, such as recipient or donor factors, might have prognostic value for predicting dropout while awaiting transplantation or recurrence after transplantation. Risk factors for dropout might enable better adjustment of transplant priority or MELD exception points.

There has been little published in regards to monitoring for recurrent disease after liver transplantation.[33] The value of monitoring is low, however, because so little can be done for patients who develop recurrent disease.

BUILDING BRIDGES

It is an exciting era in liver transplantation for HCC. Results for patients transplanted within Milan criteria are excellent. There are many critical questions still awaiting answers, however. In particular, when should bridging therapies be used? At the authors' institution, bridging therapies have been used with excellent outcomes in patients within Milan criteria. Because the mean waiting time for patients exceeds 6 months, the authors use bridging therapy for all patients with HCC amenable to treatment. Bridging therapy is delayed for patients with small HCC (2 cm) in order for those patients to receive an appealed MELD score. The authors rarely perform a biopsy of the tumor for patients with characteristic imaging findings in the proper clinical setting. Biopsies are done when there is suspicion for another malignancy, such as intrahepatic cholangiocarcinoma or metastatic disease. Which bridging therapy is best for an individual patient? TACE with chemotherapy-eluting beads designed to minimize dissemination of the chemotherapeutic agent has become the mainstay of bridging therapy at the authors' institution. Patients with a portal venous thrombus are occasionally treated with TACE but only after careful consideration of the case by the multidisciplinary team. These patients are at increased risk for widespread necrosis of the surrounding parenchyma. RFA is typically considered if there is a relative contraindication to TACE or TACE has failed due to poor visualization of the tumor. RFA carries a risk of seeding of the tumor, but this risk seems small. Radioembolization with an agent, such as yttrium 90–coated glass microspheres, has not been used at this institution a bridging therapy before transplantation although the authors have found it to be a useful modality as destination therapy in patients who are not transplant candidates.

Which patients with tumors exceeding Milan criteria can be transplanted without an increased risk of recurrence? Should bridging therapy and subsequent transplantation be restricted to patients with HCC initially within Milan criteria or is the approach appropriate to those with larger, more advanced HCC? It has been the authors' practice at Mayo Clinic to consider patients who are beyond Milan criteria but still within UCSF criteria for transplantation. These patients undergo bridge therapy and are observed for at least 6 months before transplantation. Only rarely and on a case-by-case basis after prolonged observation have patients been considered who have exceeded the UCSF criteria initially but are successfully downsized to within Milan criteria. Does successful downsizing actually predict a good outcome with transplantation? If so, what are appropriate downsizing criteria? The authors have found response to downsizing a useful surrogate marker of tumor biology. After treatment, patients undergo contrast-enhanced CT or MRI to evaluate for recurrence of disease. Rapid recurrence and enlargement of the tumor appear to be bad prognostic signs. Are there molecular characteristics of HCC that predict tumor behavior or response to bridge therapy? So far, the results have been disappointing, but if a reliable molecular signature can be found, it would be possible to make better-defined and rational decisions regarding which patients should undergo bridging therapy and which patients exceeding criteria could undergo transplantation with acceptable outcomes. Pretransplant chemotherapy could potentially have a role in patients with select molecular characteristics of the tumor.

Additional multidisciplinary research is important in rigorously answering these questions. As these questions are answered, liver transplantation will become more effective and available for more patients afflicted with HCC.

REFERENCES

1. Davila JA, Morgan RO, Richardson PA, et al. Use of surveillance for hepatocellular carcinoma among patients with cirrhosis in the United States. Hepatology 2010;52(1):132–41.
2. Penn I. Hepatic transplantation for primary and metastatic cancers of the liver. Surgery 1991;110(4):726–34 [discussion: 734–5].
3. Yoo HY, Patt CH, Geschwind JF, et al. The outcome of liver transplantation in patients with hepatocellular carcinoma in the United States between 1988 and 2001: 5-year survival has improved significantly with time. J Clin Oncol 2003; 21(23):4329–35.
4. Mazzaferro V, Regalia E, Doci R, et al. Liver transplantation for the treatment of small hepatocellular carcinomas in patients with cirrhosis. N Engl J Med 1996; 334(11):693–9.
5. Figueras J, Jaurrieta E, Valls C, et al. Survival after liver transplantation in cirrhotic patients with and without hepatocellular carcinoma: a comparative study. Hepatology 1997;25(6):1485–9.
6. Yao FY, Ferrell L, Bass NM, et al. Liver transplantation for hepatocellular carcinoma: expansion of the tumor size limits does not adversely impact survival. Hepatology 2001;33(6):1394–403.
7. Herrero JI, Sangro B, Quiroga J, et al. Influence of tumor characteristics on the outcome of liver transplantation among patients with liver cirrhosis and hepatocellular carcinoma. Liver Transpl 2001;7(7):631–6.
8. Decaens T, Roudot-Thoraval F, Hadni-Bresson S, et al. Impact of UCSF criteria according to pre- and post-OLT tumor features: analysis of 479 patients listed for HCC with a short waiting time. Liver Transpl 2006;12(12):1761–9.
9. Yao FY, Xiao L, Bass NM, et al. Liver transplantation for hepatocellular carcinoma: validation of the UCSF-expanded criteria based on preoperative imaging. Am J Transplant 2007;7(11):2587–96.

10. Mazzaferro V, Llovet JM, Miceli R, et al. Predicting survival after liver transplantation in patients with hepatocellular carcinoma beyond the Milan criteria: a retrospective, exploratory analysis. Lancet Oncol 2009;10(1):35–43.

11. Llovet JM, Bustamante J, Castells A, et al. Natural history of untreated nonsurgical hepatocellular carcinoma: rationale for the design and evaluation of therapeutic trials. Hepatology 1999;29(1):62–7.

12. Otto G, Herber S, Heise M, et al. Response to transarterial chemoembolization as a biological selection criterion for liver transplantation in hepatocellular carcinoma. Liver Transpl 2006;12(8):1260–7.

13. Yao FY, Kerlan RK Jr, Hirose R, et al. Excellent outcome following down-staging of hepatocellular carcinoma prior to liver transplantation: an intention-to-treat analysis. Hepatology 2008;48(3):819–27.

14. Zimmerman MA, Trotter JF, Wachs M, et al. Predictors of long-term outcome following liver transplantation for hepatocellular carcinoma: a single-center experience. Transpl Int 2007;20(9):747–53.

15. Graziadei IW, Sandmueller H, Waldenberger P, et al. Chemoembolization followed by liver transplantation for hepatocellular carcinoma impedes tumor progression while on the waiting list and leads to excellent outcome. Liver Transpl 2003;9(6):557–63.

16. Llovet JM, Mas X, Aponte JJ, et al. Cost effectiveness of adjuvant therapy for hepatocellular carcinoma during the waiting list for liver transplantation. Gut 2002;50(1):123–8.

17. Yao FY. Expanded criteria for hepatocellular carcinoma: down-staging with a view to liver transplantation–yes. Semin Liver Dis 2006;26(3):239–47.

18. Heckman JT, Devera MB, Marsh JW, et al. Bridging locoregional therapy for hepatocellular carcinoma prior to liver transplantation. Ann Surg Oncol 2008; 15(11):3169–77.

19. Millonig G, Graziadei IW, Freund MC, et al. Response to preoperative chemoembolization correlates with outcome after liver transplantation in patients with hepatocellular carcinoma. Liver Transpl 2007;13(2):272–9.

20. Llovet JM, Ricci S, Mazzaferro V, et al. Sorafenib in advanced hepatocellular carcinoma. N Engl J Med 2008;359(4):378–90.

21. Ringe B, Pichlmayr R, Wittekind C, et al. Surgical treatment of hepatocellular carcinoma: experience with liver resection and transplantation in 198 patients. World J Surg 1991;15(2):270–85.

22. Bismuth H, Chiche L, Adam R, et al. Liver resection versus transplantation for hepatocellular carcinoma in cirrhotic patients. Ann Surg 1993;218(2): 145–51.

23. Colella G, Bottelli R, De Carlis L, et al. Hepatocellular carcinoma: comparison between liver transplantation, resective surgery, ethanol injection, and chemoembolization. Transpl Int 1998;11(Suppl 1):S193–6.

24. Adam R, Azoulay D, Castaing D, et al. Liver resection as a bridge to transplantation for hepatocellular carcinoma on cirrhosis: a reasonable strategy? Ann Surg 2003;238(4):508–18 [discussion: 518–9].

25. Poon RT, Fan ST, Lo CM, et al. Long-term survival and pattern of recurrence after resection of small hepatocellular carcinoma in patients with preserved liver function: implications for a strategy of salvage transplantation. Ann Surg 2002;235(3): 373–82.

26. Silva M, Moya A, Berenguer M, et al. Expanded criteria for liver transplantation in patients with cirrhosis and hepatocellular carcinoma. Liver Transpl 2008;14(10): 1449–60.

27. Esnaola NF, Lauwers GY, Mirza NQ, et al. Predictors of microvascular invasion in patients with hepatocellular carcinoma who are candidates for orthotopic liver transplantation. J Gastrointest Surg 2002;6(2):224–32 [discussion: 232].

28. Pawlik TM, Gleisner AL, Anders RA, et al. Preoperative assessment of hepatocellular carcinoma tumor grade using needle biopsy: implications for transplant eligibility. Ann Surg 2007;245(3):435–42.

29. Stigliano R, Marelli L, Yu D, et al. Seeding following percutaneous diagnostic and therapeutic approaches for hepatocellular carcinoma. What is the risk and the outcome? Seeding risk for percutaneous approach of HCC. Cancer Treat Rev 2007;33(5):437–47.

30. Sakaguchi T, Suzuki S, Morita Y, et al. Impact of the preoperative des-gamma-carboxy prothrombin level on prognosis after hepatectomy for hepatocellular carcinoma meeting the Milan criteria. Surg Today 2010;40(7):638–45.

31. Taketomi A, Sanefuji K, Soejima Y, et al. Impact of des-gamma-carboxy prothrombin and tumor size on the recurrence of hepatocellular carcinoma after living donor liver transplantation. Transplantation 2009;87(4):531–7.

32. Hoshida Y, Villanueva A, Kobayashi M, et al. Gene expression in fixed tissues and outcome in hepatocellular carcinoma. N Engl J Med 2008;359(19):1995–2004.

33. Roberts JP. Tumor surveillance-what can and should be done? Screening for recurrence of hepatocellular carcinoma after liver transplantation. Liver Transpl 2005;(11 Suppl 2):S45–6.

Locoregional Therapy for Hepatocellular Carcinoma

Marcelo Guimaraes, MD*, Renan Uflacker, MD†

KEYWORDS

- Hepatocellular carcinoma • Locoregional therapy
- Chemoembolization • TACE • Liver tumor ablation
- Radioembolization

The role of the interventional radiologist (IR) in providing locoregional therapies for hepatocellular carcinoma (HCC), has grown substantially in the last 30 years, and especially in the recent decade, because of development of new techniques, improvement in existing devices, and better outcomes. However, a multidisciplinary patient management approach is critical for optimal decisions and care. HCC is usually discovered late in the course of the disease and, in general, has poor prognosis.[1] Surveillance for HCC in high-risk patients and recent improvements in surgical techniques (liver resection and transplantation) have contributed to better survival.[2] However, wide margins and the underlying cirrhosis limit the volume of liver that can be resected.[3–5] Liver transplantation offers an ~75% survival rate in early HCC at 5 years, but, if malignant vascular invasion is found in the explant, survival rates decrease significantly.[6–8] Until the introduction of sorafenib (Nexavar, Bayer Health-Care Pharmaceuticals Inc, Wayne, NJ, USA), no systemic chemotherapy showed significantly increased survival in patients with advanced HCC.[9–11] Sorafenib may be effective in shrinking HCC (**Fig. 1**) and preventing recurrence after resection or local ablation.[12] External beam radiation has had a limited role in the treatment of HCC because of radiation toxicity to the adjacent normal liver.[13] Because of these limitations and others negative factors such as tumor location, excessive number of lesions, size, presence of portal hypertension, and poor liver function, image-guided locoregional therapies were developed and present several advantages in treating HCC. Image-guided therapies are in 2 main groups: (1) endovascular catheter-based procedures using digital subtraction angiography/fluoroscopy, such as transarterial chemoembolization (TACE) and radioembolization; and (2) ultrasound (US)-assisted or computed tomography (CT)–assisted percutaneous ablative procedures, including

The authors have nothing to disclose.
† Deceased.
Division of Vascular & Interventional Radiology, Medical University of South Carolina, 25 Courtenay Drive, MSC 226, Charleston, SC 29425, USA
* Corresponding author.
E-mail address: guimarae@musc.edu

Clin Liver Dis 15 (2011) 395–421
doi:10.1016/j.cld.2011.03.013
1089-3261/11/$ – see front matter © 2011 Elsevier Inc. All rights reserved.

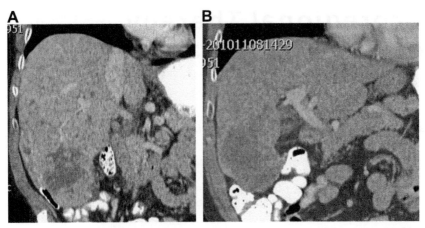

Fig. 1. Patients with Child-Turcotte-Pugh (CTP) with advanced HCC, not amenable to surgical resection. Sorafenib was effective in shrinking the HCC but, because of significant symptoms, had to be discontinued and the patient was referred for locoregional therapy. (A) Beginning of the treatment with sorafenib, and (B) follow-up in about 3 months showing significant shrinkage of the tumor.

percutaneous ethanol injection (PEI), radiofrequency ablation (RFA), microwave ablation (MWA), cryoablation, laser ablation (LA), irreversible electroporation (IRE), and high-intensity focused US (HIFU) ablation.

The interventional procedures currently performed most frequently for treatment of HCC are discussed in this article, which provides practitioners with a comprehensive understanding of the indications, treatment options, outcomes, and complications of these image-guided procedures.

PATIENT EVALUATION AND SELECTION

The best therapy for a patient diagnosed with HCC should be selected by a multidisciplinary team approach. The current options are transplantation, resection, image-guided locoregional therapies, systemic chemotherapy, and, for those with advanced disease, palliative care. The variables involved in this decision are overall tumor burden (ie, size, number, and location of HCC lesions), and the patient's clinical condition (ie, the performance status and liver function). Establishing whether the patient has developed HCC in the setting of cirrhosis is essential, because it has a great impact on determining whether resection can be performed. Liver function should be evaluated by clinical examination, laboratory testing, and cross-sectional imaging.[14] Measurement of the transjugular hepatic venous pressure gradient, to estimate the degree of portal hypertension, can aid in the choice of treatment modality because it may provide a contraindication to resection surgery.[15] CT or magnetic resonance imaging (MRI) can also show that there is portal hypertension.[14] The sensitivity and diagnostic value of preprocedural imaging by CT or MRI are ~80% except for satellite nodules of less than 1 cm. Although it is more sensitive for identifying lesions of 1 to 2 cm, MR angiography is limited for subcentimeter tumors that may or may not be HCC and that should be imaged every 3 to 6 months to detect growth suggestive of malignant transformation. The absence of growth during monitoring for 1 to 2 years implies a low likelihood of HCC, whereas enlargement in this period suggests malignancy that warrants further investigation. For nodules of 1 to 2 cm, the diagnosis of HCC is established by the presence of a characteristic vascular pattern of HCC and washout on 2 dynamic imaging studies (usually MRI and CT). If the radiological imaging features on the 2 dynamic studies do not coincide, an image-guided core biopsy can be considered.[16] Notwithstanding, there may still be no clear-cut dividing line between dysplasia and a well-differentiated tumor on small biopsy specimens.[17] Liver biopsy is not recommended routinely for lesions larger than 2 cm that have imaging characteristics compatible with HCC in patients with cirrhosis and/or a serum α-fetoprotein level greater than 200 ng/mL.[18] The positive predictive value of these clinical and radiological findings is greater than 95%. For lesions larger than 2 cm or those increasing in size and with atypical vascular patterns, an image-guided biopsy should be performed. These considerations are discussed in detail elsewhere in this issue in the article by Anis and Irshad.

The outcome of HCC is influenced by 2 key factors, namely the tumor stage, as judged by the number and sizes(s) of lesions and their spread, and the severity of the underlying liver disease as judged by measurement of Child-Turcotte-Pugh (CTP) score and class, the Model for End-stage Liver Disease (MELD) score, and the presence of portal hypertension. The general physical status of the patient as defined by the Eastern Cooperative Oncology Group (ECOG) Performance Status or similar classifications and the presence of symptoms also have prognostic value, although the cause of liver disease usually does not. Thus, the tumor burden and the severity of liver disease have to be carefully assessed in choosing the appropriate treatment.[19] Although several HCC staging systems are available, the Barcelona Clinic Liver Cancer (BCLC) scheme is the most popular choice (see the article by Sherman elsewhere in this issue).[20,21] The primary end points of most trials are overall survival, disease-free and progression-free survival time to progression, and response rates. Determination of end points other than survival can be subjective. Broadly, no more than 15% of patients are considered for surgery, 50% for nonsurgical therapies, and 35% are unsuitable for any active treatment and should receive palliative care. However, these proportions are changing as smaller tumors are diagnosed by surveillance in patients with compensated cirrhosis.[22] The BCLC staging system has been validated in European and US cohorts[23,24] and is widely endorsed, as is the multidisciplinary approach.[19]

IMAGE-GUIDED, MINIMALLY INVASIVE TREATMENT OF HCC

For treatable lesions, expectant observation should be avoided because of potential tumor size doubling in 6 months, which may decrease survival. Interruption of systemic chemotherapy usually allows the HCC to recur. On the other end of the spectrum, partial resection and liver transplantation are useful for only about 15% to 20% of the patients with good liver reserve and no portal hypertension. Transplantation offers the best survival at 5 years among all the available therapies. The minimally invasive therapies are in the middle of this spectrum and include percutaneous chemical ablation (with alcohol), thermal heat ablation (radiofrequency, microwave, laser, electroporation, high-intensity focused ultrasound), and cryoablation. The intra-arterial, catheter-based treatment modalities include bland embolization, chemoembolization, radioembolization, direct hepatic artery catheter infusion through a port device, and, more recently, direct hepatic chemotherapy saturation infusion with the help of a hepatic outflow filtering system (Delcath, New York, NY, USA). The minimally invasive vascular procedures are guided by digital subtraction angiography (DSA). In general, the main advantages of the locoregional therapies are lower morbidity and mortality, shorter hospital stays (outpatient or 1–2 days hospitalization), quicker recovery, and the advantage of access via a small nick in the skin. By now there is much information about the outcomes and survival of the patients treated with the different available locoregional therapies for HCC, although not necessarily in randomized trials (**Table 1**). Nowadays, percutaneous RFA is the only locoregional therapy that may offer complete tumor kill in patients with lesions up to 3 cm in diameter,[31] and it has comparable survival rates with partial hepatectomy[32,33] (**Table 2**) with fewer complications.[34] The main disadvantage of the less invasive treatments is that most of these therapies are limited to tumor control, although they provide an increase in survival and quality of life. Ultimately, the goals of the locoregional therapies are to prolong patients' lives, achieve complete tumor kill, and provide clinical improvement and better quality of life for symptomatic patients. A multidisciplinary tumor board should include representatives of hepatology, pathology, clinical oncology, liver and transplant surgery, interventional radiology, and radiation oncology. Currently, percutaneous ablation is the preferred locoregional therapy for nonresectable patients with 1 or several tumors up to 3 cm. Although there is no level 1 evidence that best results are achieved in lesions between 3 and 5 cm, it is clear that the level of tumor damage and kill is greater with the synergistic association of TACE and percutaneous ablation. TACE or systemic chemotherapy should be considered if the tumor burden is excessive or unsafe for ablation.

PEI

PEI is one of the oldest modalities for HCC ablation. Traditionally performed using US guidance, a fine needle (usually 20 G) is inserted into the tumor and absolute alcohol is gently injected. It is inexpensive, it has been used for the treatment of HCC of less than 2 cm even when other structures are close by, and it is not affected by the heat-sink effect of adjacent vessels (discussed later), which limits the efficacy of some thermal ablation treatments. However, the ablation zone is unpredictable, so several sessions may be needed to achieve tumor necrosis, and thus higher tumor progression rates (17%–38%) are seen than with RFA.[26,35] From 2 meta-analysis and randomized trials comparing PEI with RFA, it was concluded that RFA is better in the treatment of small HCC because it required a smaller number of sessions (threefold decrease), had lower rates of recurrence, and had about 20% higher overall survival in 3 to 4 years.[36–40]

RFA

RFA for liver tumors was developed in the early 1980s, and initial reports date from the early 1990s.[41,42] RFA may be performed using US or CT guidance and is currently by far the most popular tumor ablation technique for the treatment of HCC of 3 cm or less. Using a rapidly alternating radiofrequency current, molecular frictional heat is induced around the electrode, which leads to microvascular thrombosis and cell death. Temperatures may increase to 90 to 100°C, although at more than 60°C coagulation necrosis starts.[43] There are several RFA needle configurations, but typically the length and geometry of the probe determines the size of the ablation zone, which usually is

Table 1
Five-year survival among different locoregional therapies in heterogeneous patient populations

PEI (%)[25]	RFA (%)[26–29]	MWA (%)	Cryoablation (%)	HIFU (%)	TACE (%)	Radioembolization (%)	TACE/RFA (%)[30]
25–32	40–58	51–57	23	32	17.5–26	NA	75

Abbreviation: NA, not available.

Table 2
Studies comparing RFA with hepatic resection (HR) for HCC of 3 cm or less

			Survival (%)			Disease-Free Survival (%)			
		Studies Comparing RFA Versus HR for HCC ≤3 cm							
Author	**Treatment**	**No. of Patients**	**1 y**	**3 y**	**5 y**	**1 y**	**3 y**	**5 y**	**P-value**
Vivarelli et al[33]	RFA	22	89	—	50	70	34	—	NS
	HR	21	89	—	79	84	67	—	
Guglielmi et al[32]	RFA	32	91	50	29	72	36	36	NS
	HR	31	89	78	54	80	58	19	
Hiraoka et al[34]	RFA	105	95.1	87.8	59.3	87.5	58.7	24.6	NS
	HR	59	98.1	91.4	59.4	91.4	64.3	22.4	

Abbreviation: NS, not significant.
Data from Zhou Y, Zhao Y, Li B, et al. Meta-analysis of radiofrequency ablation versus hepatic resection for small hepatocellular carcinoma. BMC Gastroenterol 2010;10:78.

spherical and surrounded by a 1-mm to 2-mm hemorrhagic perimeter. In cirrhotic livers, the surrounding tumor tissue works as a thermal insulator, which enhances local heat retention (**Fig. 2**). The RFA technique is vulnerable to the heat-sink effect, whereby heat is dissipated by convection caused by heated blood in nearby vessels flowing away from the target zone, which reduces tissue necrosis in the proximity of large vessels. When peritumoral vessels greater than 3 mm are present, lower success rates are expected, necessitating more RFA sessions and leading to higher local recurrence (**Fig. 3**).[44–46] The greater the size and number of HCC lesions, the worse the treatment success rate. The ideal candidates for RFA treatment are patients with up to 3 HCC lesions that are less than 3 cm. In general, cancer control, but not cancer cure, is offered to cirrhotic patients because they have greater than a 10% chance annually of developing a new lesions once 1 tumor occurs. If tumor control is achieved, the outcome is defined by the progression of the liver disease. In cases of end-stage liver disease, and in patients with HCC greater than 5 cm, tumor control may be more difficult and the question of downsizing and subsequent liver transplant

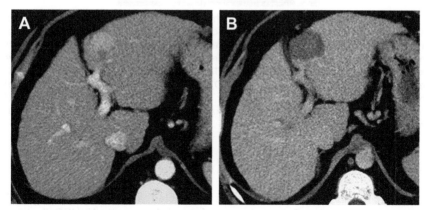

Fig. 2. (*A*) Hypervascular, 4-cm HCC in the left lobe on the arterial phase of the liver CT scan. (*B*) After radiofrequency ablation (RFA), late phase CT showing the complete ablation of the lesion.

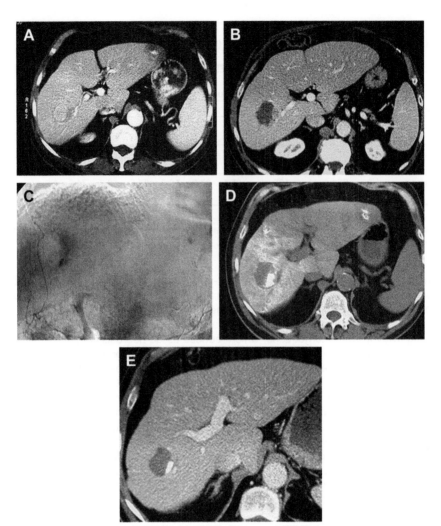

Fig. 3. (*A*) Hypervascular, 5-cm HCC in the right lobe of the liver. Note the large vessel just medial to the edge of the tumor. (*B*) CT scan of the liver after RFA shows a medial area of contrast-enhanced viable tumor, just next to the large branch of the portal vein. An additional RFA was ineffective in ablating that area. (*C*) Later phase arteriogram of the liver preceding transarterial chemoembolization (TACE) with Lipiodol and mitomycin C shows arterial enhancement of the residual tumor. (*D*) Post-TACE CT of the liver shows the residual tumor well enhanced by the Lipidol used for treatment with the chemotherapy drug. (*E*) Follow-up CT at 3 months shows overall shrinkage of the ablated tumor and of the residual tumor.

must be considered (**Fig. 4;** see the article by Masuoka and Rosen elsewhere in this issue).

In small to medium HCC, tumor necrosis is expected to be 80% after a single RFA session, and ~90% when 2 sessions are performed. The smaller the HCC, the better are the results of RFA. However, it is common to develop post–tumor ablation syndrome (PTAS), in which the patient may experience variable degrees of fever,

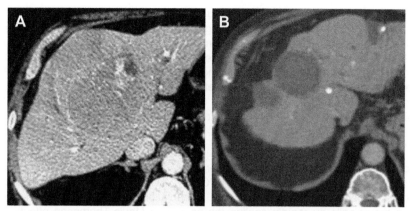

Fig. 4. (*A*) A 70-year-old man with alcoholic cirrhosis presented with a 15-cm HCC, which was deemed unresectable. Locoregional therapy was initiated with TACE and RFA. The patient responded well to the treatment and, in a period of 8 years, presented with many recurrent tumors that were treated with combination TACE and RFA. (*B*) CT scan of the liver, at 8-years follow-up, showing the residual scars of the large tumor (completely controlled) and other areas with scars of smaller, recurrent HCC nodules treated by RFA and TACE.

abdominal pain and distension, nausea, vomiting, flulike symptoms, lack of energy, anorexia, and noninfective leukocytosis. PTAS is most intense in the first 48 hours after RFA, but may last up to 2 weeks, although it is usually easily managed symptomatically. Percutaneous RFA major complication rates are low (0.9%–5.0%), namely hepatic bleeding; injuries of bowel, bile duct, and abdominal wall; and liver infection.[27,47] Liver infection can be avoided with careful sterile technique and intravenous antibiotic prophylaxis. Thrombocytopenia should be corrected, whereas correction of a prolonged prothrombin time is advocated by some but not all, and practices vary. Tumor seeding is now extremely rare because cauterization of the needle track is part of the standard technique. The most popular RFA devices in the US market are the Cool-Tip (Covidien, Mansfield, MA, USA), the RITA (AngioDynamics, Queensbury, NY, USA), and the LeVeen (Boston Scientific, Natick, MA, USA) probes. There do not seem to be significant differences among these devices in treatment success, complication rates, and patient survival.[48,49]

MWA

MWA was initially used in Japan in the early 1980s[50,51] and, like RFA, MWA may be performed using US or CT guidance. MWA also promotes tumor coagulation necrosis by molecular frictional heating generated by shorter lengths and higher-frequency electromagnetic waves than RFA (900–2450 MHz in MWA versus 300–500 kHz in RFA), which agitate water molecules and rupture cell membranes.[52,53] RFA and MWA have similar clinical applications but, for HCCs that are adjacent to structures such as main bile ducts, gallbladder, bowel, or stomach, RFA is preferred rather than MWA, because the latter generates a much broader zone of ablation with higher temperatures within the target lesion, particularly at the tip of the antenna (probe). In cases in which there are branches of the hepatic artery or the portal or hepatic veins greater than 3 mm nearby, MWA is preferable because the volume of ablation is less likely to be affected by the heat-sink effect. The prevalence of complications (0%–8%) and outcomes in small HCCs are similar when treated with MWA or RFA.[54] The theoretical advantages of MWA compared with RFA are a larger area of coagulation necrosis for the same size of needle tip, higher temperatures, shorter treatment times (typically 10 minutes for MWA and ≥20 minutes for RFA), grounding pads are not necessary, and many antennas may be used simultaneously compared with the alternating activation of RFA. Two studies of more than 200 patients each (mostly CTP B, mean tumor size 4 cm) achieved complete ablation in about 90% of the cases in a single session of MWA, and 3-year and 5-year survivals of 66% to 72% and 51% to 57% respectively in 5 years, with local recurrence of 7% to 8%.[55,56]

CRYOABLATION

Cryoablation has been used to treat tumors since the mid–nineteenth century. Then, salt solutions containing crushed ice (−18°C to −24°C) were applied to freeze cancers of the skin, cervix, and breast.[57] Modern cryoablation uses cool thermal energy to freeze tumor cells by rapidly cooling the cryoprobe (Joule-Thompson effect). The cold-induced injury creates intracellular ice crystal formation, sequesters free extracellular water, dehydrates and shrinks organelles, and disrupts plasma membranes. During thawing, extracellular ice melts before intracellular ice, creating an osmotic shift of water into damaged cells that swell and burst.[58,59] Cryoablation has not been popular in the treatment of HCC mainly because of the larger size of the cryoprobes and because the ablation zone is smaller than with RFA. Cryoablation is susceptible to cold-sink effects, and the safety margin around the ice ball varies from 4 to 10 mm, which ablates additional surrounding normal liver parenchyma to obtain free margins. Recently, the decrease in probe diameter to 17 G, now offers the option of using more than 1 probe simultaneously. Because cryoablation is painless and the ice ball can be seen by any imaging method (ie, US, CT, or MRI), it is still an attractive option.[60–64] In short-term follow-up studies with the newer cryoprobes, complete ablation was accomplished in 88% of the cases, local progression was ∼20%, and overall 3-year survival was 79%. Long-term study of medium to larger lesions (mean diameter of 4.6 cm) treated either with cryoablation or with combination TACE/cryoablation showed a 5-year survival rate of 23% and local progression rate of 24% but an increased complication rate (31%) and 2 deaths. Complications may be as high as 40% and include liver parenchyma fracture, cryoshock, biliary fistula, hemorrhage, and cold-induced lesion in nearby structure.[65,66] More studies with the newer generation cryoprobes are necessary to identify potential benefits, compared with the heat thermal ablation techniques.

LA

LA is a high temperature thermal technique in which tumors are heated beyond the threshold of protein denaturation, using low-power laser energy delivered through optical fibers. LA generates heat by laser light absorption in the tissue, which causes cell death. LA may also cause coagulate microvessels and cause progressive ischemic injury for as long as 72 hours after the procedure.[67] Using US, CT, or MRI guidance, 1 or several laser fibers can be inserted into an HCC mass, via a needle or a plastic sheath that is then retracted, exposing the laser fiber to the tumor itself. Special MRI sequences designed to evaluate thermal patterns (ie, MRI thermometry) monitor the actual formation of an ablation zone. Theoretically, this allows complete tumor ablation, and a variable tumor margin can be created in a more controlled and reproducible fashion than the hyperechoic focus that is formed when performing RFA with US guidance. The most common laser source is the continuous-wave neodymium-doped yttrium aluminum garnet (Nd:YAG) device. The laser beam is propagated through 300-μm quartz-core fiberoptics. The optical fibers are illuminated simultaneously. The wavelength and power of an Nd:YAG laser is well suited to medical applications, in which tissue scatter and absorption creates heat with an ablation zone of approximately 1 to 1.5 cm, allowing 4 simultaneous punctures to achieve a tumor ablation zone of approximately 4 cm in diameter.[68] The sheath is fitted with a diffusing tip, allowing light to diffuse 12 to 15 mm from the point of origin. HCC lesions up to 2 cm may be treated by a single applicator. HCC lesions as large as 8 cm may be ablated with 4 or 5 simultaneous laser sheaths.[69] LA offers increased efficiency because ablation is done during a period of 2 to 6 minutes compared ~20 minutes for RFA. LA is even more attractive when several lesions need to be ablated (**Fig. 5**). In some LA studies, 90% to 98% complete ablation rates were seen at 3 to 6 months on CT angiography follow-up,[70–72] with local recurrence rates of 5% to 6% that compare favorably with RFA.[73,74] LA advantages include faster ablation times than RFA and MWA, and tumor access through smaller (21 G) needles. For eye protection, operators and patients must wear safety goggles. Minor complications (pleural

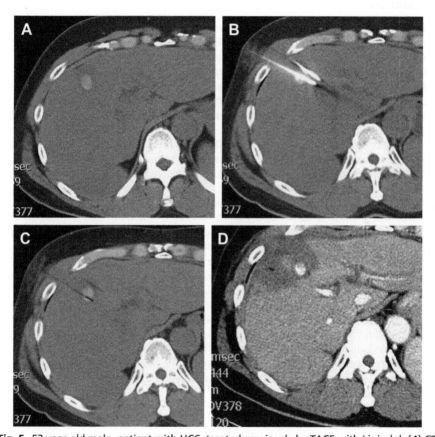

Fig. 5. 52 year-old male, patient with HCC, treated previously by TACE with Lipiodol. (*A*) CT image showing target lesion measuring 2.4 x 3 cm. (*B*) Introducer of the Visualase Laser device. Introducer stylets placed. (*C*) Laser catheter placement. Note that the catheters are radiolucent and show only a negative image due to the presence of air within the catheter. Ablation was performed with Laser at 30 W for 2 min, simultaneously. (*D*) Post-ablation contrast CT image showing wide area of ablation with an adequate margin around the tumor. Note small subcapsular bleeding without clinical consequences.

effusions and small hematomas) occurred in less than 10% of patients. Major complications occurred in less than 1% of patients, with a mortality of 0.1%, in a study that included 2520 lesions and 899 patients.[69] PTAS occurred in approximately one-third of patients.[69] In 1 study of LA treatment of HCC lesions located in critical sites, recurrence was 21.87% (7 of 32 patients) in a mean follow-up period of 24.2 months (range 6–72 months).[75] LA is advocated by some IRs because of the sharp drop in temperature from center to periphery of the tumors during the procedure, the short application time, and the use of fine needles.[70] A well-demarcated separation between necrotic and normal tissue has been described, attributed to the rapid decay of laser light from center to periphery that avoids charring that may limit the size of lesion produced (see **Fig. 5**).[76] In conclusion, LA seems to be as efficacious and safe as RFA, but with more customizable geometries of tumor kill, smaller needle calibers, and MRI compatibility. Improvements in the laser technology may position LA as the primary percutaneous tumor ablative therapy in the future.

IRE ABLATION

Electroporation, also known as electropermeabilization, describes the permeabilization of tumor cell membranes from the application of short and intense electric fields. The permeabilization can be temporary (reversible electroporation) or permanent (IRE), depending on the electrical field magnitude, and the duration and the number of pulses.[77] IRE, an innovative nonthermal ablation method designed for effective ablation of soft tissues, permanently permeabilizes cell membranes by delivering intense electrical pulses that induce nanoscale cell membrane defects.[78] It may be performed using US, CT, or MR guidance. In animal studies, IRE is effective for targeted ablation of liver tumors.[79,80] In 9 of 10 treated rats, 7 to 15 days after treatment, there was extensive necrosis and complete tumor regression.[80] Unlike conventional RFA, with IRE there is no limit in larger tumors caused by a heat-sink effect. IRE produces a distinct margin between ablated and viable tissues, where the magnitude of the electrical field is less than the lethal dose threshold. Additional potential advantages of IRE include a tumor-specific immunologic reaction, little impact on the collagen network within treated tissues, and the potential to ablate tumor tissues near large vessels without compromising them. In addition, application of the electroporation pulses during IRE requires less than 1 second, which contrasts dramatically with the duration required for RFA. Recently, the US Food and Drug Administration (FDA) approved an electroporation device (NanoKnife; AngioDynamics, Latham, NY, USA) that has electrode probes that transmit active energy from its generator to the target. The main disadvantage of IRE is the need for general anesthesia with endotracheal intubation and neuromuscular blockade (because of generalized body contractions). Some patients may develop self-limiting ventricular tachycardia that can be minimized by using electrocardiogram gating.[81] IRE has promise for liver-directed treatment of HCC, which may offer potential benefits compared with conventional ablation methods when further developed.

HIFU ABLATION

HIFU is a noninvasive method that has been used for the treatment of uterine fibroids and solid malignancies in the liver and breast.[82] The ultrasound beam penetrates deeply to reach the target and perform deep ablation. The focused acoustic energy at the target site is much higher than surrounding tissue, which is not damaged and neither is the tissue that the ultrasound traverses. HIFU exposure generates heat because of absorption of acoustic energy in the target, inducing coagulation necrosis when the tissue temperature is rapidly raised to 60°C or more for 1 second or longer.[83,84] Heat is probably the main mechanism of HIFU tumor ablation.[85] In patients with large unresectable HCC,[85–87] complete ablation was achieved with HIFU in 28% to 69% of the patients, and 1-year overall survival rates varied from 50% to 76%. In 1 study with a longer follow-up period, 5-year survival was 32%.[86] HIFU is noninvasive, but usually requires more than 1 session, which may last 4 to 5.5 hours each. Another drawback is the potential risk of minor skin burns (13%–25% of patients), and respiratory movement can cause oscillations in the target lesion site, for which respiratory gating and general anesthesia may be helpful. Another limitation is path obstruction by the overlying ribs. As of this writing, the FDA has not approved HIFU for HCC ablation.

TACE

TACE is a catheter-based angiographic technique that produces vascular occlusion from the injection of either microparticles or microspheres using fluoroscopic guidance, combined with a chemotherapeutic agent. The effectiveness of TACE in the treatment of HCC relies on the difference in the blood flow to the tumor and the non-tumorous liver. HCC is hypervascular and heavily dependent on the arterial blood supply for nutrients and oxygen. HCC uses 5 to 7 times the volume of arterial flow per unit of tissue compared with the surrounding liver, which receives 75% of its blood supply from the portal vein. Following embolization of the artery, the reduction in the arterial blood supply to the tumor causes hypoxia and cell death, typically sparing adjacent liver cells, as the portal vein remains patent.[24] However, using the ethiodized poppy seed oil (Ethiodol or Lipiodol Ultra-Fluide) chemoembolization technique some of the suspension enters the portal vein and reduces portal venous supply to the tumor. Since the 1970s, different cytotoxic chemotherapeutic agents have traditionally been injected intra-arterially, mixed with liquid oil embolic agent, as selectively as possible into the tumor-feeding vessels. For reasons that are not well understood, Ethiodol/Lipiodol adheres to the cell wall of the tumor into which it is actively transported, causing lysis.[88] Kupffer cells in the adjacent liver parenchyma phagocytize the oil and remove it in a period of days, but, because HCC does not contain Kupffer cells, there is no active HCC removal of the oil,[89] which remains in the tumor for months to years, and can be visualized on CT and MRI (**Fig. 6**). Ethiodol/Lipiodol can also be used to locate and mark an HCC when injected intra-arterially in patients with high likelihood of HCC but negative imaging results, or as a prelude to CT-guided ablation of tumors not easily seen on CT scans. When a suspension of chemotherapeutic agent and oil is injected intra-arterially, the Ethiodol/Lipiodol acts as a carrier into the hypervascular HCC, into which high concentrations of the agents are delivered. The tumoral concentration of the chemotherapeutics after TACE is many times higher than levels following systemic intravenous therapy.[90] There are several protocols using different chemotherapeutic agents such as mitomycin C, doxorubicin, and cisplatin. In the first interventional radiology study of TACE with Ethiodol/Lipiodol mixed with these agents, a tumor response rate of 85% without progression of disease was seen in all 38 patients in 1 year,[91] a finding confirmed in subsequent publications.[92] Thus, combining chemotherapy drugs with Ethiodol/Lipiodol became popular. However, because the chemotherapy agents are quickly washed through the liver into the systemic circulation, peak levels are reached within minutes of embolization and are then quickly eliminated.[93] Systemic side effects are to be expected, including hair loss, cardiac toxicity, nausea, and diarrhea, depending on the agent used, but in practice these are uncommon. The positive results of TACE are probably related to tumor hypoxia and to the high concentration of cytotoxic agents within the

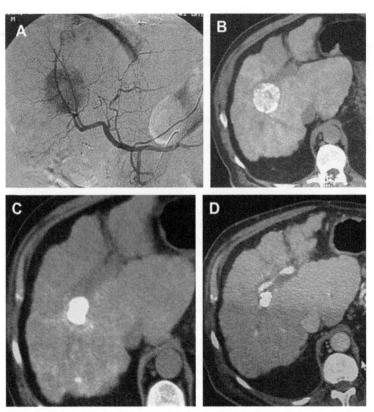

Fig. 6. Patient with hepatitis C and alcohol abuse with cirrhosis and a 4-cm HCC in the right lobe of the liver. (*A*) There is also a less defined tumor blush in the dome of the liver by angiography. TACE with Lipiodol and mitomycin C was performed. (*B*) CT scan 24 hours after TACE shows dense enhancement of the larger tumor by the Lipiodol. (*C*) Three-month follow-up CT scan shows significant response of the tumor. (*D*) Six-month follow-up CT scan shows a residual abnormality in the area of the tumor, which was persistently stable for more than 2 years. The lesion at the dome of the liver required additional RFA (not shown).

tumor.[90,94] More recently, new spherical microembolic material loaded with chemotherapeutic agent was developed in an attempt to reduce the systemic side effects. The drug-eluting beads (DEBs) available in the United States are the LC Bead microspheres (Biocompatibles International, UK) and the HepaSpheres (BioSphere Medical Inc, Rockland, MD, USA), in which the microspheres are ionically bound to negatively charged chemotherapeutics (most commonly doxorubicin). These beads have been proved in vitro and in vivo to slowly elute doxorubicin for 7 days after embolization.[93] Doxorubicin bound to DEB or Lipiodol/doxorubicin chemoembolization protocols have the same total dose (75–150 mg). Peak systemic levels of doxorubicin after DEB embolization are approximately 5% of those after doxorubicin/Lipiodol TACE, and levels remain stable for 7 to 10 days (**Fig. 7**).[93] The ischemic effect of TACE has been scrutinized for the potential negative effect of ischemia-enhancing angiogenesis in hypervascular tumors such as HCC by upregulating the expression of vascular endothelial growth factor (VEGF), implying a need for suppression of angiogenesis following TACE.[6,95]

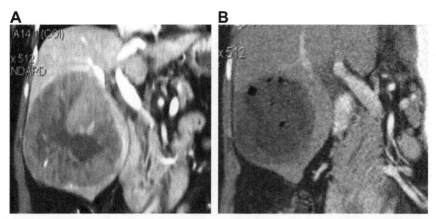

Fig. 7. Large HCC in the right lobe of the liver. (*A*) A 15-cm HCC in the right lobe of the liver was treated with LC Beads loaded with doxorubicin 150 mg embolization. (*B*) Three-month follow-up CT scan shows significant response with shrinkage of the HCC and no vascularization within the tumor, which progressively shrank with time.

Relative contraindications to chemoembolization include portal vein tumor invasion, renal insufficiency, increased bilirubin (>3 mg/dL), and greater than 50% liver involvement with tumor.[6] CO_2 angiography may be used as an alternative to liquid contrast media. Superselective HCC chemoembolization should be always attempted to preserve as much liver parenchyma as possible (**Fig. 8**), especially in patients with more advanced chronic liver disease and portal vein invasion and/or segmental occlusion. Postembolization syndrome (PES) is to be expected and can occur in up to 40% of patients, and includes right upper quadrant abdominal pain, flulike symptoms, nausea, vomiting, fatigue, abdominal distention, fever, and leukocytosis. PES is easily controlled symptomatically, is most intense in the first 48 to 72 hours after TACE, and may last up to 2 weeks. More specific complications include liver abscess (<1%), gallbladder necrosis (<1%), liver failure (1%), non–target organ embolization (<1%), and transiently increased bilirubin. Hepatic abscess is more common in diabetic patients and in those with previous biliary-enteric anastomoses (up to 5% of cases).[96] Improvement in survival after TACE has been documented in 2 major randomized controlled trials (RCTs). A 26% 3-year survival rate was obtained in the cisplatin/Lipiodol TACE group versus 3% in the symptomatic treatment group.[97,98] In a second RCT, a 63% 2-year survival rate was obtained with gelatin sponge/doxorubicin TACE versus 27% in the control group. This study was aborted early because of obvious TACE survival benefits.[96] Several meta-analyses have concluded that TACE improves survival,[99,100] with the best results in patients with well-compensated liver function (CTP class A).[101] More recently, DEB/doxorubicin and doxorubicin/Lipiodol TACE were compared in an RCT in which the systemic side effects and liver failure rates were lower in the DEB group. As expected, lower systemic doxorubicin levels correlated with lower systemic effects, but no other statistical differences were observed.[102] Results of another RCT showed improved tumor response, longer time to progression, and fewer recurrences with DEB/doxorubicin compared with bland embolization alone using similar-sized particles.[103] Regardless of the details, TACE is a safe and effective treatment of HCC in terms of tumor control. Most patients tolerate the procedure well, have good tumor responses, increased survival rates, and a higher quality of life.

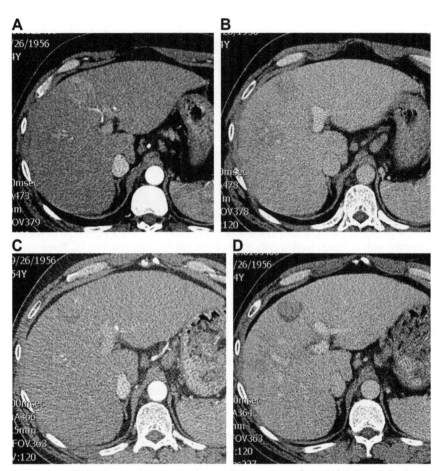

Fig. 8. (*A*) Small, hypervascular HCC in the medial segment of the left lobe of the liver on a 4-phase CT scan. (*B*) Late phase of the CT scan showing the typical washout of HCC. (*C*) The patient was treated by TACE with DC Beads loaded with doxorubicin. Note the lack of enhancement and absence of vascularity on the arterial and venous phases (*D*).

RADIOEMBOLIZATION

Yttrium-90 (^{90}Y) has emerged as the preferred radioactive agent for radioembolization. In the United States, the TheraSphere (Yttrium-90 Glass Microspheres, MDS Nordion, Ottawa, ON, Canada) and SIRSpheres (Yttrium-90 Microspheres, Sirtex Medical Ltd, Lane Cove, NSW, Australia) are the 2 preparations available. TheraSphere has FDA approval for HCC. The particles infused in radioembolization are not intended to cause arterial occlusion, thus sparing arterial flow to the adjacent liver and decreasing post-embolization symptoms.[104] The ^{90}Y is a pure β-radiation emitter, making it optimal for intra-arterial injection. β-Radiation particles are high-energy but cannot penetrate more than 11 mm in human tissue. The half-life of ^{90}Y is 64 hours; therefore 94% of the radiation is emitted within the first 11 days after treatment. Radioembolization and chemoembolization are similar because both take advantage of HCC hypervascularity and predominantly hepatic artery blood supply. A microcatheter is advanced into the hepatic artery for a target infusion of embolic material into the tumor-feeding vessels, resulting in a disproportionate distribution to the tumor, to which high doses

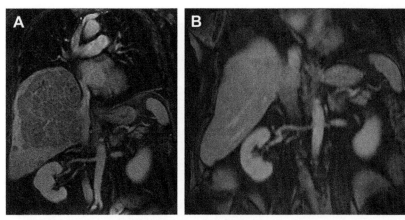

Fig. 9. (*A*) Large HCC of the right lobe of the liver. (*B*) Patient was treated with radioembolization using TheraSpheres. A follow-up CT scan at 22 months showed an excellent response with almost complete disappearance of the tumor (case kindly provided by Dr Riad Salem).

of radiation are delivered directly for 10 to 11 days.[104] In TACE, the embolism produces ischemia, whereas with TheraSpheres ischemia is minimal to nonexistent, and the effect on the tumor is almost exclusively from radiation (**Fig. 9**). Compared with TACE, a major difference is the required embolization of the gastroduodenal, right gastric, cystic, and pyloric arteries before radioembolization (although some TACE procedures performed with small beads might also benefit from preventive embolization of the same celiac trunk branches; **Fig. 10**). The severity of complications related to radioembolization is significant, and non–target organ embolization with ^{90}Y is associated with more morbidity compared with TACE. If ^{90}Y is infused into small gastric and duodenal/pancreatic branches not previously embolized, slow-healing radiation ulcers may develop in the affected bowel, in ~4% to 5% of treatments.[105] This can be prevented using mapping angiograms of the celiac and superior mesenteric arteries, followed by careful coil embolization of all the branches that are potentially threatened. Therefore a preparation procedure always precedes the treatment procedure and the celiac/superior mesenteric artery vascular bed is prepared for the ^{90}Y treatment 10 to 14 days before the treatment. The need for perfect knowledge of the vascular anatomy of the celiac branches cannot be overemphasized. Also, HCC often has small arteriovenous shunts that would allow radioactive particles from the ^{90}Y infusion to flow from the hepatic artery into the hepatic venous system and then to the lungs.[106] Immediately following the celiac/superior mesenteric artery branch vessel coil embolization, approximately 4 mCi of technetium 99 m macroaggregated albumin (^{99}Tc-MAA) is injected in the planned treatment artery (right, left, or proper hepatic artery). MAA has similar particle sizes to the ^{90}Y microspheres, so immediate planar body nuclear medicine scanning can predict distribution in the lungs, without adverse effects of ^{99}Tc, because of the different particle γ energy it emits. Radiation being emitted outside the liver correlates with the tumor shunt fraction. If the dose detected in the lungs is 20% or more than in the liver, radiosphere treatment is contraindicated because injected ^{90}Y of more than 30 Gy could cause radiation pneumonitis.[105] Radiation activity in the bowel is also a contraindication to treatment and would put the patient at risk for radiation ulcers. Radioembolization offers important benefits to some patients. Bilobar disease or extensive multifocal HCC can often be treated with 1 session, and main portal vein thrombosis does not represent a contraindication because arterial flow is preserved in the treatment area.[106] At the time of this writing, no

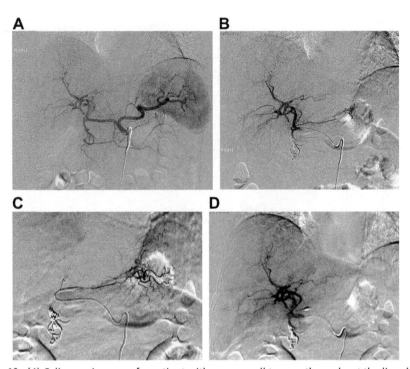

Fig. 10. (*A*) Celiac angiogram of a patient with many small tumors throughout the liver (not well depicted here). (*B*) More selective angiogram after embolization of the gastroduodenal artery, showing the right gastric artery arising from the bifurcation of the right and left hepatic arteries, directed toward the stomach body. (*C*) Selective injection of the right gastric artery, just before embolization. (*D*) Final hepatic angiogram just before radioembolization shows absence of vessels to the stomach. Note the discretely hypervascular nodules in the background.

RCT has evaluated survival in patients with HCC treated with ^{90}Y radioembolization versus medical treatments. A recent prospective study of 291 patients showed survival rates of 42% to 52% (CTP class A) in 17 months follow-up.[107] It is unclear whether ^{90}Y radioembolization is better than TACE at treating oligocentric HCC, because no RCT has compared the two treatments. A recent retrospective analysis showed no difference in tumor response or survival between TACE and ^{90}Y radioembolization in HCC.[108] Side effects from radioembolization include fatigue (57%), pain (23%), and nausea/vomiting (20%). Approximately 20% of patients have grade 3 to 4 bilirubin increase, and greater than 75% have significant lymphopenia. Major complication risks of ^{90}Y radioembolization include bowel/gastric ulcers (4%), biliary/gallbladder injury requiring surgery (<1.5%), and radiation pneumonitis (<1%).[105,107,108]

PERCUTANEOUS HEPATIC PERFUSION

Percutaneous hepatic perfusion (PHP) delivers a specific chemotherapeutic drug directly into the tumor blood supply, allowing dramatic dose escalation. The method capitalizes on the unique dual vascular supply of the liver, namely the hepatic artery and portal vein, and single venous outlet that empties directly into the inferior vena cava. Isolated hepatic perfusion reduces or eliminates systemic toxicities by isolating the circulation of the liver from the patient's general circulation, enabling treatment of

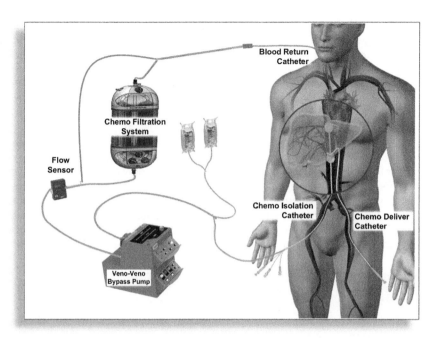

Fig. 11. PHP/CS system overview. Chemo-filtration loop on the left. Chemo-isolation & delivery on the right.

the entire liver, including micrometastases, and potentially improving tumor-killing efficacy. The original proof of concept was surgical, but that was invasive and with high morbidity. Therefore a percutaneous technique was developed including a method for liver isolation, chemotherapy saturation, and filtration of the blood collected from the hepatic vein with reinjection into the jugular vein, to allow a dose delivered to the tumor at an estimated 100-fold increase compared with systemic intravenous chemotherapy (**Fig. 11**). The filtration system removes approximately 80% of the infused drug that leaves the liver. A randomized phase III trial for treatment of metastatic melanoma in the liver was recently concluded. Results showed a significant improvement in overall survival of 300 days compared with 124 days for best available care, with similar results for hepatic progression-free survival.[109–111] A phase II trial for the treatment of HCC has recently been completed but the results are not yet available. A phase III HCC trial using PHP with doxorubicin versus sorafenib is due to start in 2011.

COMBINED THERAPIES FOR HCC TREATMENT

Combinations of locoregional therapies (PEI, RFA, MWA, and/or TACE) for the treatment of HCC have been studied recently, especially the synergistic combination of TACE and RFA. In lesions less than 3 cm, complete tumor necrosis following thermal ablation alone may vary from 76% to 100%, but it may be as low as 29% to 48% with HCC lesions larger than 3-cm,[111] probably because of the heat-sink effect from surrounding blood vessels greater than 3 mm (see **Figs. 3** and **4**).[112] Pre-RFA embolization reduces hepatic arterial blood flow and thereby perfusion-mediated heat loss, which, in turn, seems to increase the RFA zone and probability of a complete response. The decrease in blood flow through the tumor can increase the ablative zone in RFA by up to 6 or 7 cm, which should decrease recurrence rates

(Fig. 12).[112,113,114,115] Thermal ablation after TACE provides higher concentrations of cytotoxic drug(s) in the tumor and surrounding tissue and there is also increased tumor sensitization to heat-kill following TACE. Doxorubicin, even at low levels, has been shown to sensitize cells to heat kill by as much as 5°C.[116] The enhanced diameter of drug-induced and coagulation-induced necrosis increases the tumor-free margin by killing microsatellite lesions and venous tumor emboli surrounding HCC, thereby decreasing marginal recurrence.[30] For 5-cm lesions, the complete response rate of RFA after TACE has been reported to be 90% to 100% at 1 year,[117,118] similar to that for lesions of 3 cm or less. Local control and long-term survival are increased when RFA and TACE are combined compared with either procedure alone for tumors of 3 cm or less.[25,112,114] Combined therapy and hepatectomy have been compared in the treatment of HCC lesions of 3 cm or less in diameter, with similar global survivals at 1, 3, and 5 years of 98% versus 97%, 94% versus 93%, and 75% versus 81%, respectively ($P = .87$), with comparable tumor-free recurrence survivals at 1, 3, and 5 years of 92% versus 99%, 64% versus 69%, and 27% versus 26% ($P = .70$).[28] The comparative results of 5-year survival with combined therapy (75%) versus RFA alone (38%)

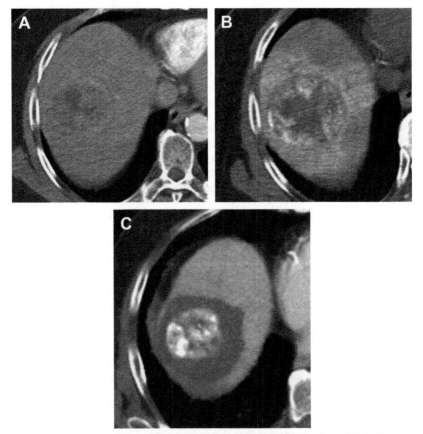

Fig. 12. (A) CT scan showing a large HCC in the right lobe of the liver. (B) TACE was performed with mitomycin C and Lipiodol. Note the heterogeneous enhancement of the tumor and the background liver. (C) CT scan at 3 months following TACE and RFA performed sequentially with the bipolar electrodes by InCircle RFA system. Note significant shrinkage of the tumor and the large area of ablation surrounding the tumor.

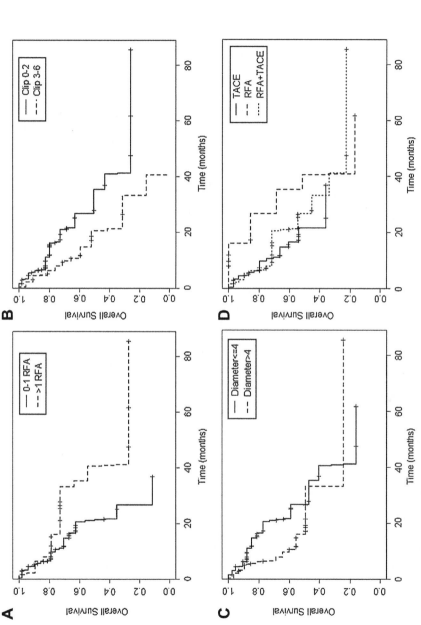

Fig. 13. (A) Overall survival by number of RFAs (N = 72; P = .0341). (B) Overall survival by Cancer of the Liver Italian Program (CLIP) score (N = 72; P = .0151). (C) Overall survival by diameter of the tumor (P = .12). Note that there is some difference in the first 20 months, but the advantage is lost after 30 months. (D) Overall survival when comparing the different treatments and combination of RFA and TACE. Note that the slight tendency of early improvement in overall survival by RFA alone did not reach significance (P = .38).

and TACE alone (8%) for HCC lesions less than 5 cm in diameter suggest that combination therapies should always be considered. However, the authors, in a recent review of their own experience in treating HCC, verified that adjusting for Cancer of the Liver Italian Program (CLIP) scores, patients who have more than 1 RFA session are at 0.35 times the risk of death at any given time compared with patients who have had 0 to 1 RFA sessions. Adjusting for number of RFAs, patients in the CLIP score 3 to 6 category are at 2.5 times the risk of death at any given time compared with patients in the CLIP score 0 to 2 category. Therefore, patients with low CLIP scores benefit the most from aggressive liver-directed therapy with marked improvement in overall survival (OS). The number of TACE sessions did not change OS in our series. The size of the lesion influenced OS improvement in the first 20 months (for lesions <4 cm) but OS was similar at 30 months and beyond for lesions greater than 4 cm. Elsewhere, the combination of TACE and RFA did not improve OS, even taking into consideration the size of the lesions (**Fig. 13**).[29]

Combined therapies may be performed on the same day or on subsequent days, as currently performed by the authors. Complications can be up to 3% but the risk of death or serious morbidity does not seem to be increased.[25] Other combined treatments, including RFA or TACE followed by systemic chemotherapy with sorafenib or bevacizumab, are being investigated.

SUMMARY

In the last decade there were significant improvements in minimally invasive therapy for treating HCC using imaging guidance, which is safe and effective. However, there are differences among the many procedures that are available in terms of advantages, disadvantages, costs, and potential complications. More RCTs are needed to compare these therapies and for devising therapeutic strategies. Notwithstanding, in the daily practice of interventional oncology, there are many situations in which individualized medicine, experience, and common sense still inform the best approach for any given patient.

REFERENCES

1. Said A, Wells J. Management of hepatocellular carcinoma. Minerva Med 2009; 100:51–68.
2. Stravitz RT, Heuman DM, Chand N, et al. Surveillance for hepatocellular carcinoma in patients with cirrhosis improves outcome. Am J Med 2008;121:119–26.
3. Pawlik TM, Delman KA, Vauthey JN, et al. Tumor size predicts vascular invasion and histologic grade: implications for selection of surgical treatment for hepatocellular carcinoma. Liver Transpl 2005;11:1086–92.
4. Otto G, Heuschen U, Hofmann WJ, et al. Survival and recurrence after liver transplantation versus liver resection for hepatocellular carcinoma: a retrospective analysis. Ann Surg 1998;227:424–32.
5. Poon RT, Fan ST, Lo CM, et al. Long-term survival and pattern of recurrence after resection of small hepatocellular carcinoma in patients with preserved liver function: implications for a strategy of salvage transplantation. Ann Surg 2002;235: 373–82.
6. Jonas S, Bechstein WO, Steinmüller T, et al. Vascular invasion and histopathologic grading determine outcome after liver transplantation for hepatocellular carcinoma in cirrhosis. Hepatology 2001;33:1080–6.

7. Figueras J, Jaurrieta E, Valls C, et al. Survival after liver transplantation in cirrhotic patients with and without hepatocellular carcinoma: a comparative study. Hepatology 1997;25:1485–9.

8. Llovet JM, Fuster J, Bruix J. Intention-to-treat analysis of surgical treatment for early hepatocellular carcinoma: resection versus transplantation. Hepatology 1999;30:1434–40.

9. Llovet JM, Ricci S, Mazzaferro V, et al. Sorafenib in advanced hepatocellular carcinoma. N Engl J Med 2008;359:378–90.

10. Burroughs A, Hochhauser D, Meyer T. Systemic treatment and liver transplantation for hepatocellular carcinoma: two ends of the therapeutic spectrum. Lancet Oncol 2004;5:409–18.

11. Davis CR. Interventional radiological treatment of hepatocellular carcinoma. Cancer Control 2010;17:87–99.

12. Peck-Radosavljevic M, Greten TF, Lammer J, et al. Consensus on the current use of sorafenib for the treatment of hepatocellular carcinoma. Eur J Gastroenterol Hepatol 2010;22:391–8.

13. Fuss M, Salter BJ, Herman TS, et al. External beam radiation therapy for hepatocellular carcinoma: potential of intensity-modulated and image guided radiation therapy. Gastroenterology 2004;127(Suppl 1):S206–17.

14. Marrero JA, Feng Z. Alpha-fetoprotein in early hepatocellular carcinoma. Gastroenterology 2010;138:400–1.

15. Bruix J, Castells A, Bosch J, et al. Surgical resection of hepatocellular carcinoma in cirrhotic patients: prognostic value of preoperative portal pressure. Gastroenterology 1996;111:1018–22.

16. Cormier JN, Thomas KT, Chari RS, et al. Management of hepatocellular carcinoma. J Gastrointest Surg 2006;10:761–80.

17. Geschwind JH, Soulen M. Interventional Oncology–principles and practice. Cambridge: Cambridge University Press; 2008. p. 146.

18. Delis SG, Dervenis C. Selection criteria for liver resection in patients with hepatocellular carcinoma and chronic liver disease. World J Gastroenterol 2008;14:3452–60.

19. Cabrera R, Nelson DR. Review article: the management of hepatocellular carcinoma. Aliment Pharmacol Ther 2009;31:461–76.

20. Llovet JM, Di Bisceglie AM, Bruix J, et al. Panel of experts in HCC-design clinical trials. Design and endpoints of clinical trials in hepatocellular carcinoma. J Natl Cancer Inst 2008;100:698–711.

21. Llovet JM, Brú C, Bruix J. Prognosis of hepatocellular carcinoma: the BCLC staging classification. Semin Liver Dis 1999;19:329–38.

22. Pleguezuelo M, Germani G, Marelli L, et al. Evidence-based diagnosis and locoregional therapy for hepatocellular carcinoma. Expert Rev Gastroenterol Hepatol 2008;2:761–84.

23. Grieco A, Pompili M, Caminiti G, et al. Prognostic factors for survival in patients with early-intermediate hepatocellular carcinoma undergoing non-surgical therapy: comparison of Okuda, CLIP, and BCLC staging systems in a single Italian centre. Gut 2005;54:411–8.

24. Marrero JA, Fontana RJ, Barrat A, et al. Prognosis of hepatocellular carcinoma: comparison of 7 staging systems in an American cohort. Hepatology 2005;41:707–16.

25. Yamakado K, Nakatsuka A, Takaki H, et al. Early-stage hepatocellular carcinoma: radiofrequency ablation combined with chemoembolization versus hepatectomy. Radiology 2008;247:260–6.

26. Koda M, Murawaki Y, Mitsuda A, et al. Predictive factors for intrahepatic recurrence after percutaneous ethanol injection therapy for small hepatocellular carcinoma. Cancer 2000;88:529–37.

27. Tateishi R, Shiina S, Teratani T, et al. Percutaneous radiofrequency ablation for hepatocellular carcinoma: an analysis of 1000 cases. Cancer 2005;103:1201–9.

28. Uflacker R, Cole S, Thomas M. Improved survival in hepatocellular carcinoma patients with low CLIP scores and liver-directed therapies: retrospective single institution study. Abstract P282, Presented at the 2010 CIRSE Annual Meeting and Postgraduate Course, Abstract book. Valencia, October 2–6, 2010. p. 405.

29. Shibata T, Isoda H, Hirokawa Y, et al. Small hepatocellular carcinoma: is radiofrequency ablation combined with transcatheter arterial chemoembolization more effective than radiofrequency ablation alone for treatment? Radiology 2009;252:905–13.

30. Veltri A, Moretto P, Doriguzzi A, et al. Radiofrequency thermal ablation (RFA) after transarterial chemoembolization (TACE) as a combined therapy for unresectable non-early hepatocellular carcinoma (HCC). Eur Radiol 2006;16:661–9.

31. Zavaglia C, Corso R, Rampoldi A, et al. Is percutaneous radiofrequency thermal ablation of hepatocellular carcinoma a safe procedure? Eur J Gastroenterol Hepatol 2008;20:196–201.

32. Guglielmi A, Ruzzenente A, Valdegamberi A, et al. Radiofrequency ablation versus surgical resection for the treatment of hepatocellular carcinoma in cirrhosis. J Gastrointest Surg 2008;12:192–8.

33. Vivarelli M, Guglielmi A, Ruzzenente A, et al. Surgical resection versus percutaneous radiofrequency ablation in the treatment of hepatocellular carcinoma on cirrhotic liver. Ann Surg 2004;240:102–7.

34. Hiraoka A, Horiike N, Yamashita Y, et al. Efficacy of radiofrequency ablation therapy compared to surgical resection in 164 patients in Japan with single hepatocellular carcinoma smaller than 3 cm, along with report of complications. Hepatogastroenterology 2008;55:2171–4.

35. Hasegawa S, Yamasaki N, Hiwaki T, et al. Factors that predict intrahepatic recurrence of hepatocellular carcinoma in 81 patients initially treated by percutaneous ethanol injection. Cancer 1999;86:1682–90.

36. Shiina S, Teratani T, Obi S, et al. A randomized controlled trial of radiofrequency ablation with ethanol injection for small hepatocellular carcinoma. Gastroenterology 2005;129:122–30.

37. Lin SM, Lin CJ, Lin CC, et al. Radiofrequency ablation improves prognosis compared with ethanol injection for hepatocellular carcinoma < or = 4 cm. Gastroenterology 2004;127:1714–23.

38. Lencioni RA, Allgaier HP, Cloni D, et al. Small hepatocellular carcinoma in cirrhosis: randomized comparison of radio-frequency thermal ablation versus percutaneous ethanol injection. Radiology 2003;228:235–40.

39. Cho YK, Kim JK, Kim MY, et al. Systematic review of randomized trials for hepatocellular carcinoma treated with percutaneous ablation therapies. Hepatology 2009;49:453–9.

40. Orlando A, Leandro G, Olivo M, et al. Radiofrequency thermal ablation versus percutaneous ethanol injection for small hepatocellular carcinoma in cirrhosis: meta-analysis of randomized controlled trials. Am J Gastroenterol 2009;104:514–24.

41. McGahan J, Browning PD, Brock JM, et al. Hepatic ablation using radiofrequency electrocautery. Invest Radiol 1990;25:267–70.

42. Rossi S, Fornari F, Pathies C, et al. Thermal lesions induced by 480 KHz localized current field in guinea pig and pig liver. Tumori 1990;76:54–7.

43. Goldberg SN, Gazelle GS, Compton CC, et al. Treatment of intrahepatic malignancy with radiofrequency ablation: radiologic-pathologic correlation. Cancer 2000;88:2452–63.

44. Kim SK, Rhim H, Kim YS, et al. Radiofrequency thermal ablation of hepatic tumors: pitfalls and challenges. Abdom Imaging 2005;30:727–33.

45. Lu DS, Yu NC, Raman SS, et al. Radiofrequency ablation of hepatocellular carcinoma: treatment success as defined by histologic examination of the explanted liver. Radiology 2005;234:954–60.

46. Bhardwaj N, Strickland AD, Ahmad F, et al. A comparative histological evaluation of the ablations produced by microwave, cryotherapy and radiofrequency in the liver. Pathology 2009;41:168–72.

47. Livraghi T, Solbiati L, Meloni M, et al. Treatment of focal liver tumors with percutaneous radio-frequency ablation: complications encountered in a multicenter study. Radiology 2003;226:441–5.

48. Lin SM, Lin CC, Chen WT, et al. Radiofrequency ablation for hepatocellular carcinoma: a prospective comparison of four radiofrequency devices. J Vasc Interv Radiol 2007;18:1118–25.

49. Shibata T, Shibata T, Maetani Y, et al. Radiofrequency ablation for small hepatocellular carcinoma: prospective comparison of internally cooled electrode and expandable electrode. Radiology 2006;238:346–53.

50. Tabuse K, Katsumi M, Kobayashi Y, et al. Microwave surgery: hepatectomy using a microwave tissue coagulator. World J Surg 1985;9:135–43.

51. Tabuse K. A new operative procedure for hepatic surgery using a microwave tissue coagulator. Nippon Geka Hokan 1979;48:160–72.

52. Goldburg N, Charboneau WJ, Dodd GD, et al. Image-guided tumour ablation: proposal for standardization of terms and reporting criteria. Radiology 2003; 228:335–45.

53. Bhardwaj N, Strickland AD, Ahmad F, et al. Liver ablation techniques: a review. Surg Endosc 2010;24:254–65.

54. Shibata T, Iimuro Y, Yamamoto Y, et al. Small hepatocellular carcinoma: comparison of radio-frequency ablation and percutaneous microwave coagulation therapy. Radiology 2002;223:331–7.

55. Dong B, Liang P, Yu X, et al. Percutaneous sonographically guided microwave coagulation therapy for hepatocellular carcinoma: results in 234 patients. AJR Am J Roentgenol 2003;180:1547–55.

56. Liang P, Dong B, Yu X, et al. Prognostic factors for survival in patients with hepatocellular carcinoma after percutaneous microwave ablation. Radiology 2005; 235:299–307.

57. Arnott J. Practical illustrations of the remedial efficacy of a very low or anesthetic temperature in cancer. Lancet 1850;2:257–9.

58. Mazur P, Rall WF, Leibo SP. Kinetics of water loss and the likelihood of intracellular freezing in mouse ova (influence of the method of calculating the temperature dependence of water permeability). Cell Biophys 1984;6: 197–213.

59. Bryant G. DSC measurement of cell suspensions during successive freezing runs: implications for the mechanisms of intracellular ice formation. Cryobiology 1995;32:114–28.

60. Callstrom MR, Charboneau JW. Technologies for ablation of hepatocellular carcinoma. Gastroenterology 2008;134:1831–5.

61. Orlacchio A, Bazzocchi G, Pastorelli D, et al. Percutaneous cryoablation of small hepatocellular carcinoma with US guidance and CT monitoring: initial experience. Cardiovasc Intervent Radiol 2008;31:587–94.

62. Shimizu T, Sakuhara Y, Abo D, et al. Outcome of MR-guided percutaneous cryoablation for hepatocellular carcinoma. J Hepatobiliary Pancreat Surg 2009;16: 816–23.

63. Morrison PR, Silverman SG, Tuncali K, et al. MRI-guided cryotherapy. J Magn Reson Imaging 2008;27:410–2.

64. Gilbert JC, Onik GM, Hoddick WK, et al. Real time ultrasonic monitoring of hepatic cryosurgery. Cryobiology 1985;22:319–30.

65. Seifert JK, Morris DL. World survey on the complications of hepatic and prostate cryotherapy. World J Surg 1999;23:109–13.

66. Pearson AS, Izzo F, Fleming RY, et al. Intraoperative radiofrequency ablation or cryoablation for hepatic malignancies. Am J Surg 1999;178:592–9.

67. Nikfarjam M, Vijayaragavan M, Malcontenti-Wilson C, et al. Progressive microvascular injury in liver and colorectal liver metastases following laser induced focal hyperthermia therapy. Lasers Surg Med 2005;37:64–7.

68. Pacella CM, Bizzarri G, Francica G, et al. Percutaneous laser ablation in the treatment of hepatocellular carcinoma with a tumor size of 4.0 cm or smaller: analysis of factors affecting the achievement of tumor necrosis. J Vasc Interv Radiol 2005;16:1447–57.

69. Vogl TJ, Straub R, Eichler K, et al. Malignant liver tumors treated with MR imaging-guided laser-induced thermotherapy: experience with complications in 899 patients (2520 lesions). Radiology 2002;225:367–77.

70. Pacella CM, Bizzarri G, Magnolfi F, et al. Laser thermal ablation in the treatment of small hepatocellular carcinoma: results in 74 patients. Radiology 2001;221: 712–20.

71. Vogl TJ, Straub R, Zangos S, et al. MR-guided laser-induced thermotherapy (LITT) of liver tumours: experimental and clinical data. Int J Hyperthermia 2004;20:713–24.

72. Stroszczynski C, Gaffke G, Gnauck M, et al. Current concepts and recent developments of laser ablation in tumor therapy. Radiologe 2004;44:320–9.

73. Curley SA, Izzo F, Ellis LM, et al. Radiofrequency ablation of hepatocellular cancer in 110 patients with cirrhosis. Ann Surg 2000;232:381–91.

74. Barnett CC, Curley SA. Ablative techniques for hepatocellular carcinoma. Semin Oncol 2001;28:487–96.

75. Caspani B, Ierardi AM, Motta F, et al. Small nodular hepatocellular carcinoma treated by laser thermal ablation in high risk locations: preliminary results. Eur Radiol 2010;20:2286–92.

76. Germer CT, Roggan A, Ritz JP, et al. Optical properties of native and coagulated human liver tissue and liver metastases in the near infrared range. Lasers Surg Med 1998;23:194–203.

77. Orlowski S, Mir LM. Cell electropermeabilization: a new tool for biochemical and pharmacological studies. Biochim Biophys Acta 1993;1154:51–63.

78. Rubinsky B, Onik G, Mikus P. Irreversible electroporation: a new ablation modality: clinical implications. Technol Cancer Res Treat 2007;6:37–48.

79. Al-Sakere B, André F, Bernat C, et al. Tumor ablation with irreversible electroporation. PLoS One 2007;2:e1135.

80. Guo Y, Zhang Y, Klein R, et al. Irreversible electroporation therapy in the liver: longitudinal efficacy studies in a rat model of hepatocellular carcinoma. Cancer Res 2010;70:1555–63.

81. Ball C, Thomson KR, Kavnoudias H. Irreversible electroporation: a new challenge in "out of operating theater" anesthesia. Anesth Analg 2010;110:1305–9.

82. Kennedy JE. High-intensity focused ultrasound in the treatment of solid tumors. Nat Rev Cancer 2005;5:321–7.

83. Hill CR, Rivens I, Vaughan M, et al. Lesion development in focused ultrasound surgery: a general model. Ultrasound Med Biol 1994;20:259–69.

84. Vaughan M, Haar G, Hill CR, et al. Minimally invasive cancer surgery using focused ultrasound: a pre-clinical, normal tissue study. Br J Radiol 1994;67:267–74.

85. Wu F, Chen WZ, Bai J, et al. Pathological changes in human malignant carcinoma treated with high-intensity focused ultrasound. Ultrasound Med Biol 2001;27:1099–106.

86. Zhang L, Zhu H, Jin C, et al. High-intensity focused ultrasound (HIFU): effective and safe therapy for hepatocellular carcinoma adjacent to major hepatic veins. Eur Radiol 2009;19:437–44.

87. Li Y, Sha W, Zhou Y, et al. Short and long term efficacy of high intensity focused ultrasound therapy for advanced hepatocellular carcinoma. J Gastroenterol Hepatol 2007;22:2148–54.

88. Chou FI, Fang KC, Chung C, et al. Lipiodol uptake and retention by human hepatoma cells. Nucl Med Biol 1995;22:379–86.

89. Kan Z, McCuskey PA, Wright KC, et al. Role of Kupffer cells in iodized oil embolization. Invest Radiol 1994;29:990–3.

90. Sasaki Y, Imaoka S, Kasugai H, et al. A new approach to chemoembolization therapy for hepatoma using ethiodized oil, cisplatin, and gelatin sponge. Cancer 1987;60:1194–203.

91. Ohishi H, Uchida H, Yoshimura H, et al. Hepatocellular carcinoma detected by iodized oil. Use of anticancer agents. Radiology 1985;154:25–9.

92. Solomon B, Soulen MC, Baum RA, et al. Chemoembolization of hepatocellular carcinoma with cisplatin, doxorubicin, mitomycin-C, Ethiodol, and polyvinyl alcohol: prospective evaluation of response and survival in a U.S. population. J Vasc Interv Radiol 1999;10:793–8.

93. Varela M, Real MI, Burrel M, et al. Chemoembolization of hepatocellular carcinoma with drug eluting beads: efficacy and doxorubicin pharmacokinetics. J Hepatol 2007;46:474–81.

94. Xiao EH, Guo D, Bian DJ. Effect of preoperative transcatheter arterial chemoembolization on angiogenesis of hepatocellular carcinoma cells. World J Gastroenterol 2009;15:4582–6.

95. Brown DB, Cardella JF, Sacks D, et al. Quality improvement guidelines for transhepatic arterial chemoembolization, embolization, and chemotherapeutic infusion for hepatic malignancy. J Vasc Interv Radiol 2009; 20(Suppl):S219–26.

96. Kim W, Clark TW, Baum RA, et al. Risk factors for liver abscess formation after hepatic chemoembolization. J Vasc Interv Radiol 2001;12:965–8.

97. Llovet JM, Real MI, Montaña X, et al. Arterial embolisation or chemoembolisation versus symptomatic treatment in patients with unresectable hepatocellular carcinoma: a randomised controlled trial. Lancet 2002;359:1734–9.

98. Lo CM, Ngan H, Tso WK, et al. Randomized controlled trial of transarterial lipiodol chemoembolization for unresectable hepatocellular carcinoma. Hepatology 2002;35:1164–71.

99. Llovet JM, Bruix J. Systematic review of randomized trials for unresectable hepatocellular carcinoma: chemoembolization improves survival. Hepatology 2003;37:429–42.

100. Cammà C, Schepis F, Orlando A, et al. Transarterial chemoembolization or unresectable hepatocellular carcinoma: meta-analysis of randomized controlled trials. Radiology 2002;224:47–54.
101. Mabed M, Esmaeel M, El-Khodary T, et al. A randomized controlled trial of transcatheter arterial chemoembolization with lipiodol, doxorubicin and cisplatin versus intravenous doxorubicin for patients with unresectable hepatocellular carcinoma. Eur J Cancer Care 2009;18:492–9.
102. Lammer J, Malagari K, Vogl T, et al. Prospective randomized study of doxorubicin-eluting-bead embolization in the treatment of hepatocellular carcinoma: results of the PRECISION V study. Cardiovasc Intervent Radiol 2010; 33:41–52.
103. Malagari K, Pomoni M, Kelekis A, et al. Prospective randomized comparison of chemoembolization with doxorubicin-eluting beads and bland embolization with Bead-Block for hepatocellular carcinoma. Cardiovasc Intervent Radiol 2010;33: 541–51.
104. Salem R, Lewandowski RJ, Atassi B, et al. Treatment of unresectable hepatocellular carcinoma with use of 90Y microspheres (Thera Sphere): safety, tumor response, and survival. J Vasc Interv Radiol 2005;16:1627–39.
105. Riaz A, Lewandowski R, Kulik L. Complications following radioembolization with yttrium-90 microspheres: a comprehensive literature review. J Vasc Interv Radiol 2009;20:1121–30.
106. Salem R, Lewandowski R, Roberts C, et al. Use of yttrium-90 glass microspheres (TheraSphere) for the treatment of unresectable hepatocellular carcinoma in patients with portal vein thrombosis. J Vasc Interv Radiol 2004;15:335–45.
107. Salem R, Lewandowski RJ, Mulcahy MF, et al. Radioembolization for hepatocellular carcinoma using yttrium-90 microspheres: a comprehensive report of long-term outcomes. Gastroenterology 2010;138:52–64.
108. Kooby DA, Egnatashvili V, Srinivasan S, et al. Comparison of yttrium-90 radioembolization and transcatheter arterial chemoembolization for the treatment of unresectable hepatocellular carcinoma. J Vasc Interv Radiol 2010;21:224–30.
109. Alexander HR Jr, Butler CC. Development of isolated hepatic perfusion via the operative and percutaneous techniques for patients with isolated and unresectable liver metastases. Cancer J 2010;2:132–41.
110. Miao N, Pingpank JF, Alexander HR, et al. Percutaneous hepatic perfusion in patients with metastatic liver cancer: anesthetic, hemodynamic, and metabolic considerations. Ann Surg Oncol 2008;3:815–23.
111. Alexander HR Jr, Libutti SK, Pingpank JF, et al. Isolated hepatic perfusion for the treatment of patients with colorectal cancer liver metastases after irinotecan-based therapy. Ann Surg Oncol 2005;12:138–44.
112. Yamakado K, Nakatsuka A, Ohmori S, et al. Radiofrequency ablation combined with chemoembolization in hepatocellular carcinoma: treatment response based on tumor size and morphology. J Vasc Interv Radiol 2002;13:1225–32.
113. Tateishi R, Shiina S, Ohki T, et al. Treatment strategy for hepatocellular carcinoma: expanding the indications for radiofrequency ablation. J Gastroenterol 2009;44(Suppl 19):142–6.
114. Lencioni R, Crocetti L, Petruzzi P, et al. Doxorubicin-eluting bead enhanced radiofrequency ablation of hepatocellular carcinoma: a pilot clinical study. J Hepatol 2008;49:217–22.
115. Ahmed M, Liu Z, Lukyanov AN, et al. Combination radiofrequency ablation with intratumoral liposomal doxorubicin: effect on drug accumulation and coagulation in multiple tissues and tumor types in animals. Radiology 2005;235:469–77.

116. Kadivar F, Soulen MC. Enhancing ablation: synergies with regional and systemic therapies. J Vasc Interv Radiol 2010;21:S251–6.
117. Gasparini D, Sponza M, Marzio A, et al. Combined treatment, TACE and RF ablation, in HCC: preliminary results. Radiol Med 2002;104:412–20.
118. Liao GS, Yu CY, Shih ML, et al. Radiofrequency ablation after transarterial embolization as therapy for patients with unresectable hepatocellular carcinoma. Eur J Surg Oncol 2008;34:61–6.

Systemic Therapy in Hepatocellular Carcinoma

Stephen H. Wrzesinski, MD, PhD[a,b], Tamar H. Taddei, MD[c,d],
Mario Strazzabosco, MD, PhD[c,e,f],*

KEYWORDS

- Systemic therapy • Chemotherapy • Hepatocellular carcinoma

Hepatocellular carcinoma (HCC) is the third leading cause of cancer-related death globally.[1] Other articles in this issue have addressed the epidemiology, screening, diagnosis, staging, and surgical and locoregional treatments. Although there have been many advances in HCC treatment, more than 60% of patients present with disease at a stage too advanced to benefit from curative modalities. In patients for whom surgical resection or curative ablation is an option, 50% experience a recurrence within 18 months, and up to 70% to 80% recur within 5 years.[2,3] Patients awaiting liver transplantation for HCC face the pressure of keeping their tumor downstaged, ie, downsized to stay within transplantable criteria. Thirty to forty percent of patients with HCC present with advanced disease amenable only to palliative locoregional therapies.[4] Although these therapies may offer prolonged median survival, the vast majority succumb to tumor progression.[5] Once advanced stage HCC has progressed through local treatment modalities, patients succumb to the disease with a median survival of about 8 months.[6] The goal of treatment, therefore, becomes focused on maintaining quality of life by slowing down the progression of disease through the administration of agents with minimal side effects.

S.H.W. and T.H.T. have nothing to disclose; M.S. received research grants from Bayer. The support of Yale University Liver Center (NIH DK 34989) to M.S. is gratefully acknowledged.

[a] Yale Comprehensive Cancer Center, Yale University School of Medicine, New Haven, CT, USA

[b] VA Connecticut Healthcare System, Comprehensive Cancer Center, 950 Campbell Avenue–111D, West Haven, CT 06516–2700, USA

[c] Department of Internal Medicine, Section of Digestive Diseases, Yale University School of Medicine, 333 Cedar Street/1080 LMP, PO Box 208019, New Haven, CT 06520–8019, USA

[d] VA Connecticut Healthcare System, Hepatitis C Resource Center (HCRC), 950 Campbell Avenue-111H, West Haven, CT 06516-2700, USA

[e] Yale Liver Center, Department of Internal Medicine, Yale University, Cedar Street 333, New Haven, CT 06520, USA

[f] Section of Digestive Diseases, University of Milan-Bicocca, Monza, Italy

* Corresponding author. Department of Internal Medicine, Section of Digestive Diseases, Yale University School of Medicine, 333 Cedar Street/1080 LMP, PO Box 208019, New Haven, CT 06520-8019.

E-mail address: mario.strazzabosco@yale.edu

HCC is a complex cancer arising in a diseased organ. All therapies must be considered with a view to the patient's liver function and performance status. Liver dysfunction is the rate-limiting step for the key components to any therapy: tolerance, efficacy, and safety. Sequelae of cirrhosis in patients with HCC include development of portal hypertension with hypersplenism leading to platelet sequestration (potentially limiting administration of myelosuppressive agents), development of varices (with their attendant risk of bleeding), and ascites formation; hypoalbuminemia, which causes peripheral edema and may interfere with drug binding (possibly altering distribution of drugs); changes in liver vascularization and capillarization of sinusoids (leading to altered pharmacokinetics); and liver dysfunction (reducing the therapeutic margin of many drugs). Collectively, these factors make it difficult to arrive at a dose that is able to provide a therapeutic benefit with minimal side effects.

Care of the patient with HCC requires a multidisciplinary approach both clinically and scientifically. The molecular biology and genetics of hepatic oncogenesis must be considered within the context of the pathobiology of cirrhosis. The intersection of these pathways will likely provide the most promising targets and will also require the most intense innovation and collaboration among investigators.

Because advanced HCC is diagnosed in most patients, there is a great clinical need to develop effective, well-tolerated targeted systemic therapies. Thomas and colleagues[7] outlined and prioritized recommendations for clinical trials research in HCC. The investigators called for trials that will identify "additional effective systemic agents, combination systemic therapies, and combined modality options." To conceive of such studies it is important to review both the failures and successes of systemic therapy for HCC and to gain an understanding of the many promising pathways for targeted therapies.

OVERVIEW OF CYTOTOXIC CHEMOTHERAPY AGENTS

There have been several cytotoxic chemotherapy regimens that have demonstrated some antitumor activity both as single agents (doxorubicin, VP-16, cisplatin, mitoxantrone, and paclitaxel) as well as in combination with other agents (**Table 1**). Among these agents, the most promising cytotoxic chemotherapy agent since the 1970s has been doxorubicin, initially evaluated in a study in Uganda with 14 patients and demonstrating an impressive 79% tumor response rate (RR).[8] Unfortunately, subsequent larger studies could not reproduce this result, with RRs in the 10% to 20% range, comparable with what has been observed with other cytotoxic agents (see **Table 1**). In terms of survival benefit, the data with doxorubicin are less clear. Although a single trial randomizing 60 patients to either doxorubicin or placebo demonstrated improved median survival in the treatment group (10.6 weeks vs 7.5 weeks),[9] there have been no additional studies to date demonstrating this limited survival benefit.

Although early clinical trials have suggested that combination therapies may improve RRs up to 27%, overall survival (OS) has not been improved by combinations of cytotoxic chemotherapies (see **Table 1**). Among the combination regimens evaluated thus far, the most promising results initially came from a Phase II study assessing a regimen consisting of cisplatin (20 mg/m^2 intravenously [IV] Days 1–4), doxorubicin (40 mg/m^2 IV Day 1), 5-fluorouracil (5-FU) (400 mg/m^2 IV Days 1–4), and the cytokine interferon (IFN)-alpha (5 MU/m^2 subcutaneously, Days 1–4) (PIAF) administered every 3 weeks for up to 6 cycles.[10] The regimen induced a partial response (PR) of 26% with 9 of 50 patients in this group initially with unresectable disease subsequently developing resectable disease. Among the 9 patients with resected disease, 4 were noted to have a pathologic complete response (CR), and alpha-fetoprotein (AFP) levels

Table 1
Summary of cytotoxic chemotherapies evaluated for HCC

Drug	Latest Stage of Clinical Development	Referenced Summary of Results
Doxorubicin	Phase III	RR up to 15%; Median OS 6.8 mo[11,71]
VP-16/Etoposide	Phase II	RR up to 18%; Median OS 6.8 mo[72]
Cisplatin	Phase II	RR up to 17%; OS unavailable[73]
Mitoxantrone	Phase II	RR 8%; Median OS 14 wk[73]
Mitoxantrone + β-IFN	Phase II	RR up to 23%; Median OS 8 mo[74]
Paclitaxel	Phase II	RR 0%; Median OS 12 wk[75]
Irinotecan	Phase II	RR up to 7%[76]
Gemcitabine	Phase II	RR 0%; Median OS 6.9 mo[77]
Capecitabine	Retrospective study	RR up to 11%; Median OS 10.1 mo[78]
Nolatrexed	Phase III	RR up to 1.5%; Median OS 22.3 wk[79]
Cisplatin , IFN-α, doxorubicin, and 5-fluorouracil	Phase II and III	Phase II RR 26%; Median OS 8.9 mo[10] Phase III RR 21% OS 8.67 mo PIAF arm vs OS 6.83 mo in single-agent doxorubicin arm[11]
Gemcitabine + Oxaliplatin	Phase II	RR up to 18%; Median OS 11.5 mo[80]
Capecitabine + Oxaliplatin	Phase II	RR up to 6%; Median OS 9.3 mo[81]
Capecitabine + Cisplatin	Cohort	RR up to 20%; Median OS 10.5 mo[82]
Cisplatin, mitoxantrone, and 5-fluorouracil	Phase II	RR up to 27%; Median OS 11.6 mo[83]
Gemcitabine, oxaliplatin, and bevacizumab	Phase II	RR up to 20%; Median OS 9.6 mo[33]

Abbreviations: IFN, interferon; OS, overall survival; RR, response rate.

decreased to within acceptable limits. In spite of these encouraging initial data, the regimen was highly myelosuppressive (up to 35% with at least grade 3 leukopenia) and patients suffered from significant gastrointestinal toxicity, including at least grade 3 diarrhea (8%) and mucositis (4%). A subsequent Phase III study enrolling 188 patients with unresectable HCC and randomized to cisplatin/IFN alpha-2b/doxorubicin/5- fluorouracil (PIAF) versus single-agent doxorubicin failed to reach the study primary end point of survival benefit with median survival of 6.83 months (95% confidence interval [CI] 4.80–9.56) and 8.67 months (95% CI of 6.36–12.00) for the doxorubicin arm and PIAF arm respectively (P = .83).[11]

A number of factors limit the efficacy of cytotoxic agents for patients with HCC. In addition to the challenges posed by cirrhosis, the resistance of HCC to many cytotoxic agents could be attributable to the tumor itself expressing the MDR gene and drug efflux pumps such as P-glycoprotein,[12] leading to efflux of the drug from the cancer cells, adding to the complexity of optimizing effective dose delivery to the tumor and its microenvironment.

Given the toxicities of multiagent chemotherapy without a reproducible clinical benefit, this approach is generally not pursued as palliative therapy in patients with advanced-stage HCC. Rather, salvage single-agent cytotoxic chemotherapies (ie, single-agent capecitabine or adriamycin) are considered after targeted therapies or clinical trial options have been exhausted.

SORAFENIB INCREASES SURVIVAL IN PATIENTS WITH HCC

In response to the lack of significant clinical benefit from cytotoxic chemotherapy, a number of agents targeting various signaling cascades in HCC (**Fig. 1**) have been evaluated in the Phase II setting, and Phase III trials are ongoing. After almost 3 decades of testing different cytotoxic chemotherapies for treating patients with HCC without demonstrating a significant clinical impact, the long-sought survival improvement was demonstrated with sorafenib.

Sorafenib is a multikinase inhibitor against the Raf1, B-Raf, vascular endothelial growth factor receptor (VEGFR)-2, platelet-derived growth factor receptor (PDGR), and c-kit pathways (see **Fig. 1**). The seminal Sorafenib HCC Assessment Randomized Protocol (SHARP) trial was a large, international, Phase III randomized placebo-controlled study of 602 patients with advanced HCC with 299 patients receiving sorafenib and 303 receiving placebo.[6] The trial was halted following a second prespecified interim analysis because of the improvement in survival in the treatment group with the hazard ratio for sorafenib/placebo being 0.69 (95% CI: 0.55, 0.86; $P = .0005$) and median survival of 10.7 months versus 7.9 months respectively. Time to progression (TTP) of disease also favored the sorafenib-treated group (5.5 months vs 2.8 months for placebo).

However, survival and TTP advantages come at a cost of a number of side effects that differ from those expected with cytotoxic chemotherapy agents. The most frequent side effects were those commonly associated with other tyrosine kinase inhibitors, including diarrhea, fatigue, hand-foot syndrome (HFS), and weight loss.

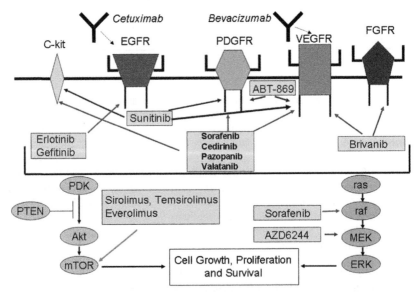

Fig. 1. Summary of converging molecular pathways in HCC inhibited by targeted agents. Antibodies listed in italics and small molecular inhibitors in shaded rectangles. EGFR, epidermal growth factor receptor; PDGFR, platelet-derived growth factor receptor; VEGFR, vascular endothelial growth factor receptor; FGFR, fibroblast growth factor receptor; PDK, phosphate-dependent kinase; PTEN, phosphatase and tensin homolog deleted in chromosomes 10; mTOR, mammalian target of rapamycin; MEK, mitogen-activated protein kinase kinase; ERK, extracellular related kinase.

Grade 3 to 4 toxicities were most common in the sorafenib arm and included diarrhea (11% vs 2% in placebo group) and HFS (8% vs 1% in placebo group).

The Asia Pacific trial confirmed the survival benefit of sorafenib.[13] This placebo-controlled study (150 subjects receiving sorafenib vs 76 receiving placebo) showed a similar improvement in survival and had an identical hazard ratio (OS 6.2 vs 4.1 months, $P = .014$, hazard ratio = 0.68). The study population differed significantly from that in the SHARP trial, as more than 70% of patients had chronic hepatitis B, and there was a higher proportion of multifocal and metastatic disease. The inclusion of subjects with more advanced disease likely explains the lower absolute survival.

Of interest, subgroup analysis from the SHARP trial identified an even greater survival benefit for patients with hepatitis C.[14] In this cohort, OS was increased to 14.0 months from 7.9 months (hazard ratio 0.58). Himmelsbach and colleagues[15] have shown that sorafenib is able to interfere with HCV replication in vitro. This intriguing observation has yet to be validated in vivo.

Most of the data available for sorafenib has been observed in patients with Child-Turcotte-Pugh (CTP) A cirrhosis; further studies will be warranted to establish whether or not a true clinical benefit can be appreciated in CTP B and C patients with HCC.

The US Food and Drug Administration (FDA) has approved sorafenib for patients with unresectable HCC and, given the lack of other agents available to treat HCC, advanced CPT B patients with HCC and good Eastern Cooperative Oncology Group (ECOG) performance status (PS) are being offered sorafenib despite lack of safety and efficacy data to date. It should be emphasized that, at the present time, there is no indication for sorafenib use in patients who are candidates for ablative treatment. Studies on the use of sorafenib as an adjuvant treatment are ongoing (see the following section).

SORAFENIB AS AN ADJUVANT THERAPY

There are growing data to suggest that intrahepatic locoregional therapies may stimulate the production of cytokines, specifically VEGF, that drive tumor angiogenesis and metastasis.[16] Because of sorafenib's antiangiogenic effect, several studies are under way to evaluate its efficacy in combination with locoregional therapies such as transarterial chemoembolization (TACE). The Sorafenib as Adjuvant Treatment in the Prevention of Recurrence of Hepatocellular Carcinoma (STORM) trial is a Phase III study of sorafenib as adjuvant treatment in the prevention of recurrence of hepatocellular carcinoma. The objective of this trial is to evaluate the efficacy and safety of sorafenib versus placebo in the adjuvant treatment of HCC after curative therapy (resection or ablation). The primary end point is recurrence-free survival. The study opened in 2008 and has completed recruitment (enrollment of 1065 patients).[17] Completion of the study is anticipated in 2014. A Phase II study is ongoing to assess the efficacy of sorafenib after TACE, namely the Sorafenib or Placebo in Combination with Transarterial Chemoembolization (SPACE) trial for intermediate-stage hepatocellular carcinoma. This is a double-blind, placebo-controlled study that has completed recruitment (307 enrolled). The primary end point is TTP. This study is expected to be completed later this year.[18] A Phase III study of TACE with or without sorafenib in unresectable HCC in patients with and without vascular invasion is actively recruiting. The purpose of the study is to assess progression-free survival (PFS). Expected enrollment is 400 patients with completion of the study anticipated in 2012. In this study, patients undergo TACE 2 weeks after a stable dose of sorafenib has been achieved.[19] Data from these studies will be pivotal in clarifying the standard of care and in driving future studies with other antiangiogenic agents.

SORAFENIB-BASED COMBINATION CYTOTOXIC CHEMOTHERAPY REGIMENS

Given the relatively modest clinical benefit of single-agent sorafenib in CPT A patients with a number of toxicities of this drug, there is a clear need for further systemic therapies for patients with HCC. To this end, sorafenib-based regimens combined with cytotoxic chemotherapy (doxorubicin, capecitabine plus oxaliplatin, or gemcitabine plus cisplatin) are being evaluated. The most mature data come from a Phase II randomized control trial evaluating doxorubicin plus placebo versus doxorubicin plus sorafenib in patients with advanced HCC. Inclusion criteria included ECOG PS 0-2, CPT A cirrhosis, and no prior systemic therapies.[20] Ninety-six patients were randomized to receive 3-week cycles of doxorubicin at 60 mg/m^2 on day 1 plus either placebo or oral sorafenib at 400 mg twice daily for up to 6 cycles of treatment. Patients were given the option to continue with sorafenib or placebo following completion of the 6 cycles of therapy. Although the initial results were encouraging (OS and TTP were 13.7 months and 8.6 months in the doublet arm vs 6.5 months and 4.8 months in the doxorubicin arm), the potential cardiotoxicity and cytopenias (grades 3–4 in up to 50% of patients in both arms) from doxorubicin raises concerns, especially when therapy in this setting is palliative.

The "control" arm was doxorubicin alone (instead of sorafenib alone); therefore, it is unclear how much, if any, benefit this specific cytotoxic agent is adding to that gained by single-agent sorafenib. Evaluation of sorafenib with other cytotoxic agents, as noted previously, will be warranted with a control arm of sorafenib alone in upcoming trials to determine whether or not combinations of this nature will lead to a clinical benefit in patients with HCC.

APPROACHES OTHER THAN CYTOTOXIC CHEMOTHERAPIES OR SINGLE-AGENT SORAFENIB FOR THE TREATMENT OF HCC

A number of targeted therapies alone and in combination with sorafenib are being evaluated, including antiestrogen/androgen agents, antiangiogenic agents, epidermal growth factor receptor (EGFR) inhibitors, mammalian target of rapamycin (mTOR) inhibitors, mitogen-activated protein (MAP) kinase kinase (MEK) inhibitors and immunotherapies with cytokines, effector cells, and antigen-presenting cells.

Hormonal Manipulation

Because HCC can express estrogen receptors and estrogens can stimulate hepatocyte proliferation in vitro and may enhance liver tumor growth in vivo, the antiestrogen, tamoxifen, has been evaluated in advanced HCC.[21–23] Unfortunately, this agent did not improve survival in patients with HCC in 6 large randomized studies, 4 of which were double-blind trials.[24] Furthermore, antiandrogen therapies, including flutamide or triptorelin, have also been shown to be ineffective at improving survival in patients with HCC in randomized studies.[25] Somatostatin receptors are also expressed by HCC, but placebo-controlled trials of a long-acting somatostatin analog have also failed to demonstrate activity in patients with advanced HCC.[26]

Antiangiogenic Agents

HCCs are vascular tumors with increased VEGF expression,[27] and VEGF signaling cascades are proposed to induce HCC. High levels of VEGF expression correlate with worse OS in patients with HCC[28]; therefore, agents blocking VEGF and its downstream signaling cascade are being evaluated in this disease.

Bevacizumab

Bevacizumab, a recombinant humanized monoclonal antibody targeting VEGF, has been developed and is approved for the treatment of a number of advanced stage solid malignancies, including metastatic lung and colon cancers.[29] Although this antibody does not have direct cytotoxic effects, its antitumor activity is thought to be attributable to several mechanisms, including direct antiangiogenic effects leading to decreased tumor vasculature production and "normalization" of existing tumor vasculature leading to increased interstitial pressure and possible improved delivery of cytotoxic or other targeted agents.[30]

Single-agent bevacizumab has been reported to demonstrate antitumor activity in 2 Phase II trials.[31,32] Both trials demonstrated an RR of 12% to 13%, and the trial conducted by Siegel and colleagues[31] reported median PFS of 6.9 months (95% CI, 6.5–9.1) and median survival of 12.4 months (95% CI, 9.4–19.9) in 46 patients. It is important to note that grade 3 or higher hemorrhage occurred in 11% of patients (5/46), with 1 fatality from variceal hemorrhage. This is notable in comparison with the SHARP trial where only one subject experienced grade 3 bleeding and no grade 4 bleeding was reported.[6]

Combinations of bevacizumab with cytotoxic chemotherapies have also been evaluated in 3 Phase II studies. Of these 3, the largest Phase II study evaluated bevacizumab in combination with gemcitabine and oxaliplatin in patients with advanced HCC.[33] Overall RR was reported to be 20% with an additional 27% of patients demonstrating stable disease for a median duration of 9 months. Median OS in patients receiving this combination was 9.6 months, which is less than that reported in the SHARP trial evaluating sorafenib alone; the median PFS approached that of single-agent sorafenib at 5.3 months.

In addition to the combination of bevacizumab and cytotoxic agents, a single-center Phase II trial has reported evaluating the combination of bevacizumab (10 mg/kg IV for 14 days) and the EGFR inhibitor, erlotinib (150 mg by mouth daily), in patients with advanced HCC.[34] The initial data are encouraging, as Thomas and colleagues[34] report a 25% RR, a median PFS of 9 months, and an OS of 15 months—all outcomes that are better than that observed with single-agent sorafenib. However, similar to the results reported by Siegel and colleagues,[31] in this study the rate of grade 3 or higher gastrointestinal hemorrhage was 12.5% (5/40 patients).

Although all of the trials suggest that bevacizumab alone and in combination with cytotoxic agents and erlotinib enhanced antitumor activity, there appears to be a significantly increased risk of bleeding compared with sorafenib. Further studies with larger cohorts will be necessary to define the safety and clinical efficacy of bevacizumab alone and in combination with the agents described previously.

Sunitinib

A number of small molecule inhibitors in addition to sorafenib have been developed that block the VEGF pathway, as well as other signaling cascades. Sunitinib is an oral multikinase inhibitor targeting VEGFR-1, VEGFR-2, PDGFR-a/b, c-kit, FLt-3, and rearranged during transfection (RET) kinases and is currently approved for the treatment of advanced renal cell cancer.[35] Two Phase II studies have evaluated this agent at different dosing schedules in patients with advanced HCC. The first study evaluated sunitinib administered orally at 37.5 mg daily for 4 weeks on, 2 weeks off, and the primary end point was PFS.[36] Among the 34 patients participating in this study, 1 patient had a PR lasting 20 months whereas an additional 10 patients had stable disease lasting at least 12 weeks. PFS was reported to be less than that observed with sorafenib at 3.9 months with OS approaching that of sorafenib at 9.8 months. The second Phase II study evaluated the administration of sunitinib at 50 mg daily for 4 weeks on and 2 weeks off in patients with unresectable HCC, with the primary end point being overall RR according to the Response Evaluation Criteria in Solid Tumors (RECIST).[37] Thirty-seven patients were enrolled and 1 patient also experienced a PR with 13 additional patients demonstrating stable disease. Median OS was reported to be 8.0 months and a PFS similar to the previous trial at 3.7 months.

When comparing the 2 dosages, as expected, the first study using the lower dosage of 37.5 mg reported lower grade 3 or 4 toxicities compared with the second study using the 50-mg higher dosage that resulted in increased grade 3 or 4 toxicities as well as a higher death rate (10%).

Although there appears to be a biologic signal from both studies demonstrating a clinical benefit from this agent, a head-to-head randomized Phase III study evaluating sunitinib at the 37.5 mg daily dosage versus sorafenib at 400 mg twice daily dosing in HCC was terminated because of a higher prevalence of serious adverse effects in the sunitinib arm.[38]

Brivanib

Like sorafenib, brivanib is also a small molecular inhibitor of VEGFR-2; however, it inhibits the fibroblast growth factor receptor (FGFR) signaling pathway (see **Fig. 1**) as well, and has been shown to inhibit HCC growth in a mouse xenograft model.[39] Recently a Phase II study was conducted to evaluate the safety and efficacy of this agent in patients with unresectable or metastatic HCC who either never received prior systemic treatment (cohort A) or progressed on one regimen of angiogenesis inhibitor (cohort B).[40] In this study, 55 patients were in cohort A and 41 patients were in cohort B and all patients received oral brivanib at 800 mg daily. The median survival of patients in cohort A was reported to be 10 months with TTP of 2.8 months with a PR observed in 5% of patients.

In both cohorts, more than 50% of patients demonstrated a greater than 40% decrease in AFP levels following initiation of this small molecule inhibitor. Of the side effects reported, the most common grade 3 or 4 events included fatigue (16%), elevated aspartate aminotransferase levels (19%), and hyponatremia (41%) in cohort A, whereas the most common grade 3 or 4 events in patients in cohort B who had previously experienced one regimen of antiangiogenesis inhibitor included hypertension (7.3%), diarrhea (4.9%), and headache (4.9%).

These clinical data have led to the development of Phase III studies of brivanib for first-line therapy (vs sorafenib in newly diagnosed patients with advanced HCC) and for patients who are sorafenib-refractory (compared with best supportive care for patients with advanced HCC).[41,42] Accrual completion is projected for February 2013 and December 2011, respectively.

AZD2171 (Cediranib)

Cediranib is a potent inhibitor of all VEGFR tyrosine kinases, with additional activity against c-kit and PDGFR (see **Fig. 1**). In a Phase II study evaluating this small molecule inhibitor dosed at 45 mg by mouth daily in patients with advanced HCC,[43,44] 16 of 19 patients developed grade 3 toxicities, with fatigue, hypertension, and anorexia accounting for most of these events. Additional cycles of this drug were refused by most patients who experienced grade 3 fatigue. Further studies are required to assess tolerability and safety of cediranib in patients with HCC.

ABT-869

ABT-869 is a selective inhibitor of both the VEGFR and PDGFR pathways (see **Fig. 1**). An interim analysis of an open-label, multicenter Phase II study of this inhibitor administered at 0.25 mg/kg daily in CPT A or once every other day in CPT B patients was recently reported.[43,45] ABT-869 was administered until disease progression or intolerable toxicities developed; the primary end point is PFS at 16 weeks. Among the 34 patients in the study for whom data were available (28 with CTP A and 6 with CTP B cirrhosis), the RR was 8.7% (95% CI, 1.1–28.0) for patients with CTP A cirrhosis, median PFS was 112 days (95% CI 61–168) and OS was 295 days (95% CI 182–333). The most common side effects were hypertension (41%), fatigue (47%), diarrhea (38%), rash (35%), proteinuria (24%), nausea/vomiting (24%), cough, and peripheral edema (24%). The most frequent grade 3 or 4 adverse events included hypertension (20.6%) and fatigue (11.8%). Unlike cediranib, the early efficacy and tolerability safety profiles of ABT-869 have encouraged additional development of this agent in patients with advanced HCC.

GW786034 (Pazopanib)

Pazopanib is a multityrosine kinase inhibitor that targets VEGFR, PDGFR, and c-kit signaling cascades (see **Fig. 1**). A Phase I study determining the maximum tolerated dose (MTD), safety, pharmacokinetics, pharmacodynamics, and antitumor effect of oral pazopanib in patients with locally unresectable or metastatic HCC was recently presented. Patients in this study were ECOG PFS 0–1, had adequate organ function, and could have received prior systemic therapy.[46] The dosing schedule included escalations of 200 mg to 800 mg daily in a 3+3 design. Of the 27 patients enrolled in this study, the MTD was 600 mg daily. There was a PR observed in 1 patient receiving 600 mg daily and 1 patient who tolerated 800 mg daily. Stable disease for greater than 4 months was reported in 11 patients (41%). Median TTP at 600 mg daily was 137.5 days (4–280 days).

PTK787/ZK222584 (Valatanib)

Valatanib targets all known VEGFR tyrosine kinases, including VEGFR/flt-1, VEGFR-2/KDR-2, and VEGFR-3/Flt-4, as well PDGFR and c-kit signaling (see **Fig. 1**). Results of an open-label, multicenter Phase I study characterizing safety, tolerability, and pharmacokinetics of valatanib administered daily at oral doses ranging from 750 to 1250 mg was reported by Koch and colleagues.[47] The MTD for valatanib was 750 mg daily. Among the 18 patients for whom efficacy data were available, 9 of 18 demonstrated stable disease with no PR or CR observed. Currently, there are no additional studies planned for this agent.

Summary of Antiangiogenic Agents

There are several antiangiogenic agents being evaluated for the treatment of advanced HCC, including a monoclonal antibody and small molecule inhibitors in addition to sorafenib that demonstrate some clinical efficacy. However, the trials evaluating these agents comprise small Phase I or II studies and, therefore, further studies enrolling larger numbers of patients and comparing these agents to the standard of care (sorafenib) are warranted. Given the large number of agents in this class of drugs relative to the number of patients available to enroll, careful consideration of the relative efficacy (ie, RRs, rates of stable of disease) versus the toxicities of each agent will be essential before initiating additional, larger Phase III trials that could take years to complete.

EPIDERMAL GROWTH FACTOR–RECEPTOR INHIBITION

The importance of EGFR/human epidermal growth factor receptor (HER)1 signaling following binding to EGFR and TGF-α in hepatocarcinogenesis[48] has provided the rationale for evaluating inhibitors of these pathways to treat patients with HCC. The small molecule inhibitors, erlotinib and gefitinib, as well as a chimeric monoclonal antibody against EGFR, cetuximab, have been studied as potential treatments for patients with advanced HCC.

Erlotinib and Gefitinib

Erlotinib and gefitinib are small molecule inhibitors of the phosphorylation of the tyrosine kinase associated with EGFR (see **Fig. 1**). Two Phase II clinical studies evaluating the safety and clinical efficacy of erlotinib at 150-mg daily dosing have demonstrated that this drug as a single agent has comparable clinical activity to the antiangiogenic agents described previously.[49,50] In the Phase II study reported by Philip and colleagues,[49] 3 (9%) of 38 patients with advanced HCC who received erlotinib experienced a PR; 12 (32%) of 38 patients demonstrated PFS at 6 months with a median OS of 13 months for this group. In another Phase II study reported by Thomas and colleagues[50] in which 40 patients with advanced HCC were enrolled, 17 patients (43%) had PFS at 16 weeks and 28% patients had PFS at 24 weeks. No PR or CR was observed in the patients enrolled in this study.

An ECOG Phase II study (E1203) evaluated gefitinib, administered at 250 mg daily, with a planned 2-stage design.[51] Unfortunately, the clinical activity of this agent did not reflect that observed in the previously discussed erlotinib studies. Of 31 patients with advanced HCC enrolled in the first stage, 1 patient experienced a PR and 7 patients demonstrated stable disease. Median PFS was 2.8 months (95% CI 1.5–3.9); median OS was 6.5 months (95% CI, 4.4–8.9). Given the data and because the preestablished criteria for enrolling patients in the second stage were not met, the investigators concluded that this agent was not active in HCC.

Cetuximab

Cetuximab is a chimeric monoclonal antibody that is FDA approved for the treatment of advanced head and neck cancers and a subset (*kras* WT) of advanced colorectal cancers.[52] Two Phase II trials have evaluated cetuximab as a single agent in CTP A and B patients with advanced HCC.[53,54] Both trials reported no objective response in any of the patients participating in either study. Zhu and colleagues[53] observed a median OS of 9.6 months (95% CI of 4.3–12.1 months) and PFS of 1.4 months (95% CI of 1.2–2.6) in the 30 patients enrolled in their study. Grünwald and colleagues[54] reported that 12 of 27 patients enrolled in their Phase II study achieved stable disease; median TTP was reported to be 8 weeks.

Combinations of this biologic agent with cytotoxic chemotherapies have also been evaluated in 2 Phase II studies. The first Phase II study evaluated the combination of cetuximab administered at 400 mg/m^2 loading dose followed by weekly administration at 250 mg/m^2 with gemcitabine administered at 1000 mg/m^2 on day 1 with oxaliplatin administered at 100 mg/m^2 on day 2 of a 14-day cycle until the development of disease progression or intolerable side effects.[55] A 20% RR among the 45 patients enrolled in this study was reported with PFS and median OS being 4.7 months and 9.5 months respectively. The 1-year survival rate was 40%. Gemcitabine/oxaliplatin doublet chemotherapy has reported antitumor activity; however, cetuximab did not demonstrate antitumor activity as a single agent. Therefore, the overall contribution of weekly cetuximab therapy to this combination regimen requires further elucidation.

A second Phase II study evaluating cetuximab with loading and weekly doses as described previously with the oral fluoropyrimidine, capecitabine, administered at 850 mg/m^2 twice daily for 14 days and oxaliplatin administered at 130 mg/m^2 IV on day 1 of a 21-day cycle has reported a RR of 10% (95% CI of 1–33) and TTP of 4.3 months (95% CI 2.3–5.0) in 20 of 25 enrolled patients with HCC with evaluable efficacy data.[56]

In summary, the efficacy of EGFR signaling inhibitors alone, and in the case of the cetuximab experience in combination with cytotoxic chemotherapy, has been modest at best. Further trials evaluating erlotinib in combination with sorafenib or bevacizumab are under way.

MEK INHIBITION

HCC frequently demonstrates MEK/extracellular signal-regulated kinase (ERK) activation. A MEK inhibitor, AZD6244, was recently evaluated in a multicenter Phase II study using RR as its primary end point in patients with advanced HCC receiving 100 mg administered by mouth twice daily. Unfortunately, although this drug was well tolerated, there was minimal clinical efficacy observed in the treated groups with no RRs reported in the 16 patients with evaluable data. Stable disease was observed in 37.5% of patients; median TTP was a dismal 8 weeks (95% CI 6.6–11.1).[57]

MTOR INHIBITION

mTOR regulates protein translation, angiogenesis, and cell-cycle progression in many cancers including HCC, and several mTOR inhibitors are used clinically (temsirolimus, everolimus, and sirolimus). Furthermore, retrospective studies evaluating liver transplant patients noted that those receiving sirolimus immunosuppression had a lower prevalence of developing HCC when compared with those receiving calcineurin inhibitors, providing the rationale for evaluating these agents in patients with HCC.[58]

The clinical studies evaluating this approach are in early phases. A pilot study evaluating sirolimus in 14 patients with advanced HCC reported a 40% RR (5 patients with PR, 1 patient with CR)[59] and global studies evaluating sirolimus and everolimus are under way.

SUMMARY OF "TARGETED" AGENTS IN ADDITION TO SORAFENIB

Thus far, the results from a number of Phase II studies have yielded disappointing results with many of the targeted agents when evaluated as single agents. Many agents did not demonstrate a RR or significant improvement in survival over that observed with single-agent sorafenib. These studies have been hampered by low enrollment numbers and, given the difficulties in accruing large numbers to these types of studies, there have been too many competing studies between various agents.

It is imperative to prioritize studies evaluating agents that have strong preclinical evidence demonstrating antitumor effects in preclinical models of HCC. These drugs must be compared with sorafenib as the control arm in the first-line setting. In addition, more agents with novel mechanisms of action should be considered high priority, given the relative ineffective clinical activity of many of the older "targeted" agents. Although sorafenib has sparked a renewed hope that systemic agents can improve clinical outcomes in patients with advanced HCC, there is certainly a great need for additional approaches for the treatment of this devastating disease.

IMMUNOTHERAPIES

Given the lack of effective targeted therapies and cytotoxic therapies for advanced HCC, novel approaches evaluating the use of cytokine-based, adoptive effector cell–based, and vaccine-based immunotherapeutic approaches have been evaluated. Of interest, results of preclinical and clinical studies have demonstrated that these tumors are not classically immunogenic in mice or humans,[60] warranting the use of immunotherapy to elicit antigen presentation to develop and maintain antitumor responses in the host.

Cytokines

Among the cytokines evaluated, IFN-α was initially evaluated in 2 randomized trials, as interferons have immunomodulatory, antiproliferative, and antiangiogenic effects that may inhibit mechanisms critical for HCC development and progression.[61,62] Unfortunately, whereas one trial performed in the 1980s demonstrated a marginal survival advantage in patients with HCC receiving IFN-α (14.5 vs 7.5 weeks, $P = .047$),[61] a second randomized European trial did not report a survival benefit and the treatment was poorly tolerated.[62] Mazzaferro and colleagues[63] conducted a randomized control trial of IFN-α for prevention of HCC recurrence after liver resection in patients with hepatitis C. Although there were no differences in recurrence-free survival in the control and treatment arms, the subgroup of patients with hepatitis C alone (in contrast to hepatitis B and C coinfection) who were adherent to therapy had far fewer late recurrences. Further study is required to understand the potential benefit of IFN-α in this group.

In addition to single-agent IFN-α, combinations of this cytokine with cytotoxic chemotherapy agents, including PIAF, have also been evaluated, as previously discussed. A subset analysis of patients with HCC receiving the PIAF regimen who were considered "good-risk patients" with preserved liver function and a bilirubin level lower than 0.6 mg/dL, demonstrated RRs of 50%.[10] Therefore, although this regimen can be highly toxic, it may be appropriate for patients with adequate liver function in which downstaging of disease may enable subsequent surgical resection.

Several cytokine-based approaches have been studied for advanced HCC. These include TACE with IFN-γ plus interleukin (IL)-2,[64] IFN-γ plus recombinant granulocyte-macrophage colony-stimulating factor (GMCSF),[65] and intratumoral injection of an adenoviral vector expressing IL-12.[66] The small number of patients enrolled in these studies (up to 20 patients were enrolled in the TACE study) and the lack of significant numbers responding to the latter two approaches, suggest that further evaluation both at the bench and the bedside is required to determine the best candidate cytokines for further clinical development.

Effector Cells

The rationale for the isolation and expansion of effector cells responsible for clearing tumors in cancer patients has been well established in preclinical and clinical studies, including those for metastatic melanoma,[67] suggesting that this approach may be viable for other solid tumors, such as HCC. The use of lymphocyte-activated killer (LAK) cells, transfer of ex vivo expanded tumor-infiltrating lymphocytes, and IL-2 and anti-CD3 activated peripheral blood lymphocytes have been evaluated in patients with HCC with largely disappointing and conflicting results.

These studies have been reviewed recently by Giglia and colleagues.[66] In an early study, decreased rates of HCC recurrence were reported in patients who underwent resection of their primary tumor followed by infusion of LAK cells generated from peripheral blood lymphocytes obtained by leukapheresis and treated with IL-2 therapy. However, a subsequent study performed 4 years later demonstrated no clinical benefit to this approach.

The generation of tumor-infiltration lymphocyte (TIL)-based approaches has been established in patients with metastatic melanoma, resulting in excellent durable RRs.[67] This approach is time and resource intensive, requiring the isolation of TILs from tumor samples and expansion of the lymphocytes ex vivo for several weeks followed by the subsequent infusion of expanded lymphocytes. Although there is one report from more than 10 years ago detailing an improved recurrence-free rate in 10 patients receiving this therapy following tumor resection,[68] further studies are warranted to determine if this therapy merits further development. To date, there are no data published evaluating this approach in patients with unresectable or advanced hepatocellular carcinoma.

Finally, the use of IL-2 and anti-CD3 activated peripheral blood lymphocytes (PBLs) has been evaluated in patients with HCC by Takayama and colleagues.[69] Although statistically significant improvements in the risk of recurrence and recurrence-free survival were reported, OS was not statistically significant.[69]

In summary, although the expansion of effector cell populations to augment anti-tumor responses in HCC has been evaluated, the lack of significant clinical benefit (ie, OS) and the requirement for significant resources to isolate and expand these lymphocyte populations limits further clinical development of this strategy.

Use of Antigen-Presenting Cells

A number of groups have evaluated dendritic cell (DC)-based vaccines and reported variable clinical responses. In these studies, DCs are harvested from patients with HCC, pulsed with HCC tumor antigens, and subsequently reinfused into the patient. Among the studies currently published, the largest one involved 31 patients treated with autologous DCs pulsed with tumor lysate.[70] Four patients receiving the DC-vaccine demonstrated a PR; 17 patients had stable disease. Furthermore, 1-year survival in the 17 patients receiving monthly boosts of vaccine was reported to be 63%. All treated patients demonstrated a 1-year survival rate of 40% when compared with historical controls (20%), suggesting that the DC approach should be further evaluated in a larger cohort of patients.

In summary, immunotherapy with cytokines, effector cells, and DC-based vaccines has demonstrated limited clinical activity. The DC-based vaccines and IFN-based biochemotherapies have resulted in the largest RRs in patients with HCC. The biologic "signals" demonstrated in the trials detailed previously suggest that immunotherapeutic approaches may be a viable strategy alone and in combination with either cytotoxic chemotherapies or targeted therapies in this patient population. However, the results are limited to small clinical trials in heterogeneous populations. These approaches, developed in parallel with an improved understanding of other immunosuppressive factors in the HCC tumor microenvironment, are promising, but much work remains to be done before immunotherapy becomes standard of care for patients afflicted with this disease.

SUMMARY

Many potential systemic therapies are being investigated for the treatment of hepatocellular carcinoma. HCC is a heterogeneous disease that occurs among very heterogeneous populations. The incidence of this malignancy is rising sharply and the vast majority of patients present at advanced stages. Studies must be prioritized to be of the highest quality and yield. Although the earlier dismal results with cytotoxic chemotherapies made way for the development of locoregional therapies that provided improved overall survival, truly personalized therapy will require the selection of phenotypically similar stages of disease and populations, an understanding of the complex molecular and genetic pathways leading HCC, and a keen understanding of the pathobiology of cirrhosis. Only then will we understand how to offer a particular patient at a specific stage of disease the appropriate therapy to truly prolong survival.

Until then, treatment of HCC will continue to blend science and art, and require experience and a multidisciplinary approach. Many treatments are available, often for very similar patients. These treatments are provided by physicians working in different subspecialties and departments. In our experience, the use of multidisciplinary boards is needed to guide the best plan of therapy. Until recently, HCC treatment was restricted to surgical resection, liver transplantation, and ablative treatments. The advent of drugs able to target specific signaling pathways involved in HCC progression bear the promise to change our approach to HCC treatment. It is important to emphasize, however, that at this time (1) only sorafenib and mTOR inhibitors (the latter used to reduce post–liver transplant recurrence) have entered the clinical arena; (2) sorafenib and similar drugs are not considered first-line treatment, except in advanced, unresectable HCC; and (3) objective criteria must be devised to judge tumor response (decrease in vascularization vs decrease in mass diameter) to have objective and uniform measures of success in upcoming clinical trials.

With new drugs in the pipeline and information on the use of sorafenib as an adjuvant treatment, it is very likely that the indications for systemic treatment of HCC will significantly increase, moving from a sequential to a combination treatment strategy. As alluded to in the introduction, there are several clinical conditions that eagerly await solutions and will likely become the main indications for systemic treatment. In addition to the patient with advanced stage HCC, patients treated with surgery, ablation, or TACE may benefit from systemic treatment to reduce the recurrence of their disease and/or mitigate the effects of cytokines released after locoregional treatment. Patients listed for transplantation who are not amenable to ablative treatment may also benefit from systemic treatment.

Clinical trials designed to understand these questions are being performed; until the results are available, we should refrain from routinely administering systemic therapy in the absence of strong evidence. Furthermore, before embarking on costly treatments with drugs characterized by a narrow therapeutic margin, it is mandatory to consider their impact on quality of life and their place in the overall plan of care.

REFERENCES

1. Bosch FX, Ribes J, Diaz M, et al. Primary liver cancer: worldwide incidence and trends. Gastroenterology 2004;127(5 Suppl 1):S5–16.
2. Llovet JM, Schwartz M, Mazzaferro V. Resection and liver transplantation for hepatocellular carcinoma. Semin Liver Dis 2005;25(2):181–200.
3. Livraghi T, Meloni F, Di Stasi M, et al. Sustained complete response and complication rates after radiofrequency ablation of very early hepatocellular carcinoma in cirrhosis: is resection still the treatment of choice? Hepatology 2008;47(1):82–9.
4. Bruix J, Llovet JM. Major achievements in hepatocellular carcinoma. Lancet 2009;373(9664):614–6.
5. Bruix J, Sala M, Llovet JM. Chemoembolization for hepatocellular carcinoma. Gastroenterology 2004;127(5 Suppl 1):S179–88.

6. Llovet JM, Ricci S, Mazzaferro V, et al. Sorafenib in advanced hepatocellular carcinoma. N Engl J Med 2008;359(4):378–90.

7. Thomas MB, Jaffe D, Choti MM, et al. Hepatocellular carcinoma: consensus recommendations of the National Cancer Institute Clinical Trials Planning Meeting. J Clin Oncol 2010;28(25):3994–4005.

8. Olweny CL, Toya T, Katongole-Mbidde E, et al. Treatment of hepatocellular carcinoma with adriamycin. Preliminary communication. Cancer 1975;36(4):1250–7.

9. Lai CL, Wu PC, Chan GC, et al. Doxorubicin versus no antitumor therapy in inoperable hepatocellular carcinoma. A prospective randomized trial. Cancer 1988; 62(3):479–83.

10. Leung TW, Patt YZ, Lau WY, et al. Complete pathological remission is possible with systemic combination chemotherapy for inoperable hepatocellular carcinoma. Clin Cancer Res 1999;5(7):1676–81.

11. Yeo W, Mok TS, Zee B, et al. A randomized phase III study of doxorubicin versus cisplatin/interferon alpha-2b/doxorubicin/fluorouracil (PIAF) combination chemotherapy for unresectable hepatocellular carcinoma. J Natl Cancer Inst 2005; 97(20):1532–8.

12. Kato A, Miyazaki M, Ambiru S, et al. Multidrug resistance gene (MDR-1) expression as a useful prognostic factor in patients with human hepatocellular carcinoma after surgical resection. J Surg Oncol 2001;78(2):110–5.

13. Cheng AL, Kang YK, Chen Z, et al. Efficacy and safety of sorafenib in patients in the Asia-Pacific region with advanced hepatocellular carcinoma: a phase III randomised, double-blind, placebo-controlled trial. Lancet Oncol 2009;10(1):25–34.

14. Bolondi L, Caspary W, Bennouna J, et al. Clinical benefit of sorafenib in hepatitis C patients with hepatocellular carcinoma (HCC): subgroup analysis of the sharp trial. J Clin Oncol 2008;26(Suppl):A129.

15. Himmelsbach K, Sauter D, Baumert TF, et al. New aspects of an anti-tumour drug: sorafenib efficiently inhibits HCV replication. Gut 2009;58(12):1644–53.

16. Schoenleber SJ, Kurtz DM, Talwalkar JA, et al. Prognostic role of vascular endothelial growth factor in hepatocellular carcinoma: systematic review and meta-analysis. Br J Cancer 2009;100(9):1385–92.

17. Available at: http://www.clinicaltrials.gov/ct2/show/NCT00692770. Accessed April 1, 2011.

18. Available at: http://www.clinicaltrials.gov/ct2/show/NCT00855218. Accessed April 1, 2011.

19. Available at: http://www.clinicaltrials.gov/ct2/show/NCT01004978?term= NCT01004978. Accessed April 1, 2011.

20. Abou-Alfa GK, Johnson P, Knox JJ, et al. Doxorubicin plus sorafenib vs doxorubicin alone in patients with advanced hepatocellular carcinoma: a randomized trial. JAMA 2010;304(19):2154–60.

21. Castells A, Bruix J, Bru C, et al. Treatment of hepatocellular carcinoma with tamoxifen: a double-blind placebo-controlled trial in 120 patients. Gastroenterology 1995;109(3):917–22.

22. Liu CL, Fan ST, Ng IO, et al. Treatment of advanced hepatocellular carcinoma with tamoxifen and the correlation with expression of hormone receptors: a prospective randomized study. Am J Gastroenterol 2000;95(1):218–22.

23. Chow PK, Tai BC, Tan CK, et al. High-dose tamoxifen in the treatment of inoperable hepatocellular carcinoma: a multicenter randomized controlled trial. Hepatology 2002;36(5):1221–6.

24. Nowak AK, Stockler MR, Chow PK, et al. Use of tamoxifen in advanced-stage hepatocellular carcinoma. A systematic review. Cancer 2005;103(7):1408–14.

25. Manesis EK, Giannoulis G, Zoumboulis P, et al. Treatment of hepatocellular carcinoma with combined suppression and inhibition of sex hormones: a randomized, controlled trial. Hepatology 1995;21(6):1535–42.
26. Becker G, Allgaier HP, Olschewski M, et al. Long-acting octreotide versus placebo for treatment of advanced HCC: a randomized controlled double-blind study. Hepatology 2007;45(1):9–15.
27. Miura H, Miyazaki T, Kuroda M, et al. Increased expression of vascular endothelial growth factor in human hepatocellular carcinoma. J Hepatol 1997;27(5): 854–61.
28. Poon RT, Ho JW, Tong CS, et al. Prognostic significance of serum vascular endothelial growth factor and endostatin in patients with hepatocellular carcinoma. Br J Surg 2004;91(10):1354–60.
29. Jenab-Wolcott J, Giantonio BJ. Bevacizumab: current indications and future development for management of solid tumors. Expert Opin Biol Ther 2009;9(4): 507–17.
30. Jain RK. Antiangiogenic therapy for cancer: current and emerging concepts. Oncology (Williston Park) 2005;19(4 Suppl 3):7–16.
31. Siegel AB, Cohen EI, Ocean A, et al. Phase II trial evaluating the clinical and biologic effects of bevacizumab in unresectable hepatocellular carcinoma. J Clin Oncol 2008;26(18):2992–8.
32. Malka D, Dromain C, Farace F. Bevacizumab in patients with advanced hepatocellular carcinoma (HCC): preliminary results of a phase II study with circulating endothelial cell (CEC) monitoring. J Clin Oncol 2007;25(Suppl 18):4570.
33. Zhu AX, Blaszkowsky LS, Ryan DP, et al. Phase II study of gemcitabine and oxaliplatin in combination with bevacizumab in patients with advanced hepatocellular carcinoma. J Clin Oncol 2006;24(12):1898–903.
34. Thomas MB, Morris JS, Chadha R, et al. Phase II trial of the combination of bevacizumab and erlotinib in patients who have advanced hepatocellular carcinoma. J Clin Oncol 2009;27(6):843–50.
35. Faris JE, Michaelson MD. Targeted therapies: sunitinib versus interferon-alpha in metastatic RCC. Nat Rev Clin Oncol 2010;7(1):7–8.
36. Zhu AX, Sahani DV, Duda DG, et al. Efficacy, safety, and potential biomarkers of sunitinib monotherapy in advanced hepatocellular carcinoma: a phase II study. J Clin Oncol 2009;27(18):3027–35.
37. Faivre S, Delbaldo C, Vera K, et al. Safety, pharmacokinetic, and antitumor activity of SU11248, a novel oral multitarget tyrosine kinase inhibitor, in patients with cancer. J Clin Oncol 2006;24(1):25–35.
38. Available at: http://clinicaltrials.gov/ct2/show/NCT00699374. Accessed April 1, 2011.
39. Huynh H, Ngo VC, Fargnoli J, et al. Brivanib alaninate, a dual inhibitor of vascular endothelial growth factor receptor and fibroblast growth factor receptor tyrosine kinases, induces growth inhibition in mouse models of human hepatocellular carcinoma. Clin Cancer Res 2008;14(19):6146–53.
40. Raoul J, Finn R, Kang Y, et al. An open-label phase II study of first- and second-line treatment with brivanib in patients with hepatocellular carcinoma (HCC). J Clin Oncol 2009;27(15S):4577.
41. Available at: http://clinicaltrials.gov/ct2/show/NCT00858871. Accessed April 1, 2011.
42. Available at: http://clinicaltrials.gov/ct2/show/NCT00825955. Accessed April 1, 2011.
43. Zhu AX. Systemic treatment of hepatocellular carcinoma: dawn of a new era? Ann Surg Oncol 2010;17(5):1247–56.
44. Alberts S, Morlan B, Kim G. NCCTG phase II trial (N044J) of AZD2171 for patients with hepatocellular carcinoma (HCC): interim review of toxicity. American Society

of Clinical Oncology 2007 Gastrointestinal Cancers Symposium. Orlando (FL), June 1–5, 2007 [abstract A-186].

45. Toh H, Chen P, Carr B, et al. A phase II study of ABT-869 in hepatocellular carcinoma (HCC): interim analysis. J Clin Oncol 2009;27(15S):4581.

46. Yau C, Chen P, Curtis C, et al. A phase I study of pazopanib in patients with advanced hepatocellular carcinoma. J Clin Oncol 2009;27(15S):3561.

47. Koch I, Baron A, Roberts S. Influence of hepatic dysfunction on safety, tolerability, and pharmacokinetics (PK) of PTK787/ZK 222584 in patients (pts) with unresectable hepatocellular carcinoma (HCC). J Clin Oncol 2007;23(Suppl):4134.

48. Whittaker S, Marais R, Zhu AX. The role of signaling pathways in the development and treatment of hepatocellular carcinoma. Oncogene 2010;29(36):4989–5005.

49. Philip PA, Mahoney MR, Allmer C, et al. Phase II study of Erlotinib (OSI-774) in patients with advanced hepatocellular cancer. J Clin Oncol 2005;23(27):6657–63.

50. Thomas MB, Chadha R, Glover K, et al. Phase 2 study of erlotinib in patients with unresectable hepatocellular carcinoma. Cancer 2007;110(5):1059–67.

51. O'Dwyer P, Giantonio B, Levy D. Gefitinib in advanced unresectable hepatocellular carcinoma: results from the Eastern Cooperative Oncology Group's study E1203 [abstract]. J Clin Oncol 2006;24(18S):A-4143.

52. Markman B, Capdevila J, Elez E, et al. New trends in epidermal growth factor receptor-directed monoclonal antibodies. Immunotherapy 2009;1(6):965–82.

53. Zhu AX, Stuart K, Blaszkowsky LS, et al. Phase 2 study of cetuximab in patients with advanced hepatocellular carcinoma. Cancer 2007;110(3):581–9.

54. Grünwald V, Wilkens L, Gebel M, et al. A phase II open-label study of cetuximab in unresectable hepatocellular carcinoma: final results. J Clin Oncol 2007; 25(Suppl):4598.

55. Asnacios A, Fartoux L, Romano O, et al. Gemcitabine plus oxaliplatin (GEMOX) combined with cetuximab in patients with progressive advanced stage hepatocellular carcinoma: results of a multicenter phase 2 study. Cancer 2008; 112(12):2733–9.

56. O'Neil B, Bernard S, Goldberg R. Phase II study of oxaliplatin, capecitabine, and cetuximab in advanced hepatocellular carcinoma. J Clin Oncol 2008; 26(Suppl):4604.

57. O'Neil B, Williams-Goff L, Kauh J, et al. A phase II study of AZD6244 in advanced or metastatic hepatocellular carcinoma. J Clin Oncol 2009;27(15S):e15574.

58. Geissler EK. The impact of mTOR inhibitors on the development of malignancy. Transplant Proc 2008;40(Suppl 10):S32–5.

59. Decaens T, Luciani A, Itti E. Pilot study of sirolimus in cirrhotic patients with advanced hepatocellular carcinoma. Gastrointestinal Cancers Symposium. San Francisco (CA), January 15–17, 2009 [abstract 244].

60. Overwijk WW, Theoret MR, Finkelstein SE, et al. Tumor regression and autoimmunity after reversal of a functionally tolerant state of self-reactive CD8+ T cells. J Exp Med 2003;198(4):569–80.

61. Lai CL, Lau JY, Wu PC, et al. Recombinant interferon-alpha in inoperable hepatocellular carcinoma: a randomized controlled trial. Hepatology 1993;17(3): 389–94.

62. Llovet JM, Sala M, Castells L, et al. Randomized controlled trial of interferon treatment for advanced hepatocellular carcinoma. Hepatology 2000;31(1): 54–8.

63. Mazzaferro V, Romito R, Schiavo M, et al. Prevention of hepatocellular carcinoma recurrence with alpha-interferon after liver resection in HCV cirrhosis. Hepatology 2006;44(6):1543–54.

64. Lygidakis NJ, Kosmidis P, Ziras N, et al. Combined transarterial targeting locoregional immunotherapy-chemotherapy for patients with unresectable hepatocellular carcinoma: a new alternative for an old problem. J Interferon Cytokine Res 1995;15(5):467–72.

65. Reinisch W, Holub M, Katz A, et al. Prospective pilot study of recombinant granulocyte-macrophage colony-stimulating factor and interferon-gamma in patients with inoperable hepatocellular carcinoma. J Immunother 2002;25(6): 489–99.

66. Giglia JL, Antonia SJ, Berk LB, et al. Systemic therapy for advanced hepatocellular carcinoma: past, present, and future. Cancer Control 2010;17(2):120–9.

67. Rosenberg SA, Dudley ME. Adoptive cell therapy for the treatment of patients with metastatic melanoma. Curr Opin Immunol 2009;21(2):233–40.

68. Wang Y, Chen H, Wu M, et al. Postoperative immunotherapy for patients with hepatocarcinoma using tumor-infiltrating lymphocytes. Chin Med J (Engl) 1997; 110(2):114–7.

69. Takayama T, Sekine T, Makuuchi M, et al. Adoptive immunotherapy to lower postsurgical recurrence rates of hepatocellular carcinoma: a randomised trial. Lancet 2000;356(9232):802–7.

70. Lee WC, Wang HC, Hung CF, et al. Vaccination of advanced hepatocellular carcinoma patients with tumor lysate-pulsed dendritic cells: a clinical trial. J Immunother 2005;28(5):496–504.

71. Chlebowski RT, Brzechwa-Adjukiewicz A, Cowden A, et al. Doxorubicin (75 mg/m2) for hepatocellular carcinoma: clinical and pharmacokinetic results. Cancer Treat Rep 1984;68(3):487–91.

72. Melia WM, Johnson PJ, Williams R. Induction of remission in hepatocellular carcinoma. A comparison of VP 16 with adriamycin. Cancer 1983;51(2):206–10.

73. Falkson G, Ryan LM, Johnson LA, et al. A random phase II study of mitoxantrone and cisplatin in patients with hepatocellular carcinoma. An ECOG study. Cancer 1987;60(9):2141–5.

74. Colleoni M, Buzzoni R, Bajetta E, et al. A phase II study of mitoxantrone combined with beta-interferon in unresectable hepatocellular carcinoma. Cancer 1993; 72(11):3196–201.

75. Chao Y, Chan WK, Birkhofer MJ, et al. Phase II and pharmacokinetic study of paclitaxel therapy for unresectable hepatocellular carcinoma patients. Br J Cancer 1998;78(1):34–9.

76. O'Reilly EM, Stuart KE, Sanz-Altamira PM, et al. A phase II study of irinotecan in patients with advanced hepatocellular carcinoma. Cancer 2001;91(1):101–5.

77. Fuchs CS, Clark JW, Ryan DP, et al. A phase II trial of gemcitabine in patients with advanced hepatocellular carcinoma. Cancer 2002;94(12):3186–91.

78. Patt YZ, Hassan MM, Aguayo A, et al. Oral capecitabine for the treatment of hepatocellular carcinoma, cholangiocarcinoma, and gallbladder carcinoma. Cancer 2004;101(3):578–86.

79. Gish RG, Porta C, Lazar L, et al. Phase III randomized controlled trial comparing the survival of patients with unresectable hepatocellular carcinoma treated with nolatrexed or doxorubicin. J Clin Oncol 2007;25(21):3069–75.

80. Louafi S, Boige V, Ducreux M, et al. Gemcitabine plus oxaliplatin (GEMOX) in patients with advanced hepatocellular carcinoma (HCC): results of a phase II study. Cancer 2007;109(7):1384–90.

81. Boige V, Raoul JL, Pignon JP, et al. Multicentre phase II trial of capecitabine plus oxaliplatin (XELOX) in patients with advanced hepatocellular carcinoma: FFCD 03-03 trial. Br J Cancer 2007;97(7):862–7.

82. Shim JH, Park JW, Nam BH, et al. Efficacy of combination chemotherapy with capecitabine plus cisplatin in patients with unresectable hepatocellular carcinoma. Cancer Chemother Pharmacol 2009;63(3):459–67.
83. Ikeda M, Okusaka T, Ueno H, et al. A phase II trial of continuous infusion of 5-fluorouracil, mitoxantrone, and cisplatin for metastatic hepatocellular carcinoma. Cancer 2005;103(4):756–62.

Liver Neoplasia in Children

Nedim Hadzic, MD, MSc[a],*, Milton J. Finegold, MD[b]

KEYWORDS

- Liver neoplasia • Pediatric liver tumors
- Hepatocellular carcinoma • Hepatoblastoma

Routine use of ultrasonography in general pediatric practice, even following very mild and nonspecific abdominal symptoms, has dramatically increased the detection of focal hepatic lesions. They range from entirely benign incidental lesions to malignant tumors (**Box 1**) and on most occasions warrant further diagnostic work-up, including axial radiological imaging (multiphasic computed tomography [CT], magnetic resonance imaging [MRI]), and specific serologic tumor markers.

EPIDEMIOLOGY
Malignant Tumors

Primary liver tumors in childhood are rare and account for approximately 1% of all pediatric malignancies.[1–4] The National Cancer Institute estimated that in 2010, 24,120 individuals would be diagnosed with a tumor of the liver and/or biliary tract in the United States (http://seer.cancer.gov/csr/1975_2007/). Of those, approximately 1.1% were expected to be younger than 20 years. Two-thirds of hepatic neoplasms in children are malignant. The 2 main malignant tumors are hepatoblastoma (HB), affecting around 80% of children, and hepatocellular carcinoma (HCC).[2] In children younger than 5 years, HB accounts for 91% of the malignant tumors.[5] Additional rare malignant liver tumors in children are sarcoma, including its 3 variants—rhabdomyosarcoma, embryonal or undifferentiated sarcoma, and angiosarcoma—predominantly presenting in early childhood.[6] Also included is the exceedingly uncommon cholangiocarcinoma, which can present at any age, often in the context of chronic biliary disease.[7] Common pediatric malignancies, such as acute lymphoblastic leukemia and neuroblastoma, can initially present with liver infiltrates and dysfunction, mimicking multifocal liver tumors.[8]

Some changes in the incidence of malignant tumors in the US children were observed between 1973 and 1977 and 1993 and 1997. While HCC rates decreased (from 0.45 to 0.29 cases per 1 million population), HB rates increased (from 0.6 to 1.2 cases per 1 million population).[5] The decline in HCC may be attributed to

---

[a] King's College Hospital Denmark Hill, London SE5 9RS, UK
[b] Baylor College of Medicine, Texas Children's Hospital, 6621 Fannin Street, TX, USA
* Corresponding author.
E-mail address: nedim.hadzic@kcl.ac.uk

Clin Liver Dis 15 (2011) 443–462
doi:10.1016/j.cld.2011.03.011
1089-3261/11/$ – see front matter © 2011 Elsevier Inc. All rights reserved.

Box 1
Pediatric liver masses

- Malignant Tumors
  - Hepatoblastoma (43% of all tumors)
    - (Rhabdoid tumor)
  - Hepatocellular Carcinoma (23%)
    - (Fibrolamellar carcinoma)
  - Embryonal Sarcoma
  - Rhabdomyosarcoma
  - Angiosarcoma
  - Epithelioid hemangio-endothelioma
  - Nested Stromal–Epithelial Tumor
  - Endocrine tumor
  - Germ cell–yolk sac tumor
  - Megakaryoblastic leukemia
- Benign Tumors
  - Mesenchymal hamartoma (beware sarcoma)
  - Focal nodular hyperplasia
  - Hemangioma, hemangioendothelioma (beware angiosarcoma)
  - Kaposiform hemangioendothelioma
  - Adenoma
  - Nodular regenerative hyperplasia
  - Teratoma
  - Angiomyolipoma–PEComa (perivascular epithelioid tumor)
- Other Masses
  - Vascular malformations
  - Congenital cysts
    - Simple
    - Polycystic liver disease
  - Parasitic cysts
  - Abscess
    - Pyogenic
    - Amebic
- Metastases
  - Wilms'
  - Neuroblastoma
  - Lymphoma
  - Germ cell
  - Desmoplastic small cell
  - Pancreaticoblastoma

immunization of infants against perinatal transmission of hepatitis B virus (HBV) infection[9] and the routine use of nitizinone for tyrosinemia type 1, whereas improved survival rates of extremely premature babies (birth weight <1500 g), has led to a new population of children having increased susceptibility to develop HB.[10] The incidence of HB is also increased in Beckwith-Wiedemann syndrome[11] and familial adenomatous polyposis.[12,13]

There are 2 distinct groups of HCC patients in childhood: those developing HCC in the context of advanced chronic liver disease (CLD) (**Box 2**), and children who develop sporadic HCC without preceding liver disease. The latter group typically affects older children, Their clinical behavior and biologic behavior are similar to HCC in adults. Approximately 26% of cases are histologically of a fibrolamellar type,[14] which does not appear to make a prognostic difference. Sporadic HCC in children has a relatively poor outcome,[15] while the several small series that report on HCC developing in CLD do so in the context of liver transplantation (LT).[16–19]

Some biologic differences may exist between HCCs developing in adults and children. One study reported an unusually high radiological response (49%) to chemotherapy in pediatric HCC.[15] Kim and colleagues[20] have compared expression of G1 phase regulatory proteins (cyclin D1, cyclin E, and cdk4) and loss of heterozygosity (LoH) on chromosomal arms 8p, 13q, and 17p between 9 pediatric and 9 adult HBV-related HCCs. They have observed that expression of cyclin 1 was lower and LoH higher at 13q in pediatric malignancies.

Benign Tumors

The spectrum of benign liver tumors in children is more diverse than in adults. They include: infantile hemangioendothelioma (IHE), mesenchymal hamartoma, adenoma, nodular regenerative hyperplasia (NRH), focal nodular hyperplasia (FNH), and inflammatory pseudotumor (see **Box 1**). About 50% of the benign tumors present within the first 2 years of life. Some of the focal lesions such as FNH develop in the background of primary vascular/perfusion anomalies,[21,22] becoming more clinically significant with growth of the child. They may mimic malignant tumors, and their clinical diagnosis rests on radiological features and the histopathological picture,[23] if the tissue is available.

Box 2
Metabolic disease and HCC

- Children
  - Hereditary tyrosinemia, type 1 (FAH deficiency)
  - Glycogen storage diseases; especially, type 1a (glucose-6- phosphatase deficiency)
  - Chronic cholestasis syndromes: PFIC 2 (BSEP deficiency); Alagille syndrome (JAGGED-1 deficiency); chronic total parenteral nutrition
  - Mitochondrial—"Navajo" hepatopathy (MPV 17 mutation)
- Adults
  - Hereditary hemochromatosis
  - Alpha-1 anti-trypsin deficiency
  - Wilson's disease (ATP7B mutation)
  - Non-alcoholic steatohepatitis

Some of the benign tumors, such as adenomas or FNH, develop in association with various endocrine stimuli such as precocious puberty, virilization, or use of high-estrogen content oral contraceptive pills. Elevation of serum alphafetoprotein (AFP) in benign tumors is exceptional, but given the potential for HCC to emerge in a background of adenomatosis in metabolic diseases, such as glycogen storage disease (GSD), one would hope that serum AFP would serve as a reliable screening tool along with ultrasonography during follow-up. However, 1 recent series reported that AFP was not elevated in 6 out of 8 young adults with GSD type 1 and HCC.[24]

Physiologically elevated serum levels of this protein in the first year of life, in both term and prematurely born infants, must be accounted for during clinical work-up of a liver mass.[25] The differential diagnostic consideration should also always include low AFP variants of HB.

CLINICAL PRESENTATION AND DIAGNOSIS

Hepatic tumors in children most commonly present insidiously with nonspecific abdominal discomfort, feeding difficulties, and abdominal distension. Chronic fatigue secondary to anemia and lack of appetite are often reported. Jaundice and biochemical derangement are signs of advanced neoplastic change. Occasionally, the child may present acutely with vomiting, fever and clinical signs of abdominal irritation, often suggestive of tumor rupture with intraperitoneal spread. Very rarely HB can present with signs of precocious puberty/virilization due to β-HCG secretion by the tumor. Serum AFP remains the key clinical marker of malignant neoplastic change, response to the treatment, and relapse. However, there are some variants of both HB and HCC that have low or normal AFP. These variants may have distinct histologic features and poorer prognoses.

Abdominal ultrasonography usually demonstrates a large mass, possibly with some satellite lesions and areas of hemorrhage within the tumor. The next diagnostic step is multiphase CT or MRI, depending on local radiological availability and expertise. Hypervascularized hepatic lesions with delayed contrast excretion are highly suspicious of a malignant tumor. Tissue diagnosis of the tumor is essential, although some advocate that in the presence of very high AFP in a young child (6 months to 3 years)[26] this may not be necessary, as avoiding the biopsy theoretically reduces the risks of the tumor seeding. The practice in the United States is not to treat without a tissue sample except under the most urgent life-threatening circumstances, such as tumor growth into the right atrium.[27] The rationale for this recommendation is provided in the section on pathology and in the article by Roskams.

Segmental assessment of the extent of the tumor and its relation with the main hepatic vessels is of foremost importance for planning the intensity of chemotherapy and eventual surgery. In Europe, The Childhood Liver Tumor Study Group of the International Society of Pediatric Oncology (SIOPEL) has developed a preoperative evaluation of the tumor extent (PRETEXT) grading system, which appears to provide a valuable tool for the risk stratification,[28] although the system has not been formally evaluated for prognostic accuracy. Formal staging of the tumor should include chest and brain CT and bone scanning.

Benign hepatic tumors are usually diagnosed incidentally. IHE can have an acute presentation, typically within the first couple of weeks or months of life. Dramatic abdominal distension can lead to major respiratory distress, prompting the need for assisted ventilation and intensive care support. Nowadays some IHEs may be detected on routine antenatal ultrasonography, due to their characteristic vascular multichannel appearance. They are often associated with other cutaneous vascular lesions "birth marks" and high-output cardiac failure.[3] Some children may develop the Kasabach-Merritt phenomenon, a triad of coagulopathy, hemolytic anemia and thrombocytopenia due to intralesional pooling of the blood. A proportion of children develop a bizarre secondary hypothyroidism[29] that is thought to be secondary to tumor production of the enzyme iodothyronine deiodinase, which stimulates the conversion of thyroxine to reverse triiodothyronine and of triiodothyronine to 3,3'-diiodothyronine, leading to a biochemical picture of hypothyroidism, requiring thyroxin supplementation.[30] This phenomenon resolves once the tumor is removed or significantly decreases in size, usually within the first 2 years of life.[29]

PATHOLOGY

The great variety of neoplasms that arise in the livers of children reflects not only the intrinsically diverse population of mature resident cells, but the potential for disorderly differentiation of the cells during development (see **Box 1**). The increased incidence of HB in children born before 28 weeks gestation (with birth weight <1500 g) compared with term gestations, may be explained by the exposure of rapidly dividing hepatoblasts to endogenous metabolites and hormones as well as exogenous chemicals that would normally be eliminated via the placenta. Inefficiency and compromise of the immature detoxification mechanisms could produce multiple somatic mutations and epigenetic (ie, methylation) modifications of the genome.[31,32] Also, the liver's crucial role in metabolism could account for the several metabolic and cholestatic diseases listed in **Box 2** as precursors to HCC. The occurrence of both hepatoblastoma (**Figs. 1** and **2**) and adenomas (**Fig. 3**) in some of these same conditions offers

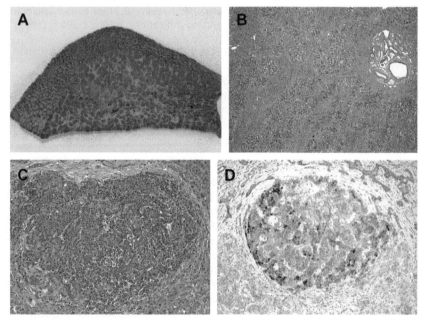

Fig. 1. Explanted liver of 10-month-old boy with severe intestinal insufficiency and failure to thrive due to neurogenin 3 mutation (A). Lifelong parenteral nutrition kept him alive, but biliary cirrhosis (B) led to liver transplantation. Two random sections from the left lobe contained embryonal hepatoblastoma (C), showing nuclear beta-catenin positivity (D) (original magnifications: B-50×, C-100×, D-125×).

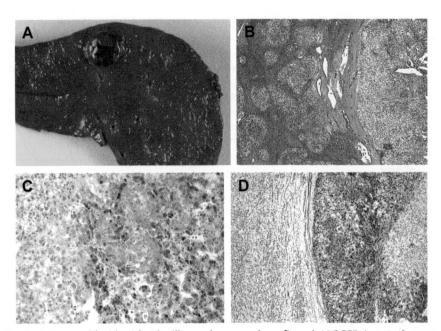

Fig. 2. A 1-year-old girl with Alagille syndrome and confirmed *JAGGED*-1 mutation progressed unusually rapidly to biliary cirrhosis. She had serum alphafetoprotein of 1667 ng/nL. The explant contained 1 large circumscribed nodule (*A*) plus multiple smaller regenerative nodules of cirrhosis (*B*). Nuclear beta-catenin was present in some cells of the largest nodule (*C*), and glypican 3 was positive in the cytoplasm of many cells (*D*). These immunostains indicate an early hepatocellular carcinoma (original magnifications: B-50×, C-200×, D-80×).

testimony to the vulnerability of hepatocytes at varying stages of differentiation to acquired genomic alterations.[33]

The gross and microscopic features of hepatic neoplasms in children have been well illustrated in recent texts.[34,35] The article by Roskams also provides an update on the importance of pathologic assessment to prognosis. Therefore, the discussion of pathology in this article is limited to some of the unique aspects of pediatric liver tumors, using specific patient examples.

Case 1

An HB was resected from an 11-year-old boy with constitutional familial adenomatous polyposis and an elevated serum AFP (see **Fig. 3**A). The tumor was composed solely of well-differentiated fetal hepatoblasts with low mitotic activity. This histologic designation reflects the resemblance of the neoplastic hepatocytes to developmental stage precursors[36] and will be significantly enhanced by molecular analyses of gene expression and genomic modifications.[37] According to the protocol used by the US Children's Oncology Group (COG),[35] the child was cured by surgery alone, without prior or subsequent chemotherapy. In the tissue between the HB and the healthy host liver, there was a region of uncertain nature (see **Fig. 3**A, B) that proved to be an adenoma, using immunohistochemistry with antibodies to β-catenin and glypican-3 (see **Fig. 3**C, D).

Comment

This case illustrates the rare phenomenon of HB arising in an older child, outside of its peak incidence between 2 and 3 years of age, and provides a good example of the

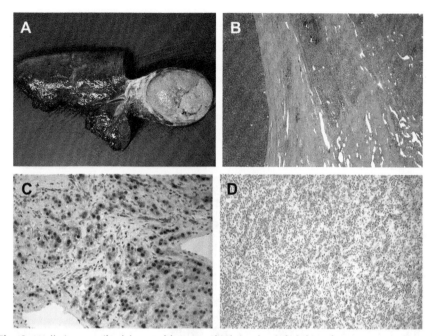

Fig. 3. Well-circumscribed hepatoblastoma (HB) in the left lobe of an 11-year-old with familial adenomatosis polyposis (*A*). The spongy tissue between the tumor and healthy host liver proved to be a hepatocellular adenoma histologically (*B* - HB left, adenoma, right) and immunohistochemically. Beta-catenin is positive in the nuclei of both the adenoma (*C*) and the HB. Glypican-3 was positive only in the HB (*D*) (original magnifications: B-25×, C-250×, D-100×).

importance of surveillance in instances of a well-known constitutional propensity to neoplasia,[12] as well as the potential for multiple and diverse histologies.

Case 2

A 1-month-old girl with hemihypertrophy and cardiac malformations (Beckwith-Wiedemann syndrome) was found to have a multicystic mass in the liver. AFP was 62,000 ng/mL. Biopsy was diagnosed as mesenchymal hamartoma (**Fig. 4**A). A second biopsy at 3 months revealed a capillary hemangioma (see **Fig. 4**B). One year later, imaging showed many complex masses (see **Fig. 4**C), and the AFP was 1306 ng/mL. Because growth of the masses began to compromise respiration (see **Fig. 4**D), resection was performed at age 3 years, at which time AFP was 12,000 ng/mL. Thorough histologic examination revealed persistence of the original benign tumor with biliary cysts and maturation of the myxoid stroma into mature collagen (**Fig. 5**A), plus multiple neoplastic foci including embryonal HB (see **Fig. 5**B), HCC (see **Fig. 5**C), and cholangiocarcinoma (see **Fig. 5**D). Review of the original biopsy revealed epithelial cell clusters consistent with fetal HB.

Comment

This child with Beckwith-Wiedemann syndrome, a well-known precursor to malignancy, not only illustrates the multipotentiality of neoplastic transformation, but the necessity of thorough tissue examination. Tumors like HB are typically highly variegated (**Box 3**), so that small samples obtained by biopsy may fail to reveal all

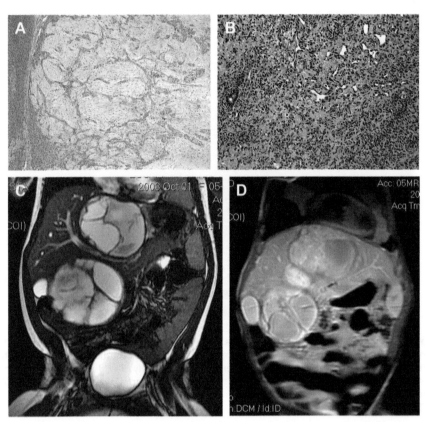

Fig. 4. Multicystic mass in the liver was biopsied at 1 month of age. It consisted of loose myxoid stroma blending with host parenchyma and containing a few clusters of immature hepatocytes and bile ducts (*A*). Biopsy 2 months later revealed multiple nests of small capillaries with bland endothelium, consistent with benign hemangioendothelioma (*B*). Magnetic resonance imaging 1 year later showed multiple heterogenous masses (*C*). Two years later imaging showed further expansion of the masses with elevation of the right hemidiaphragm, compromising respiration (*D*) (original magnifications: A-25×, B-100×). (*Courtesy of Dr Stacey Berry, Banner Desert Medical Center, Mesa, AZ.*)

diagnostic components, some of which may be life-threatening (**Fig. 6**). Another caveat from this case is that molecular analyses of tumors with such diverse histology, especially when intimately intermingled, can be misleading or inconclusive with respect to pathogenesis. Therefore, careful attention to histology and tissue selection, using laser capture microdissection if necessary to assure uniformity, is critical if one is to comprehend the consequences of specific molecular alterations.[37,38]

Other instances of the simultaneous presence of both HB and HCC have been observed in relation to perinatally-acquired HBV infection[34] or as sequential findings in relation to chemotherapy,[39] as illustrated in **Fig. 7**. Around 70% of HBs are unresectable at presentation (stage 3) or have metastasized to the lungs (stage 4), so chemotherapy is required.[35] If resection can then be achieved, the histology typically shows extensive tumor necrosis, even of intravenous tumor, abundant osteoid, and ductular transformation or reaction.[39] Maturation or persistence of fetal HB is more likely than more primitive embryonal cells, possibly because the latter are much

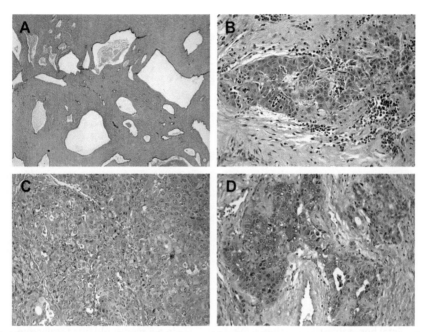

Fig. 5. Resection at age 3 revealed diverse histology. The mesenchymal hamartoma has persistent biliary cysts embedded in a collagenous stroma (*A*). Foci of small poorly differentiated cells with high nuclear-cytoplasmic ratio typical of embryonal hepatoblastoma (*B*) were strikingly different from much larger, more pleomorphic and actively dividing cells typical of hepatocarcinoma (*C*), and from neoplastic ductal elements representing a cholangiocarcinoma (*D*) (original magnifications: A-25×, B–D -200×).

Box 3
Hepatoblastoma histology

- Epithelial
  - Fetal
    - Well-differentiated—uniform, round nuclei, cords (EMH)
    - "Crowded"—mitotically active; usually less glycogen
    - "Anaplastic"—nuclear atypia (pleomorphism, hyperchromasia)
    - Cholangioblastic—bile duct-like—often at periphery of fetal nodules
  - Embryonal: small, high N/C, angular, primitive tubules (EMH)
    - (Macrotrabecular—a pattern of 20+ cells in a cluster with epithelial cytology—resembling HCC)
  - Small undifferentiated cell: no pattern, ± mitoses
  - Rhabdoid: discohesive; eccentric irregular nuclei, prominent nucleoli; abundant cytoplasmic filaments
- Mixed
  - Stromal derivatives; spindle cells ("blastema"), osteoid, skeletal muscle, cartilage
  - Teratoid: mixed, plus primitive endoderm; neural, melanin

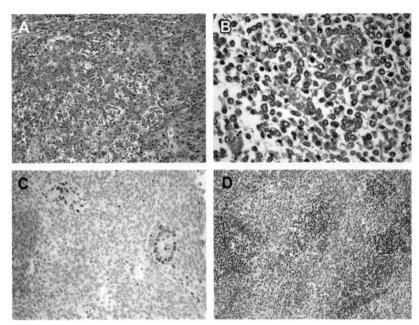

Fig. 6. Fetal hepatoblastoma with low mitotic activity in a 6-month-old was totally resected (stage 1) (*A*). Six months later, despite chemotherapy, there was a recurrence, and the histology was suggestive of a small cell undifferentiated HB (*B*). Metastasis to the lungs was fatal within the year. This occurred before current protocols and the recognition of integrase interactor (INI or switch/sucrase nonfermentable {SWI/SNF}-related matrix-associated actin-dependent regulator of chromatin subfamily B1 [SMARC B1]) immunohisto-chemistry as a critical modality in understanding the behavior of such cells.[42] In this case, the small cell nuclei are INI negative, whereas the entrapped bile duct nuclei are stained (*C*). In other hepatoblastomas, indistinguishable small undifferentiated cells may be INI positive (*D*), so their behavior is predicted to be less ominous (original magnifications: A-200×, B-400×, C-200×, D-160×).

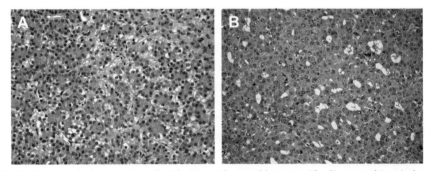

Fig. 7. Six-year-old boy presented with stage 4 hepatoblastoma. The liver was biopsied and a well-differentiated fetal hepatoblastoma was found (*A*). Resection of a lung metastasis following chemotherapy revealed hepatocellular carcinoma (*B*) (original magnifications: A, B-250×).

more mitotically active, or because of intrinsic or acquired resistance to the usually effective agents. This has been pointed out in a recent review of Boston Children's Hospital experience; 25% of their 22 patients had HCC-like morphology after chemotherapy, which was more often associated with metastatic disease.[39]

These examples lead to the question of a transitional liver cell tumor (TLCT), raised by SIOPEL colleagues.[40] They reported on 7 older children with stage 3 or 4 disease and elevated serum AFP, only 1 of whom responded to conventional chemotherapy that should have cured at least 4 more patients if the tumors had behaved like the suspected HB. However, the original tumor histology in 3 patients was consistent with HCC, and the positive nuclear expression of β-catenin (see **Fig. 3**C) suggested a new and aggressive category of neoplasia to these investigators.

In the situation in which a patient with mesenchymal hamartoma has a concurrent or more typically a second neoplasm, it is more likely to be an undifferentiated (embryonal) sarcoma (**Fig. 8**). Several such patients have been reported, prompting increasing tendency for elective resection of these histologically benign liver tumors.[41]

Case 3

A 6-month-old child presented with an elevated serum AFP and resectable HB. Histologically, it was judged to be a pure fetal tumor. (see **Fig. 6**A) This occurred before the current COG protocol, so chemotherapy with cisplatinum and doxorubicin was given. Within 6 months there was a recurrence that consisted exclusively of small undifferentiated cells (see **Fig. 6**B), foci of which were found by retrospective review of the original resection. The cells were negative for nuclear integrase interactor (INI) immunostaining (see **Fig. 6**C), therefore manifesting a rhabdoid-like variant.[42] The loss of INI expression reflects mutations in the switch/sucrase non-fermentable {SWI/SNF}-related matrix-associated actin-dependent regulator of chromatin subfamily B1 (SMARCB1) locus and/or chromosome 22 deletions.

Comment

From this unfortunate infant, much has been learned about unfavorable histology and the requirement for alternative therapeutic agents.[43–45] When the majority of an infant's HB is composed of small undifferentiated cells, the serum AFP is typically normal or minimally elevated.[46] For the more common instances, when small undifferentiated cells comprise a small proportion of an otherwise typical HB, immunostaining for INI may be positive (see **Fig. 6**D), and the usual chemotherapy regimen may be

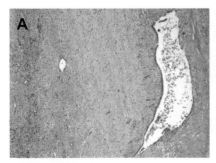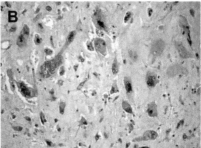

Fig. 8. Mesenchymal hamartoma in an 8-year-old boy who came to attention because of abdominal trauma (*A*). Serum alpha-fetoprotein was normal. Cytogenetic analysis revealed a 19q13.4 translocation. Thorough histologic examination revealed areas of embryonal sarcoma, with the classic cytologic atypia and cytoplasmic protein globules (*B*) (original magnifications: A-50×, B-400×).

adequate. Completion of current clinical trials may provide a definitive answer to this question.

Case 4

A 16-year-old girl presented with Cushing syndrome and a mass in the liver (**Fig. 9**). Right hepatic lobectomy revealed a nested stromal–epithelial tumor, with a characteristic lobular pattern of growth and intimate association with bile ductules. Immunohistochemistry demonstrated adrenocorticotrophic hormone (ACTH) in the tumor cells. This tumor is another example of unusual behavior and unresolved origin and pathogenesis. One year after the lobectomy, it recurred, necessitating curative LT.

Comment

The authors are aware of 24 cases, aged 2 to 33 years at diagnosis, 13 of whom were under 20 years and 17 of whom were female.[47–49] Eight patients had hepatic calcification/ossification detected incidentally several years earlier. Including this patient, 5 patients had Cushing syndrome, 4 of whom were female, and all resolved by surgery. There have been 5 recurrences among the 22 patients 1 to 6 years later; one had a local lymph node metastasis, and one 16-year-old girl has had lung metastases after 1 year.[49]

These illustrative cases demonstrate the value of immunohistochemistry in differential diagnosis, as well as molecular characterization of the various hepatic neoplasms.[50–52]

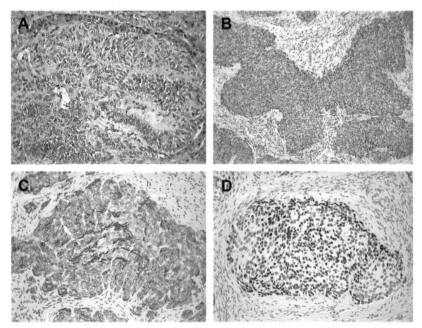

Fig. 9. Sixteen-year-old girl presented with Cushing syndrome and hepatic mass. Right hepatic lobectomy revealed a nested stromal–epithelial tumor, with a characteristic lobular pattern of growth and intimate association with bile ductules (*A*). Immunohistochemistry demonstrated adrenocorticotrophic hormone (ACTH) in the tumor cells (*B*). The relationship between the tumor and biliary epithelial cells is seen with CD56 neutral cell adhesive molecule (NCAM) antibody (*C*). The epithelial component was strongly positive for Wilms tumor gene (WTI) (*D*), thought to reflect its origin from a mesodermal precursor and an abnormality in the transition to epithelium (original magnifications: A,C,D-200×, B-80×).

In adults, Bióulac-Sage and colleagues[53,54] have provided a series of elegant applications of this technique, combined with RNA expression analyses, to hepatocellular neoplasms, especially adenomas, using antibodies to β-catenin, liver fatty acid binding protein (LFAB), glutamine synthetase, and serum amyloid A, to classify adenomas and predict potential for HCC to develop.

MANAGEMENT
Malignant Tumors

The key to successful treatment of malignant liver tumors in children is surgical removal, either by tumor resection/partial hepatectomy or LT. The approach to hepatic resection differs in North America and Europe. SIOPEL recommends initial chemotherapy,[55,56] while the American guidelines from COG require primary resection if possible, followed by chemotherapy,[57] unless the tumor is pure fetal type HB stage 1, when the chemotherapy is not given. Both strategies have been successful in increasing the 5-year survival rates in HB to approximately 80% due to effective chemotherapy (cisplatinum in combination with doxorubicin or vincristine). Moreover, the timing and nature of surgical interventions are better defined for HB, and they are well-placed within the management protocols. For HCC, however, chemotherapy is not effective, and complete surgical excision or transplantation are essential for cure.

The Childhood Liver Tumor Strategy Group in Europe has demonstrated a partial response to chemotherapy in HCCs at 49% and an overall 5-year survival rate of 28% in SIOPEL-1 study.[15] Thirty-six percent of the tumors were resectable.[15] COG reports that 17% of HCCs were resectable at presentation,[58] similar to the 18.2% reported from a large Taiwanese study.[59] Their overall 5-year event-free survival was only 19%.[58] All studies report that accompanying cirrhosis makes the resection technically even more challenging. Clearly, the results of chemotherapy and resection for HCC were disappointing, and the option of LT needed to be explored earlier and more vigorously. In one of the earliest studies, Reyes and colleagues[60] reported overall 1-year, 3-year, and 5-year disease-free survival rates for HCC of 79%, 68%, and 63%, respectively. The main risk factors for recurrence were vascular invasion, presence of distant metastases, lymph node involvement, tumor size, and male gender. More recently, Austin and colleagues[61] reported 1-, 5-, and 10-year survival rates from the United Network for Organ Sharing (UNOS) database to be 86%, 63%, and 58%, respectively.

Adjunctive therapy for HCC in children plays a very limited role due to ineffectiveness of the present chemotherapy regimens and lack of experience in alternative methods such as chemoembolization, radiofrequency ablation, or ethanol injections. Results of one study showed that intrahepatic chemoembolization (IHCE) with cisplatinum and doxorubicin could be considered as adjuvant treatment before LT.[62,63] IHCE did not affect resectability of HCC in those children.[62]

As formal criteria for LT in cases of HCC in children do not exist, many centers have been developing local guidelines. Conventional criteria for LT for HCC in adults have been criticized for being relatively conservative, particularly in the pediatric context.[64] Several series reported that Milan criteria (MC), which are based on the overall number and size of the neoplastic lesions, were not helpful in determining the recurrence and prognosis of the children receiving LT for HCC.[16–18,60] It has been reported that even children with larger tumors, clearly exceeding MC but transplanted on compassionate grounds, had a good short-to-medium term outcome.[16–18,60] It was also pointed out that the pediatric patients often have an additional option of living-related left lobe transplantation, which shortens waiting time. Another challenging concept is whether the children who developed a HCC in the background of CLD should be considered for LT using even more liberal criteria, based on the argument that the potential for additional neoplastic transformation will be eliminated. Unfortunately, studies addressing this question are lacking at present. The prospective trials on HCC in children, including the last launched by the SIOPEL group in 2005, have addressed management of sporadic HCC, while the reported LT series have included a mixture of both subgroups.[16–18,60] Therefore, management of HCC related to CLD, including consideration of LT, still remains, to some extent, intuitive.

Benign Tumors

The most important step in the management of benign tumors in children is confirmation of their genuine benign nature. Multiphase contrast CT imaging and, less frequently, direct angiography are required for the radiological diagnosis. Some of the benign tumors, including IHE, mesenchymal hamartoma, and FNH, would have characteristic radiological features, not always requiring a tissue diagnosis. For example, on contrast CT, FNH often has a characteristic central scar and frequently is associated with vascular abnormalities such as arterio-venous shunts, congenital absence of portal vein (Abernethy malformation, which was first reported in 1793 by John Abernethy [1764–1831], an English surgeon) or patent ductus venosus. Mesenchymal hamartoma characteristically has a well-demarcated, cystic, nonprogressive appearance, typically affecting younger children with negative tumor serum markers (however, see Case 2). In some centers, determining the size of the hepatic artery in IHE on Doppler ultrasound is the initial but very important screening test, as its elective ligation may be a simple and very effective therapeutic measure for the uncomplicated tumors.[65]

Differentiation between NRH adenomas and HCC is not simple in children and may, in addition to sequential CT imaging, require tissue diagnosis. Biopsying these lesions remains controversial due to potential sampling error and seeding of the tumor. Expert histopathology review is often required in ambiguous cases. In addition to allowing a specific histologic diagnosis, biopsies yield tissues for molecular analyses that are beginning to play an increasing role in the diagnosis of both benign and malignant neoplasms.[37,38,53,66] In the current absence of simple and noninvasive clinical means of interval change monitoring, it is hoped that novel radiological methods such as microbubble contrast-enhanced ultrasonography[67] could lead to better follow-up of focal lesions in children with non-end stage CLD.

In IHE, abdominal distension secondary to massive hepatomegaly may be so dramatic as to require ventilation and multiorgan support, including urgent consideration for LT. In less acute presentations the medical treatment options include corticosteroids,[68] interferon-α,[69] vincristine,[70] and propranolol.[71] In a recent prospective study, the nonspecific beta-blocker propranolol (2 mg/kg/d) was shown to be very effective in 8 infants with diffuse multifocal IHEs.[71] The proposed pharmacologic mechanisms for the beneficial effects of propranolol in regression of IHE include vasoconstriction due to decreased release of nitric oxide, blocking of proangiogenic signals (vascular endothelial growth factor, basic fibroblast growth factor, matrix metalloproteinase 2/9), and induction of apoptosis.[72] Recently, propranolol-induced changes in angiotensin-converting enzyme activity in the proliferating endothelial progenitor cells of the microvasculature have also been documented in an in vitro model of IHE.[73] Treatment with interferon-alpha seems to have become obsolete due to concerns about its safety early in infancy and described spastic diplegias developing following its use in about 20% of children.[74] In IHEs, persistent thrombocytopenia and anemia often require ongoing but cautious blood product support due to sudden deterioration in abdominal distension following the transfusions. Due to commonly present high-output congestive cardiac failure and hypothyroidism, some infants additionally require digoxin/diuretics and thyroxin, respectively. Nonmedical approaches include hepatic artery ligation, chemoembolization, resection, and LT. Hepatic artery ligation is a relatively simple operation that could lead to dramatic improvement in bilobar tumors with a large single feeding vessel.[65] Liver replacement is an effective modality, but it may be deemed extreme for smaller, regressing, and non life-threatening tumors. Refinement of laser therapy may offer additional option for IHE in the future. However, both medical and surgical approaches to management of IHE differ considerably between centers, and some international collaboration for management of these rare tumors appears warranted.

MEDICAL ISSUES RELATED TO CURRENT CHEMOTHERAPY

Children with malignant tumors treated with combination of LT and chemotherapy have been treated with less aggressive immunosuppressive regimens, based on the belief that they remain relatively immunosuppressed secondary to chemotherapy. Indeed, some studies have shown that the rate of episodes of acute cellular rejection in those children is reduced when compared with other LT indications.[75,76]

Routine assessment of hearing, renal, and cardiac function is standard during treatment for pediatric malignancies. It is no surprise that most of the toxicity data stem from HB treatment survivors, while information from the HCC setting is lacking. Chronic dose-related nephrotoxicity remains a significant long-term issue for both chemotherapy for malignant liver tumors and calcineurin inhibitor-based immunosuppression. Therefore, early use of calcineurin inhibitor-sparing agents, such as mycophenolate mofetil or sirolimus, is recommended for children after LT for liver tumors. Post-chemotherapy neutropenia rarely represents additional concerns during the surgical treatment. Nevertheless, it is prudent not to give chemotherapy 2 weeks before or after resection or LT. Platinum compounds (cisplatin and carboplatin), which have been a backbone of the successful treatment for pediatric liver tumors, are also quite ototoxic. Around 40% of children develop significant hearing loss, which typically affects high-register tones, and could be delayed.[77] COG has recently reported results of a randomized prospective study where amifostine, an organic thiophosphate thought to have cytoprotective effects, failed to reduce significant hearing loss after chemotherapy (<40 db).[78] The observed overall ototoxicity rate was 40%, more prevalent in stage 3/4 (48%) than in stage 1/2 (19%) HB patients.[78] Sodium thiosulfate has been reported to have certain otoprotective effects and is presently being tested in a randomized prospective trial for HB in Europe (SIOPEL-6).

Novel strategies are required for management of metastatic and relapsing malignancies. HB is one of the few pediatric malignancies where the presence of metastases does not necessarily imply a poor outcome. Surgical resection of isolated pulmonary metastases has been reported as a successful supplementary method in management of children with HB. Meyers and colleagues[79] have reported that 8 out of 9 children with stage 4 HB are long-term survivors following resection of pulmonary metastases. Alternative medications such as irinotecan and thalidomide are being investigated for patients with relapse, where other forms of conventional chemotherapy have been exhausted due to toxicity.

SCREENING

Hepatic neoplasms develop in a myriad of chronic liver disorders of childhood, often without or with minimal symptoms. Therefore, regular screening with abdominal ultrasound and serum AFP measurement should be in place for all children with CLD at least annually. Some of the conditions with known increased propensity to develop malignancies such as tyrosinemia type 1 (even on nitizinone treatment) or bile salt export pump (BSEP) deficiency should be assessed every 6 months (see **Box 2**). Children with chronic hepatitis B should be also regularly checked, but because communities in which immunization has yet to be provided are typically impoverished and medically underserved, recommendations for screening have not yet been implemented.

HB is dramatically more common in ex-premature babies but arranging effective screening programs could prove to be difficult because of their increasing numbers and fact that their long term care is typically provided outside hepatology clinics. Monitoring much smaller cohorts of children with Beckwith-Wiedemann syndrome for HB is more feasible, and one study has suggested abdominal ultrasonography and serum AFP every 3 months until 4 years of age.[80]

SUMMARY AND FUTURE ISSUES

Management of pediatric liver tumors has significantly improved over the last 2 decades. The principal reasons are that efficient chemotherapy and established medico-surgical treatment algorithms for HB have now integrated LT as a very valuable complementary treatment option. The management options for HCC are less effective and not well defined, broadly mirroring the therapeutic guidelines in adults, except for a more cautionary approach to neoadjuvant and loco-regional methods.

In the pediatric context the main clinical aims are to reduce chemotherapy toxicity (predominantly ototoxicity and nephrotoxicity) in children treated for HB and to investigate additional modes of treatment for HCC. An increasing number of children develop HCC in the background of CLD, and screening methods need to be better observed, particularly in increased-risk conditions such as tyrosinemia type 1, BSEP deficiency, and other chronic cholestatic disorders.

Improved understanding of HB and HCC biology may improve risk stratification at presentation and direct the treatment at specific molecular targets in the future (see article by Wrzenski and colleagues). Management of less common benign and malignant tumors should benefit from establishing international collaborative pediatric networks such as the Pediatric Liver Unresectable Tumor Observatory (PLUTO).[81]

REFERENCES

1. Litten JB. Tomlinson GE.Liver tumors in children. Oncologist 2008;13:812–20.
2. Finegold MJ, Egler RA, Goss JA, et al. Liver tumors: pediatric population. Liver Transpl 2008;14:1545–56.
3. Emre S, McKenna GJ. Liver tumors in children. Pediatr Transplant 2004;8:632–8.
4. Available at: http://seer.cancer.gov/csr/1975_2007/. Accessed October 2010.
5. Darbari A, Sabin KM, Shapiro CN, et al. Epidemiology of primary hepatic malignancies in US children. Hepatology 2003;38:560–6.
6. Awan S, Davenport M, Portmann B, et al. Angiosarcoma of the liver in children. J Pediatr Surg 1996;31:1729–32.
7. Scheimann AO, Strautnieks SS, Knisely AS, et al. Mutations in bile salt export pump (ABCB11) in two children with progressive familial intrahepatic cholestasis and cholangiocarcinoma. J Pediatr 2007;150:556–9.
8. Litten JB, Rodríguez MM, Maniaci V. Acute lymphoblastic leukemia presenting in fulminant hepatic failure. Pediatr Blood Cancer 2006;47:842–5.

9. Chang MH. Cancer prevention by vaccination against hepatitis B. Recent results. Cancer Res 2009;181:85–94.

10. McLaughlin CC, Baptiste MS, Schymura MJ, et al. Maternal and infant birth characteristics and hepatoblastoma. Am J Epidemiol 2006;163:818–28.

11. DeBaun MR, Tucker MA. Risk of cancer during the first four years of life in children from the Beckwith-Wiedemann Syndrome Registry. J Pediatr 1998;132: 398–400.

12. Kingston JE, Draper GJ, Mann JR. Hepatoblastoma and polyposis coli. Lancet 1982;1(8269):457.

13. Giardiello FM, Petersen GM, Brensinger JD, et al. Hepatoblastoma and APC gene mutation in familial adenomatous polyposis. Gut 1996;39:867–9.

14. Katzenstein HM, Krailo MD, Malogolowkin MH, et al. Fibrolamellar hepatocellular carcinoma in children and adolescents. Cancer 2003;97:2006–12.

15. Czauderna P, Mackinlay G, Perilongo G, et al. Liver Tumors Study Group of the International Society of Pediatric Oncology. Hepatocellular carcinoma in children: results of the first prospective study of the International Society of Pediatric Oncology group. J Clin Oncol 2002;20:2798–804.

16. Arikan C, Kilic M, Nart D, et al. Hepatocellular carcinoma in children and effect of living-donor liver transplantation on outcome. Pediatr Transplant 2006;10: 42–7.

17. Beaunoyer M, Vanatta JM, Ogihara M, et al. Outcomes of transplantation in children with primary hepatic malignancy. Pediatr Transplant 2007;11:655–60.

18. Sevmis S, Karakayali H, Ozçay F, et al. Liver transplantation for hepatocellular carcinoma in children. Pediatr Transplant 2008;12:52–6.

19. Hadzic N, Quaglia A, Portmann B, et al. Hepatocellular carcinoma in children with biliary atresia; King's College Hospital Experience. J Pediatr 2011, in press.

20. Kim H, Lee MJ, Kim MR, et al. Expression of cyclin D1, cyclin E, cdk4 and loss of heterozygosity of 8p, 13q, 17p in hepatocellular carcinoma: comparison study of childhood and adult hepatocellular carcinoma. Liver 2000;20:173–8.

21. Fischer HP, Zhou H. Nodular lesions of liver parenchyma caused by pathological vascularisation/perfusion. Pathologe 2006;27:273–83.

22. Citak EC, Karadeniz C, Oguz A, et al. Nodular regenerative hyperplasia and focal nodular hyperplasia of the liver mimicking hepatic metastasis in children with solid tumors and a review of literature. Pediatr Hematol Oncol 2007;24:281–9.

23. Paradis V. Benign liver tumors: an update. Clin Liver Dis 2010;14:719–29.

24. Franco LM, Krishnamurthy V, Bali D, et al. Hepatocellular carcinoma in glycogen storage disease type Ia: a case series. J Inherit Metab Dis 2005;28:153–62.

25. Blohm ME, Vesterling-Hörner D, Calaminus G, et al. Alpha 1-fetoprotein (AFP) reference values in infants up to 2 years of age. Pediatr Hematol Oncol 1998; 15:135–42.

26. Czauderna P, Otte JB, Aronson DC, et al. Childhood Liver Tumour Strategy Group of the International Society of Paediatric Oncology (SIOPEL). Guidelines for surgical treatment of hepatoblastoma in the modern era–recommendations from the Childhood Liver Tumour Strategy Group of the International Society of Paediatric Oncology (SIOPEL). Eur J Cancer 2005;41:1031–6.

27. Finegold MJ. Chemotherapy for suspected hepatoblastoma without efforts at surgical resection is a bad practice. Med Pediatr Oncol 2002;39:484–6.

28. Roebuck DJ, Aronson D, Clapuyt P, et al. International Childhood Liver Tumor Strategy Group 2005 PRETEXT: a revised staging system for primary malignant liver tumours of childhood developed by the SIOPEL group. Pediatr Radiol 2007;37:123–32.

29. Ayling RM, Davenport M, Hadzic N, et al. Hepatic hemangioendothelioma associated with production of humoral thyrotropin-like factor. J Pediatr 2001;138: 932–5.

30. Huang SA, Tu HM, Harney JW, et al. Severe hypothyroidism caused by type 3 iodothyronine deiodinase in infantile hemangiomas. N Engl J Med 2000;343:185–9.

31. Honda S, Haruta M, Sugawara W, et al. The methylation status of RASSF1A promoter predicts responsiveness to chemotherapy and eventual cure in hepatoblastoma patients. Int J Cancer 2008;5:1117–25.

32. Sakamoto LH, DeCamargo B, Cajaiba M, et al. MT1G hypermethylation: a potential prognostic marker for hepatoblastoma. Pediatr Res 2010;67:387–93.

33. Jain S, Singhal S, Lee P, et al. Molecular genetics of hepatocellular neoplasia. Am J Transl Res 2010;2:105–18.

34. Finegold MJ. Hepatic tumors in childhood. In: Russo P, Ruchelli ED, Piccoli DA, editors. Pathology of pediatric gastrointestinal and liver disease. New York: Springer-Verlag; 2004. p. 300–46.

35. Lopez-Terrada DH, Finegold MJ. Tumors of the liver. In: Suchy FJ, Sokol RJ, Balistreri WF, editors. Liver disease in children. 3rd edition. New York: Cambridge University Press; 2007. p. 943–74.

36. Zimmermann A. Pediatric liver tumors and hepatic ontogenesis: common and distinctive pathways. Med Pediatr Oncol 2002;39:492–503.

37. Lopez-Terrada DH, Gunaratne PH, Adesina AM, et al. Histologic subtypes of hepatoblastoma are characterized by differential canonical Wnt and Notch pathway activation in DLK+ precursors. Hum Pathol 2009;40:783–94.

38. Luo J-H, Ren B, Keryanov S, et al. Transcriptonic and genomic analysis of human hepatocellular carcinomas and hepatoblastomas. Hepatology 2006;44:1012–24.

39. Wang LL, Filippi RZ, Zurakowski D, et al. Effects of neoadjuvant chemotherapy on hepatoblastoma: a morphologic and immunohistochemical study. Am J Surg Pathol 2010;34:287–99.

40. Prokurat A, Kluge P, Kosciesza A, et al. Transitional liver cell tumors (TLCT) in older children and adolescents: a novel group of aggressive hepatic tumors expressing beta-catenin. Med Pediatr Oncol 2002;39:510–8.

41. Shehata B, Gupta NA, Katzenstein H, et al. Undifferentiated embryonal sarcoma of the liver is associated with mesenchymal hamartoma and multiple chromosomal abnormalities: a review of eleven cases. Pediatr Dev Pathol 2010. [Epub ahead of print].

42. Al Nassan A, Sughayer M, Ismail M, et al. INI1 (BAF47) is an essential diagnostic tool for children hepatic tumors and low alpha-feto protein. J Pediatr Hematol Oncol 2010;32:e79–81.

43. Haas JE, Feusner JH, Finegold MJ. Small cell undifferentiated histology in hepatoblastoma may be unfavorable. Cancer 2001;92:3130–4.

44. Jayaram A, Finegold MJ, Parham DM, et al. Successful management of rhabdoid tumor of the liver. J Pediatr Hematol Oncol 2007;29:406–8.

45. Trobaugh-Lotrario AD, Finegold MJ, Feusner JH. Rhabdoid tumors of the liver: rare, aggressive, and poorly responsive to standard cytotoxic chemotherapy. Pediatr Blood Cancer 2010. [Epub ahead of print].

46. De Ioris M, Brugieres L, Zimmermann A, et al. Hepatoblastoma with a low serum alpha feto protein level at diagnosis: the SIOPEL group experience. Eur J Cancer 2008;44:545–80.

47. Heerema-McKenney A, Leuschner I, Smith N, et al. Nested stromal epithelial tumor of the liver: six cases of a distinctive pediatric neoplasm with frequent

calcifications and association with Cushing syndrome. Am J Surg Pathol 2005;29: 10–20.

48. Makhlouf HR, Abdul-Al MM, Wang G, et al. Calcifying nested stromal-epithelial tumors of the liver. Am J Surg Pathol 2009;33:976–83.

49. Grazi GL, Vetrone G, d'Errico A, et al. Nested stromal-epithelial tumor (NSET) of the liver. Pathol Res Pract 2010;206:282–6.

50. Yang XR, Shi GM, Fan J, et al. Cytokeratin 10 and cytokeratin 19: predictive markers for poor prognosis in hepatocellular carcinoma patients after curative resection. Clin Cancer Res 2008;14:3850–9.

51. Yu B, Yang X, Xu Y, et al. Elevated expression of DKK1 is associated with cytoplasmic/nuclear beta-catenin accumulation and poor prognosis in hepatocellular carcinomas. J Hepatol 2009;50:948–57.

52. Nassar A, Cohen C, Siddiqui MT. Utility of Glypican-3 and survivin in differentiating hepatocellular carcinoma form benign and preneoplastic hepatic lesions and metastatic carcinomas in liver fine-needle aspiration biopsies. Diagn Cytopathol 2009;37:629–35.

53. Bióulac-Sage P, Laumonier H, Couchy G, et al. Hepatocellular adenoma management and phenotypic classification: the Bordeaux experience. Hepatology 2009; 50:481–9.

54. Bióulac-Sage P, Rebouissou S, Thomas C, et al. Hepatocellular adenoma subtype classification using molecular markers and immunohistochemistry. Hepatology 2007;46:740–8.

55. Perilongo G, Maibach R, Shafford E, et al. Cisplatin versus cisplatin plus doxorubicin for standard-risk hepatoblastoma. N Engl J Med 2009;361:1662–70.

56. Zsíros J, Maibach R, Shafford E, et al. Successful treatment of childhood high-risk hepatoblastoma with dose-intensive multiagent chemotherapy and surgery: final results of the SIOPEL-3HR study. J Clin Oncol 2010;28:2584–90.

57. Meyers RL, Rowland JR, Krailo M, et al. Predictive power of pretreatment prognostic factors in children with hepatoblastoma: a report from the Children's Oncology Group. Pediatr Blood Cancer 2009;53:1016–22.

58. Katzenstein HM, Krailo MD, Malogolowkin MH, et al. Hepatocellular carcinoma in children and adolescents: results from the Pediatric Oncology Group and the Children's Cancer Group intergroup study. J Clin Oncol 2002;20:2789–97.

59. Chen JC, Chen CC, Chen WJ, et al. Hepatocellular carcinoma in children: clinical review and comparison with adult cases. J Pediatr Surg 1998;33:1350–4.

60. Reyes JD, Carr B, Dvorchik I, et al. Liver transplantation and chemotherapy for hepatoblastoma and hepatocellular cancer in childhood and adolescence. J Pediatr 2000;136:795–804.

61. Austin MT, Leys CM, Feurer ID, et al. Liver transplantation for childhood hepatic malignancy: a review of the United Network for Organ Sharing (UNOS) database. J Pediatr Surg 2006;41:182–6.

62. Arcement CM, Towbin RB, Meza MP, et al. Intrahepatic chemoembolization in unresectable pediatric liver malignancies. Pediatr Radiol 2000;30:779–85.

63. Czauderna P, Zbrzeziniak G, Narozanski W, et al. Preliminary experience with arterial chemoembolization for hepatoblastoma and hepatocellular carcinoma in children. Pediatr Blood Cancer 2006;46:825–8.

64. Otte JB. Should the selection of children with hepatocellular carcinoma be based on Milan criteria? Pediatr Transplant 2008;12:1–3.

65. Moazam F, Rodgers BM, Talbert JL. Hepatic artery ligation for hepatic hemangiomatosis of infancy. J Pediatr Surg 1983;18:120–3.

66. Marquardt JU, Factor VM, Thorgeirsson SS. Epigenetic regulation of cancer stem cells in liver cancer: current concepts and clinical implications. J Hepatol 2010; 53:568–77.

67. Zhou X, Liu JB, Luo Y, et al. Characterization of focal liver lesions by means of assessment of hepatic transit time with contrast-enhanced US. Radiology 2010; 256:648–55.

68. Zarem HA, Edgerton MT. Induced resolution of cavernous hemangiomas following prednisolone therapy. Plast Reconstr Surg 1967;39:76–83.

69. Ezekowitz RAB, Mulliken JB, Folkman J. Interferon alfa-2a therapy for life-threatening hemangiomas of infancy. N Engl J Med 1992;326:1456–63.

70. Payarols JP, Masferrer JP, Bellvert CG. Treatment of life-threatening infantile hemangiomas with vincristine. N Engl J Med 1995;333:69.

71. Mazereeuw-Hautier J, Hoeger PH, Benlahrech S, et al. Efficacy of propranolol in hepatic infantile hemangiomas with diffuse neonatal hemangiomatosis. J Pediatr 2010;157:340–2.

72. Storch CH, Hoeger PH. Propranolol for infantile haemangiomas: insights into the molecular mechanisms of action. Br J Dermatol 2010;163:269–74.

73. Itinteang T, Brasch HD, Tan ST, et al. Expression of components of the renin–angiotensin system in proliferating infantile haemangioma may account for the propranolol-induced accelerated involution. J Plast Reconstr Aesthet Surg 2010. [Epub ahead of print].

74. Barlow CF, Priebe CJ, Mulliken JB, et al. Spastic diplegia as a complication of interferon alfa-2a treatment of hemangiomas of infancy. J Pediatr 1998;132: 527–30.

75. Al-Qabandi W, Jenkinson HC, Buckels JA, et al. Orthotopic liver transplantation for unresectable hepatoblastoma: a single center's experience. J Pediatr Surg 1999;34:1261–4.

76. Faraj W, Dar F, Marangoni G, et al. Liver transplantation for hepatoblastoma. Liver Transpl 2008;14:1614–9.

77. Grewal S, Merchant T, Reymond R, et al. Auditory late effects of childhood cancer therapy: a report from the Children's Oncology Group. Pediatrics 2010;125: e938–50.

78. Katzenstein HM, Chang KW, Krailo M, et al. Children's Oncology Group. Amifostine does not prevent platinum-induced hearing loss associated with the treatment of children with hepatoblastoma: a report of the Intergroup Hepatoblastoma Study P9645 as a part of the Children's Oncology Group. Cancer 2009;115:5828–35.

79. Meyers RL, Katzenstein HM, Krailo M, et al. Surgical resection of pulmonary metastatic lesions in children with hepatoblastoma. J Pediatr Surg 2007;42: 2050–6.

80. Tan TY, Amor DJ. Tumour surveillance in Beckwith-Wiedemann syndrome and hemihyperplasia: a critical review of the evidence and suggested guidelines for local practice. J Paediatr Child Health 2006;42:486–90.

81. Otte JB, Meyers R. PLUTO first report. Pediatr Transplant 2010;14:830–5.

Index

Note: Page numbers of article titles are in **boldface** type.

Clin Liver Dis 15 (2011) 463–471
doi:10.1016/S1089-3261(11)00024-9
1089-3261/11/$ – see front matter © 2011 Elsevier Inc. All rights reserved.

liver.theclinics.com

Printed and bound by CPI Group (UK) Ltd, Croydon, CR0 4YY

03/10/2024

01040448-0006

Moving?

Make sure your subscription moves with you!

To notify us of your new address, find your **Clinics Account Number** (located on your mailing label above your name), and contact customer service at:

Email: journalscustomerservice-usa@elsevier.com

800-654-2452 (subscribers in the U.S. & Canada)
314-447-8871 (subscribers outside of the U.S. & Canada)

Fax number: 314-447-8029

Elsevier Health Sciences Division
Subscription Customer Service
3251 Riverport Lane
Maryland Heights, MO 63043

*To ensure uninterrupted delivery of your subscription, please notify us at least 4 weeks in advance of move.

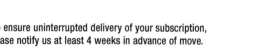
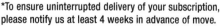